About the publisher

BPP Learning Media is dedicated to supporting aspiring professionals with top quality learning material. BPP Learning Media's commitment to success is shown by our record of quality, innovation and market leadership in paper-based and e-learning materials. BPP Learning Media's study materials are written by professionally-qualified specialists who know from personal experience the importance of top quality materials for success.

About The BMJ

The BMJ (formerly the British Medical Journal) in print has a long history and has been published without interruption since 1840. The BMJ's vision is to be the world's most influential and widely read medical journal. Our mission is to lead the debate on health and to engage, inform, and stimulate doctors, researchers, and other health professionals in ways that will improve outcomes for patients. We aim to help doctors to make better decisions. BMJ, the company, advances healthcare worldwide by sharing knowledge and expertise to improve experiences, outcomes and value.

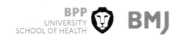

Contents

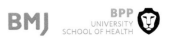

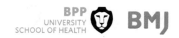

About the editors

Professor Adrian Hunnisett is a biomedical scientist specialising in clinical biochemistry and haematology. He completed his initial BMS training at Gloucester Royal Hospital and then graduated from Oxford Brookes University, completing research training in Oxford and London. He has worked in a variety of roles within the NHS and private medical sectors, most recently as Head of Clinical R&D at Southampton General Hospital. He is now Professor of Evidence-Based Healthcare at BPP University.

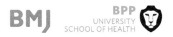

Introduction to Research Methods and Reporting series

As a healthcare worker, you are working in an "evidence-based" or "evidence-informed" professional environment whatever your professional discipline, whether you are doctors, nurses, physiotherapists, occupational therapist or part of the emerging plethora of allied professions. The evidence you use, the research base, is being generated constantly and that is impacting on clinical practice at all levels. The information you all learned in your clinical training has rapidly, and inevitably, become outdated. As a result there is a clear need to understand the principles of research and research methods to help you make decisions about the mass of new knowledge and integrating it into your practice whilst discontinuing the "old traditions".

Over recent years, the teaching of clinical research methods, research practice and the evaluation of clinical evidence has become a core addition to undergraduate and postgraduate curricula across all healthcare disciplines. In addition, many clinical journals have articles and sections concentrating on continuing education providing tools for reading and critiquing the vast amount of emerging research. Such material is considered so important in the development of evidence-based practice that they may attract credits toward the CPD portfolios required by many of the professional registration bodies today.

The BMJ Research Methods & Reporting books bring together a collection of review articles first published in The BMJ. They are not designed to replace the basic knowledge of research methods and evaluation, but rather to answer some of the key questions that researchers at all levels ask along with updates in the reporting structures and regulations for articles in the medical press. Each of the articles is written by acknowledged experts in their fields and they offer a broad update on many aspects of research, research methodology and guidelines for undertaking and reporting research. They are written in a user-friendly way that is easy to follow and understand by the non-specialist. In addition, each article is fully referenced with links to further information and evidence to support the statements made in the article. The collections are aimed at non-specialist doctors, general practitioners, research nurses and healthcare practitioners. They can also be used by individuals who may be preparing for any postgraduate examinations that have a research element.

There are two separate volumes, each concentrating on a different aspect of the research process. The first volume examines some key messages about the basics of research along with up to date articles on statistical approaches, methods and interpretation. The topics covered concentrate on subjects such as confidence intervals, p values, sample size calculations, use of patient reported outcome measures, conundrums in the application of RCT and more complex statistical analysis. It also highlights implementation research and prognostic research. The second is more specific with articles on the reporting requirements for research. It examines guidelines such as CONSORT, SPIRIT, GPP2, PRISMA and the IDEAL framework for surgical innovation. It also gives some guidance on economic evaluations, policy and service interventions and publication guidelines, as well as providing useful tips on preparing data for publication.

Each book is a stand-alone volume, but together they will give the reader a comprehensive overview of the commoner research issues and guidelines.

Adrian Hunnisett (November 2015).

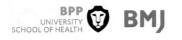

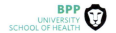

The routine use of patient reported outcome measures in healthcare settings

Jill Dawson, senior research scientist[1], visiting professor[2], Helen Doll, senior medical statistician[1], Ray Fitzpatrick, professor of public health[1], Crispin Jenkinson, professor of health services research[1], Andrew J Carr, Nuffield professor of orthopaedic surgery[3]

Department of Public Health, University of Oxford, Oxford OX3 7LF

Oxford Brookes University, School of Health and Social Care, Oxford OX3 0BP

Nuffield Department of Orthopaedics, Rheumatology and Musculoskeletal Sciences, University of Oxford, Oxford OX3 7LD

Correspondence to: J Dawson jill.dawson@dphpc.ox.ac.uk

Cite this as: BMJ 2010;340:c186

DOI: 10.1136/bmj.c186

http://www.bmj.com/content/340/bmj.c186

ABSTRACT

The use of patient reported outcome measures might seem to be quite straightforward; however, a number of pitfalls await clinicians with limited expertise. Jill Dawson and colleagues provide a guide for individuals keen to use patient reported outcome measures at a local level

Patient reported outcome measures (PROMs) are standardised, validated questionnaires that are completed by patients to measure their perceptions of their own functional status and wellbeing. Many such measures were originally designed for assessing treatment effectiveness in the context of clinical trials,[1] but are now used more widely to assess patient perspectives of care outcomes. This outcomes based definition of PROMs distinguishes them from questionnaires used to measure patients' experience of the care process.

PROMs are designed to measure either patients' perceptions of their general health ("generic" health status) or their perceptions of their health in relation to specific diseases or conditions. The short form 36 (SF-36) health survey,[2] for example, is a generic questionnaire that assesses self perceived health status by using 36 questions relating to eight broad areas (or "domains") of wellbeing. Examples of condition specific questionnaires include the Parkinson's disease questionnaire (PDQ-39),[3] which assesses quality of life in patients with Parkinson's disease; the visual function questionnaire (VF-14),[4] which uses 14 questions to measure various aspects of visual function affected by cataracts; and the Oxford hip score,[5] which uses 12 questions to assess hip pain and function in relation to outcomes of hip replacement surgery.

Patients complete PROMs by rating their health in response to individual questions. These responses are scored (from 0 to 4, for example) according to the level of difficulty or severity reported by the patient. When PROMs are analysed, the individual ratings are combined to produce an overall score to represent an underlying phenomenon or "construct," such as "perceived level of pain" or anxiety. The analysis of PROMs tends to focus on the amount of change that has occurred in the patients' condition or their general health related quality of life, as represented by a change in PROM score following an intervention.

To date, PROMs have been used in clinical trials,[6][7] national audits,[8] and registers for joint replacement[9][10] and other conditions.[11] However, the routine use of PROMs has become widespread in heath care at a local level.[12] Interest is also rapidly growing in the application of PROMs in the context of audit and "registers," to inform individual care and manage the performance of healthcare providers.[12][13][14][15][16] Indeed, in the specific areas of hip and knee replacement, inguinal hernia repair, and varicose vein surgery, the routine collection of PROMs has, since April 2009, been introduced throughout the NHS to measure and improve clinical quality.[17] Government led initiatives such as this are likely to encourage more widespread use of PROMs at both a national and a local level.

Specific guidance on methods for collecting baseline PROM data are provided in guidelines for the recent NHS-wide PROMs initiative,[18] in which subsequent data collection and handling are undertaken by private contractors. This article, however, is aimed at individuals who are keen to use PROMs at a local level, who may have limited research experience or access to expertise and advice on relevant research methods, and who may be unaware of a number of pitfalls that could undermine their aim of ultimately producing useful, meaningful data. In addition, there are very few published examples of the application of PROMs in the context of clinical governance and quality assurance,[19] with this form of application being largely unevaluated. Evidence of the impact of using PROMs on routine practice is also lacking.

Using an appropriate validated measure

When choosing a PROM to use, careful consideration should be given to the content of the questionnaire and its relevance to the intended form of usage and patient group. An appropriate measure is one that is supported by published evidence demonstrating that it is acceptable to patients, reliable, valid, and responsive (sensitive to change).[1] In addition, evidence for these properties needs to have been obtained in a similar context and on similar types of patients (in terms of age range, sex, and diagnostic or surgical category) to those whom the PROM is now to be applied. Using a PROM that meets these criteria is likely to maximise the response rate.

Choosing the right PROM for a particular purpose can be challenging because there may be a number of relevant questionnaires from which to choose. Alternatively, none

SUMMARY POINTS

- Patient reported outcome measures (PROMs) are standardised, validated questionnaires that are completed by patients to measure their perceptions of their own functional status and wellbeing

- An appropriate and validated measure that is suitable for both the particular study population and the reason for collecting the PROMs data should be chosen

- PROMs data need to be obtained from relevant patients at the same point in time relative to the date of an intervention or event of interest (for example, within four weeks pre-intervention, then at six months following the intervention) and recorded in association with the date of completion (not the date of data entry)

- The intensity with which follow-up information is sought and obtained is known to greatly influence study results; every effort should thus be made to minimise missing data and the biases that might otherwise occur

- Poor data cannot be "fixed" in an analysis by a statistician. Advice should be sought from those with relevant expertise from the very beginning of the study.

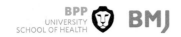

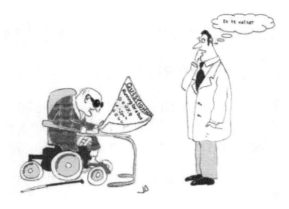

Illustration by Jill Dawson, with additional technical assistance by Phillip Saunders

may seem entirely appropriate as potential measures may include a number of questions irrelevant to the study sample—questions about sports participation or vigorous physical activity, for example, may not suit most elderly people. Listings of available measures[20] and systematic reviews of available instruments can assist in selecting an appropriate PROM.

Once a seemingly appropriate instrument has been identified, it is advisable to pilot the questionnaire on a small number of patients. This process can reveal whether or not the questionnaire truly is appropriate for the intended purpose. For instance, a questionnaire will be unsuitable if the questions address the patients' state of mind "today" and patients are likely to complete the questionnaire on the day that they are admitted for treatment—a time when they may be unusually anxious.

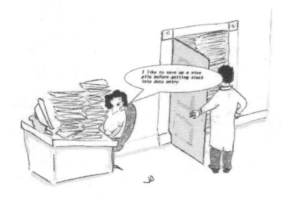

Illustration by Jill Dawson, with additional technical assistance by Phillip Saunders

It is important to note that the wording of a validated PROM should not be changed because even relatively small alterations can make a considerable difference to the meaning of the questions and consequently to the measurement properties of a questionnaire.

Data collection and storage

PROMs are generally applied in longitudinal studies that have at least one follow-up survey planned. Good research practice requires investigators to clearly identify the purpose of the study, and data should be collected at prespecified time points so that particular questions (for example, how successful a procedure is at one year after a particular

intervention) can be addressed. In the absence of a precise research question (for example, in exploratory research or descriptive audits), a reason for collecting PROMs data, preferably in relation to an event (for example, a particular intervention with a date), and any follow-up period still need to be specified before commencing data collection. This approach will help guide and standardise methods of data collection and aid the design of any associated database for storing data, as well as inform consideration of inclusion and exclusion criteria. If PROMs are collected to monitor long term conditions (for example, diabetes) where there is no specific "event," or in situations where there is no prospect of obtaining both pre-intervention and post-intervention assessments (for example, shortly after a stroke), a different rationale for the timing of regular assessments is required.[21]

Plans for long term data collection may naturally lead to other considerations for data gathering and storage. For instance, conditions and interventions that can affect bilateral structures (such as joints, eyes, or breasts), or that may require subsequent therapy revision or more than one course of treatment, can create complexity at every stage of data collection and storage and, indeed, when commencing analysis. The unit of analysis (that is, patient v right or left joint, eye, or breast) should preferably be decided upon in advance and any database designed accordingly.

Dates are crucial to longitudinal outcomes analysis, but they need to be the right ones. PROM questionnaires need to be obtained and responses recorded with the date of completion—not the date of data entry, which may involve a time lag—and with reference (labelled with and/or linked) to the date of an intervention or event of interest (for example, date of surgery, admission for rehabilitation, or start (or end) of a course of chemotherapy). Staff conducting data entry will need to be trained in relation to the importance of these issues.

Methods of data collection should be piloted and reviewed at an early stage. Once practicable methods have been tried and tested, they should be written down and adhered to. All these steps, as well as detailing methods for informing patients about the project and obtaining their written consent to participate, will be necessary if the approval of an institutional or external research ethics committee is required.

PROMs are meant to represent the patients' perspective and be independent of the views of the clinical team providing their care. The method of data collection should, therefore, ensure that patients self complete their questionnaire unobserved and unaided by members of the clinical team. Assistance with questionnaire completion from a relative or friend, however, is occasionally unavoidable and indeed helpful. Nevertheless, a patient's inability to understand a questionnaire, for reasons of impaired cognition or difficulty with the language in which it is available, should constitute an exclusion criterion.

Translation of PROMs into other languages involves establishing conceptual and semantic equivalence, a task not to be undertaken lightly. This process should include forward and backward translation methods, plus an assessment of the translated questionnaire's measurement properties. The accepted method of translating and re-evaluating a PROM is both demanding and costly, so most PROMs are not available in a variety of different languages. This can prove to be problematic in healthcare settings

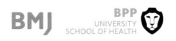

that serve populations with diverse language preferences. Asking a relative or friend to translate the questionnaire for the patient is not acceptable, as a faithful translation that maintains the correct meaning cannot be guaranteed.

Data should be stored in a database or spreadsheet in a manner that allows for immediate statistical analysis without the need for detective work and complex data programming—that is, stored in an unambiguous fashion and with variables appropriately labelled. The aim should be to minimise complexity—for example, by avoiding the use of relational databases, which can add additional complexity to an already complicated process. In addition, methods for downloading data and conducting some simple analyses should be piloted before too many cases (no more than, say, 20) have been entered.

Minimising missing and duplicated data

The most successful trials that use PROMs are undoubtedly those that achieve very high questionnaire response rates at the prespecified times.[22] Nevertheless, systems to maximise the number of questionnaire returns carry cost implications,[22][23] and a balance has to be struck between maximising response and alienating patients.

Responders may differ systematically from non-responders in ways that matter—for example, they may have poorer general health or represent a particular age band or socioeconomic group.[24][25] Thus every effort should be made to address such potential biases. Where PROM data are to be obtained by post, sending patients a reminder letter if questionnaires are not returned within two or three weeks (with a contact telephone number in case patients need to request a second questionnaire) is generally essential to obtain satisfactory response rates from a representative sample of the population (box 1).

BOX 1 IS THE SAMPLE REPRESENTATIVE?

A response rate of 80% at baseline sounds very acceptable, particularly if the response to the first follow-up survey is also 80%. If the non-responders at each stage are different people, however, these values would equate to only a 60% overall response rate for measures of change (which require the presence of both pre-intervention and post-intervention measures of outcome). This rate would not be considered adequate in terms of sample representativeness.

Collecting follow-up data when patients attend outpatient appointments is inadvisable because of the risk of introducing bias. Outpatient appointments can rarely be organised to occur at precise time points after a hospital based procedure or course of treatment, and are frequently changed by the hospital or the patient. Also, patients who experience continuing problems are more likely to attend, or attend more often, than other patients, which could mean extra data are obtained from patients with poorer outcomes. It is in any case much easier to regularise and monitor the collection of follow-up data if questionnaires are sent out to patients' homes from one office on relevant dates, with the dates when questionnaires were sent out and returned then recorded in a database.

Follow-up times should be the same for all patients in relation to the intervention or other key event. Collecting data continuously but irregularly after an intervention (that is, not at particular time points) will seriously limit the usefulness of the data (for an example, see Saleh et al[23]). This can easily happen if follow-up data are collected when patients attend outpatient appointments.

Thinking about data analysis

Before commencing data collection, serious consideration should be given to the way in which data will ultimately be analysed. This process will help to identify other pieces of information that may need to be collected to place the PROMs data in an appropriate context and to interpret the data correctly. For instance, outcomes might be expected to suggest that an intervention is less successful for some patients than for others—for example, hip replacement may not fully restore a patient's mobility if the patient has another coexisting condition that affects walking ability. In this example, details about other conditions that might affect walking must be obtained during follow-up to allow adjustment to be made for such factors in the analysis, in addition to collecting outcomes data specific to the hip operation (box 2).

BOX 2 WHAT IS THE INFLUENCE OF CASE MIX ON PROMS?

The analysis and interpretation of results from PROMs used in an audit or study with a non-randomised design is complex because it is difficult to control for all the possible "case mix" factors that may influence outcomes. Some examples are presence of other comorbidities, severity of the condition before treatment commenced, period of time since start (or end) of treatment, between-subject variation in treatment (such as drug dosages), and previous or concurrent other forms of treatment.

The importance of obtaining additional information from patients needs to be weighed carefully against the risk of missing data owing to patients feeling overburdened by a lengthy questionnaire and not completing it fully.

If data collection has occurred over a number of years, a large amount of data will be available. It is important to recognise, however, that a large amount of data does not necessarily equate with good data. Poor (that is, biased) data cannot be "fixed" in an analysis, even by the cleverest of statisticians. Indeed, leading geneticist and statistician R A Fisher (1890-1962) once said: "To consult the statistician after an experiment is finished is often merely to ask him to conduct a postmortem examination. He can perhaps say what the experiment died of."[26] We would, therefore, advocate seeking advice from those with relevant expertise from the beginning of the data collection period.

Conclusions

Overall, many clinicians are very positive about the usefulness of collecting PROMs; this consensus is reflected in the widespread use of such measures. PROMs can be used to assess the impact healthcare interventions have on patients, assist with guiding resource allocation, evaluate the effects of changes to services, and provide feedback to consultants to assist clinical governance. The systematic use of PROMs may result in improvements to patient outcomes in a number of ways—for example, by providing patient centred information and thus facilitating improved communication between doctors and their patients. Patients may also feel that healthcare personnel are more involved in their care because professionals are showing an interest in obtaining their perspective on their health and wellbeing.

The analysis of PROMs data may also reveal important differences in outcomes between different patient groups, which can trigger a subsequent more focused investigation. PROMs that are routinely collected are unlikely to reliably reveal the reasons underlying any such differences, however, given the difficulty of adjusting for all relevant

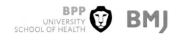

confounders. In addition, it is important to be aware of the limitations of this new approach in influencing health care. The incautious application of PROMs may produce meaningless or misleading and potentially harmful results. Many of the points raised in this paper represent pitfalls that are easy to fall into, but that are also largely avoidable if sufficient time and thought occur at the planning stage.

We acknowledge the additional technical assistance with illustrations that was provided by Phillip Saunders, Unit Administrator, Department of Public Health (Health Services Research Unit), University of Oxford.

Contributors: All the authors have considerable experience in developing, evaluating, and applying questionnaires for patients and are currently involved in long term multicentre trials where patient reported outcomes are the main end points. JD and AJC have chiefly worked in the area of patient reported outcomes in the context of orthopaedic surgery. HD is a senior statistician specialising in the development and application of patient reported outcome measures and on randomised controlled trials of complex interventions. RF has worked on both patient reported outcomes and patient experience of care relating to a wide range of conditions and interventions, both surgical and long term medical. CJ has worked on both patient reported outcomes and patient experience of care, the latter related to his work with the Picker Institute Europe, Oxford, UK. All authors contributed to the writing of this paper. JD is the guarantor.

Competing interests: All authors have completed the Unified Competing Interest form at www.icmje.org/coi_disclosure.pdf (available on request from the corresponding author) and declare (1) No financial support for the submitted work from anyone other than their employer; (2) No financial relationships with commercial entities that might have an interest in the submitted work; (3) No spouses, partners, or children with relationships with commercial entities that might have an interest in the submitted work; (4) No non-financial interests that may be relevant to the submitted work.

Provenance and peer review: Commissioned, externally peer reviewed.

1   Fitzpatrick R, Davey C, Buxton MJ, Jones DR. Evaluating patient-based outcome measures for use in clinical trials. *Health Technol Assess* 1998;2:1-74.
2   Ware-JE J, Sherbourne CD. The MOS 36-item short-form health survey (SF-36). I. Conceptual framework and item selection. *Med Care* 1992;30:473-83.
3   Jenkinson C, Fitzpatrick R, Peto V, Greenhall R, Hyman N. The Parkinson's Disease Questionnaire (PDQ-39): development and validation of a Parkinson's disease summary index score. *Age Ageing* 1997;26:353-7.
4   Steinberg EP, Tielsch JM, Schein OD, Javitt JC, Sharkey P, Cassard SD, et al. The VF-14: An index of functional impairment in patients with cataract. *Arch Ophthalmol* 1994;112:630-8.
5   Dawson J, Fitzpatrick R, Carr A, Murray D. Questionnaire on the perceptions of patients about total hip replacement. *J Bone Joint Surg [Br]* 1996;78:185-90.
6   Silverman LR, Demakos EP, Peterson BL, Kornblith AB, Holland JC, Odchimar-Reissig R, et al. Randomized controlled trial of azacitidine in patients with the myelodysplastic syndrome: a study of the Cancer and Leukemia Group B. *J Clin Oncol* 2002;20:2429-40.
7   Grant AM, Wileman SM, Ramsay CR, Mowat NA, Krukowski ZH, Heading RC, et al for the REFLUX Trial Group. Minimal access surgery compared with medical management for chronic gastro-oesophageal reflux disease: UK collaborative randomised trial. *BMJ* 2008;337:a2664.
8   Williams O, Fitzpatrick R, Hajat S, Reeves BC, Stimpson A, Morris R, et al. Mortality, morbidity, and 1-year outcomes of primary elective total hip arthroplasty. *J Arthroplasty* 2002;17:165-71.
9   Malchau H, Garellick G, Eisler T, Herberts P. Presidential guest address: the Swedish Hip Registry: Increasing the sensitivity by patient outcome data. *Clin Orthop Rel Res* 2005.
10   New Zealand Joint Registry. *The New Zealand Joint Registry Nine Year Report January 1999 to December 2007*. Department of Orthopaedic Surgery and Musculoskeletal Medicine, Christchurch Hospital, 2008. www.cdhb.govt.nz/njr/.
11   Zanoli G, Nilsson LT, Stromqvist B. Reliability of the prospective data collection protocol of the Swedish Spine Register: test-retest analysis of 119 patients. *Acta Orthop* 2006;77:662-9.
12   Appleby J, Devlin N. *Measuring success in the NHS. Using patient-assessed health outcomes to manage the performance of healthcare providers*. The King's Fund, 2004.
13   Wasson J, Keller J, Rubenstein L, Hays R, Nelson E, Johnson D. Benefits and obstacles of health status assessment in ambulatory settings: the clinician's point of view. *Med Care* 1992;30:MS42-MS49.
14   Greenhalgh J, Long AF, Flynn R. The use of patient reported outcome measures in routine clinical practice: lack of impact or lack of theory? *Soc Sci Med* 2005;60:833-43.
15   Haywood K, Marshall S, Fitzpatrick R. Patient participation in the consultation process: a structured review of intervention strategies. *Patient Educ Couns* 2006;63:12-23.
16   Timmins N. Assessing patient care—NHS goes to the PROMS. *BMJ* 2008;336:1464-5.
17   Department of Health. *Our NHS, our future: NHS next stage review. Interim report*. 2007. http://www.dh.gov.uk/en/Publicationsandstatistics/Publications/PublicationsPolicyAndGuidance/DH_079077.
18   Department of Health. *Guidance on the routine collection of Patient Reported Outcome Measures (PROMs)*. 2009. http://www.dh.gov.uk/en/Publicationsandstatistics/Publications/PublicationsPolicyAndGuidance/DH_092647.
19   Vallance-Owen A, Cubbin S, Warren V, Matthews B. Outcome monitoring to facilitate clinical governance: experience from a national programme in the independent sector. *J Public Health* 2004;26:187-92.
20   MAPI Research Trust. Patient reported outcome and quality of life instruments database. 2009. http://www.proqolid.org.
21   Black N, Jenkinson C. Measuring patients' experiences and outcomes. *BMJ* 2009;339:b2495
22   Ganz PA, Gotay CG. Use of patient-reported outcomes in phase III cancer treatment trials: lessons learned and future directions. *J Clin Oncol* 2007;25:5063-9.
23   Saleh KJ, Bershadsky B, Cheng E, Kane R. Lessons learned from the hip and knee musculoskeletal outcomes data evaluation and management system. *Clin Orthop Rel Res* 2004;429:272-8.
24   Bracken M. Reporting observational studies. *Br J Obstet Gynaecol* 1989;96:383-8.
25   Matthews FE, Chatfield M, Freeman C, McCracken C, Brayne C. Attrition and bias in the MRC cognitive function and ageing study: an epidemiological investigation. *BMC Public health* 2004;4:12.
26   Edwards AWF. Some quotations from R A Fisher. http://www.economics.soton.ac.uk/staff/aldrich/fisherguide/quotations.htm.

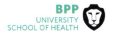

Strengths and weaknesses of hospital standardised mortality ratios

Alex Bottle, lecturer in medical statistics, Brian Jarman, emeritus professor, Paul Aylin, clinical reader in epidemiology and public health

Foster Unit, Department of
imary Care and Public Health,
nperial College London, London
C1A 9LA

orrespondence to: A Bottle robert.
ottle@imperial.ac.uk

te this as: BMJ 2010;341:c7116

OI: 10.1136/bmj.c7116

ctp://www.bmj.com/content/342/
mj.c7116

ABSTRACT

Hospital standardised mortality ratios are fairly easy to produce and, as the example of Mid Staffordshire shows, can help identify hospitals with poor performance. However, they are not without problems

Hospital standardised mortality ratios (HSMRs) are intended as an overall measure of deaths in hospital, a proportion of which will be preventable. High ratios may thus suggest potential problems with quality of care. Although a growing number of countries are using HSMRs, they are controversial, especially if the figures are made public, as in England and Canada.[1][2][3]

The HSMR is complex but cheap and relatively easy to calculate from national or other benchmark data that allow calculation of patients' predicted risks of death. However, there are a number of methodological challenges in their construction and interpretation, which we discuss below. Although there are other versions of the HSMR, we focus on the Jarman one.[4] Full methodological details of its construction in England are given on bmj.com. A few of the finer points that we discuss are specific to English hospital data, but most of the methodological concerns are relevant to HSMRs (or other composite hospital mortality measures) in any developed country.

What is an HSMR?

The HSMR is derived from administrative data commonly used for billing purposes from hospital information systems such as Hospital Episode Statistics in England. It is the ratio of the observed to expected deaths, multiplied by 100, with expected deaths derived from statistical models that adjust for available case mix factors such as age and comorbidity.

The HSMR is meant as an overall measure of adjusted in-hospital mortality and serves as a screening tool. Some of the deaths in the numerator will be preventable. Thus some of the variation in HSMRs between hospitals will be due to important variation in preventable deaths, although much will be due to other factors. Estimates of the number of preventable in-hospital deaths vary; in the UK it is estimated to be in the thousands.[5] Nevertheless, two English hospital groups, Mid Staffordshire NHS Trust and Basildon and Thurrock NHS Trust, had high HSMRs when they were investigated by the national healthcare regulator and found to have substandard care (box).

How they are used

HSMRs are used as a small part of our system for monitoring quality of care.[6] Some hospitals also use them as part of quality improvement efforts.[7][8] Their boards monitor the HSMR alongside other indicators such as mortality for individual diagnosis groups, infections, and patient experience. In England, Dr Foster Intelligence, a private company and joint venture with the NHS Information Centre, includes HSMRs in its annual *Hospital Guide,* and the figures are publicly available on the NHS Choices website.

We envision the role of HSMRs as part of a suite of measures for hospitals' internal use. The figures can be broken down by diagnosis group, and any potential problems investigated by checking the data and analysing processes, often going as far as a case note review.[9] This is considered the gold standard method for deciding whether an individual death was preventable but has inherent difficulties such as inter-rater reliability.[10]

Methodological uncertainties

We have divided the uncertainties into those relating to the numerator, denominator, risk modelling, interpretation, and coding.

Numerator

Most hospital administrative databases capture only deaths that occur in hospital. The choice is then between including all in-hospital deaths or only those that occur within a set number of days since admission. Inclusion of all in-hospital deaths will capture long stay patients, perhaps with more chronic disease or complications from treatment; in surgery research, the follow-up length is often 30 days postoperatively to try to attribute any death to the surgery rather than the patient's underlying condition.

The English HSMR has no limit to the length of follow-up. Transfers to other hospitals are linked together so that deaths occurring after the transfer are allocated to all the hospitals to which the patient was admitted preceding death. An alternative approach would be to allocate the death to only one hospital (first, last, or that accounting for most bed days). Although linking these transfers is desirable, some administrative systems do not allow this, in which case transfers can affect a unit's estimated performance.[11] Linkage of hospital admissions to death registrations is possible in some countries, but in England currently incurs a considerable time lag, limiting its utility.

Denominator

Hospital administrative data generally use the International Classification of Diseases (ICD) to code diagnostic information, which is typically divided into the primary diagnosis (main problem treated) and various secondary diagnoses (including comorbidities and complications).

SUMMARY POINTS

- HSMRs are intended as an overall measure of in-hospital mortality
- They are used as a screening tool in increasing numbers of countries
- Case mix adjustment, admissions consisting of multiple care episodes and inter-hospital transfers, and patients with multiple admissions complicate their construction

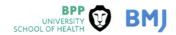

CASE STUDY: MID STAFFORDSHIRE NHS TRUST

In its annual assessment of every UK healthcare provider the Healthcare Commission (now replaced by the Care Quality Commission) gave Mid Staffordshire NHS Trust a good-fair rating in 2006-7 and a good-good rating in 2007-8. The rating is based largely on self assessment, however. An investigation was carried out between March 2008 and October 2008 and, prompted by a large number of reports of high mortality from both our monitoring system and their own, focused on emergency admissions. The hospital was found to have poor standards of care, resulting in unnecessary patient deaths, and the rating was downgraded to weak. The commission's report[21] noted that:

"In April 2007, Dr Foster's Hospital Guide showed that the trust had an HSMR of 127 for 2005/06, in other words more deaths than expected. The trust established a group to look into mortality, but put much of its effort into attempting to establish whether the high rate was a consequence of poor recording of clinical information."

This response, and a campaign by local people about the quality of care, led the commission to proceed with a full investigation. The commission noted that the trust began to monitor clinical outcomes only after the publication of the high HSMR by Dr Foster in 2007, but it was not until after the investigation that it undertook various remedial actions such as recruitment of extra nurses. What can the HSMR tell us about its mortality during this time? Figure 1 shows the HSMR by financial quarter with a one year moving average up to December 2009.

The HSMR had been above 100 for several years before falling steadily from a peak of 138 in the first quarter of 2006. This is despite a slight increase in the crude death rate from the fourth quarter of 2005 to the first quarter of 2008 (fig 2).

Figure 3 shows the expected death rate over time, which rose from the second quarter of 2006 to the first quarter of 2008. This increase seems to have driven the first part of the fall in HSMR over this period. Some of the increase seems to be due to changes in coding, as the mean comorbidity score for HSMR records rose from 2.8 in 2006-7 to 4.7 in 2008-9 (and is still at 4.7 in 2009-10); real changes in the case mix of admitted patients, although unlikely, would have the same effect. Expected deaths then plateaued.

The rest of the fall in the HSMR from the second quarter of 2008 is due to a large reduction in observed deaths and hence also crude death rates (with no significant change in numbers of admissions). This coincided with the launch of the Healthcare Commission's investigation in March 2008 and its demand for immediate action to improve emergency care in May 2008. This fall is probably too large and occurred during too short a period to be attributed solely to quality improvements, though these may have contributed. Other explanations include changes in admission or discharge policies (we do not yet have the out of hospital deaths linked with Hospital Episode Statistics for this period), a sudden and large failure to record some in-hospital deaths (which seems unlikely), and changes in case mix that are not captured by the risk adjustment models and therefore by the expected deaths.

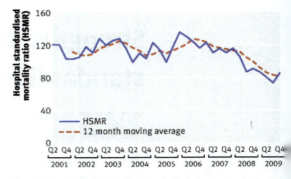

Fig 1 HSMR trend for Mid Staffordshire by financial quarter, April 2001 to December 2009

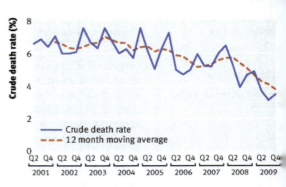

Fig 2 Crude death rate trend for Mid Staffordshire, April 2001 to December 2009

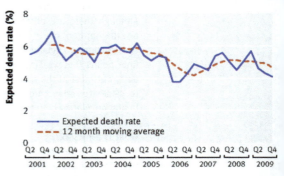

Fig 3 Expected death rate trend for Mid Staffordshire, April 2001 to December 2009

It could be argued that palliative care and not-for-resuscitation patients (some US but not UK data can identify the latter) should be excluded, providing that this was based on intention to treat on admission. However, if the HSMRs are used for judgment (by the regulator or in a pay for performance scheme) this creates the potential for gaming.

Another approach would seek diagnoses for which it is recognised that mortality is one of the most useful markers of quality of care, ideally with documented variations between hospitals. The Agency for Healthcare Research and Quality produced a patient safety indicator, death in diagnosis related groups with low mortality (<0.5%). Death in patients with these conditions would be considered unusual and hence these might represent preventable deaths. This indicator will of course have a small numerator, hampering inter-hospital comparisons, but would be practical for clinical audit. However, this indicator would exclude frail and elderly people, who are most vulnerable to deficiencies in care.

A further consideration is whether to count patients or admissions. Administrative databases count admissions or discharges. In England, the basic units are "finished

The Agency for Healthcare Research and Quality's Clinical Classification System is one way of grouping ICD codes, and is intended to be clinically meaningful for health services research, but other groupings exist. The HSMR is based on admissions with a primary diagnosis belonging to one of the Clinical Classification System groups that cover a combined total of 80% of in-hospital deaths. In England, 56 of the 259 groups achieve this, but this varies by country. 80% is chosen because of the Pareto principle (80% of the effects come from 20% of the causes). All diagnoses could be included, though, with simplified risk models in groups with few deaths.

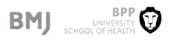

consultant episodes" (time spent under the care of a given senior doctor), which need to be linked to form admissions. In 2008-9, 15.5% of the overall total and 28.7% of HSMR admissions had more than one consultant episode. As each episode can contain different diagnostic information, this raises the question of which to use. In some hospitals, the first episode can be short, covering a preadmission or observation ward. The primary diagnosis may be simply "chest pain" or "abdominal pain." Diagnoses in subsequent episodes may represent complications rather than the reason for admission, and we would argue the diagnosis recorded in earlier episodes is preferable for monitoring. However, none of these episode diagnoses may equal the cause of death, which may also be of interest.

HSMRs use the first episode (or second if the first has only a symptom code as its primary diagnosis). An extension of this multiepisode phenomenon is the admission consisting of one or more hospital transfers (called a superspell). In the UK the ability to capture and link all the transfers varies regionally, resulting in the "loss" of an unknown number of deaths, which also varies by diagnosis. With a patient based measure, however, assuming a suitable patient identifier exists in the dataset, we also need to decide which admission for chronic obstructive pulmonary disease, for example, to include for each patient. Options include the first, last, or randomly chosen admission. However, since each admission is an opportunity for the hospital to save the patient's life, it could be argued that all admissions should be included. HSMRs count all admissions, partly for practical reasons, with an adjustment for each patient's number of unplanned admissions within the previous 12 months. This clearly imperfect method tries to take some account of hard to quantify factors such as disease severity and admission thresholds. Another option would be to exclude chronic conditions liable to repeat admissions. Limiting the set of diagnoses to first time events—for example, acute myocardial infarction and stroke—would minimise this problem but be less inclusive.

As well as varying admission thresholds, the definition of what constitutes an admission as opposed to an emergency department attendance or time spent in an assessment unit may change or differ between hospitals or countries. The proportion of patients in England admitted and discharged on the same day has shown a large, steady increase, from 5.9% of all inpatients in 1996-7 to 15.4% in 2008-9. We could therefore exclude these records as not "proper" admissions, but poor emergency care can result in death and therefore any deaths in these admissions should not be excluded. HSMRs currently include all unplanned as well as planned inpatient admissions.

Risk modelling

The expected deaths in an HSMR are derived from sets of logistic regression models, one for each diagnosis group, that include available case mix factors. An ideal risk adjustment model would capture all important patient factors and fully adjust for them. Two commonly used proxies for health status are socioeconomic deprivation and age. These can be problematic if, for example, the deprivation score captures factors related to life expectancy such as smoking and diet better in some areas of the country than in others.[12] Adjusting for deprivation may also remove some of the effect of quality of care if one hospital is less able to deal with the needs of its disadvantaged patients than another hospital.

A few studies have combined patient administrative data with information from laboratory systems and found that a few variables such as serum creatinine can improve the model fit,[13] but unfortunately doing this often remains technologically difficult.

The surgery a patient had can give useful risk information not captured elsewhere, but adjustment for procedure is not straightforward and is not done with HSMRs. The degree to which the surgery reflects the surgeon's choice (which relates to quality of care and should not be adjusted for) will vary and may be hard to ascertain. We would not recommend using systems of grouping patients for billing purposes such as diagnosis related groups or healthcare resource groups in the risk models, as they are based on the treatment given and also include complications, which again partly relate to quality. Furthermore, redo or revision procedures often involve greater risk, but if they were as a result of difficulties during the original procedure, adjusting for the revision will obscure this quality element.

Other factors outside the control of the hospital but not the healthcare system include the provision of community services and the proportion of deaths occurring in the community. Jarman et al originally found factors such as the number of general practitioners and NHS facilities per head of population to be statistically significant (although not necessarily important) explanatory factors of in-hospital mortality.[4] Investigations into a high HSMR may show problems that lie beyond the hospital.

In-hospital case fatality rates have been falling in England for several years, partly reflecting a fall in total mortality (5.4% reduction in females and 4.0% in males in 2009 compared with 2008[14]) but also potentially due to an increase in total admissions (inflating the denominator) and coding practice changes. The HSMR risk models therefore include adjustment for financial year, meaning that hospitals are compared with the national average for the relevant year. This recalibration is done annually, but in the second half of the year, the continuing fall in mortality means that hospitals will typically have apparently falling HSMRs. More frequent recalibration than annual is possible given adequate resources but, for less common diagnoses, can be impeded by small numbers.

All hospitals are used to derive the predicted risks, but an alternative would be to exclude "atypical" trusts, as is done in the Netherlands, for example.[15] Hospitals could be defined as "atypical" according to case mix, data quality, or even performance. Around 94% of the admissions and deaths used in HSMRs are to acute non-specialist trusts, so the numerical difference is likely to be small.

Interpretation

HSMRs are typically published annually, but this may not be the most appropriate timeframe for monitoring. Quarterly and monthly figures will be timelier and may detect changes that an annual summary may miss, but are more subject to chance fluctuations, which can be considerable. A hospital will not have the same number of admissions in each diagnosis group every month, and case mix adjustment is more successful in some groups than others. Consequently, temporal variation in patient mix can affect the HSMR.

Alternatively, hospitals may want to track the progress of their HSMR over time after implementing improvement efforts[16] rather than compare themselves with the contemporaneous national average. To do this, they base

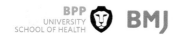

all their expected deaths on some previous year so their performance is relative to that year instead of the current one. This also reduces the interpretation problems with diagnostic coding varying between hospitals.

"Unacceptable" or outlying performance needs to be defined. With nearly 150 acute non-specialist hospital trusts in England and many more in other countries, the type I error rate with 95% confidence intervals is not negligible. Funnel plots with 99.8% control limits are therefore increasingly common. With simple random variation in the HSMRs, just 0.2% of hospitals with average rates would be expected to lie outside the control limits just by chance. However, 59 (40%) out of 149 English HSMRs lay outside the 99.8% control limits in 2008-9. If the intention is to detect outliers, the control limits may be widened to adjust for the extra variation.[17] Unfortunately, it is impossible to tell from the plot whether the greater than random variation is due to signal (differences in quality of care) or noise.

Coding

The accuracy of diagnostic coding is clearly vital and is the direct responsibility of the hospital administration. UK clinical coders are checked regularly by the Audit Commission.[18] In 2001 Campbell et al investigated the accuracy of hospital data in the UK through systematic review of studies comparing routinely collected data with case note review.[19] Median coding accuracy rates for primary diagnostic codes were 91% in England or Wales and 82% in Scottish studies. These figures will have improved since that study but still vary by hospital.

Patients transferred from another hospital can be very ill, but it can be hard to capture their high risk using administrative data. We now adjust for "source of admission," which includes from home or other hospitals, though anecdotal evidence suggests that this field is not well coded.

Secondary diagnosis coding in hospital data includes comorbidites and is likely to vary between hospitals more than primary diagnosis coding, though in elderly patients with multiple problems deciding which should be the primary can be hard. The possibility of distinguishing conditions present on admission from complications developed during the admission exists only in some countries. Several comorbidity indices (the HSMR uses Charlson,[20] for example) have been developed for administrative systems that lack flags for conditions present at admission and try to include only chronic conditions that could not be developed during the hospital stay. Adjustment for comorbidity in risk models is advisable but can incur measurement error.[12] However, the discovery that a hospital's HSMR is artificially high because of poor coding can be a spur to improve recording, which may have other benefits for that hospital from reimbursement systems. Some specific theoretical concerns have been raised about some of the information used in our risk model, including comorbidities,[1][3][12] but it is important to see how influential they are in practice. England now has a list of diagnoses that are mandatory to code for on patient records. The list includes many of the diagnoses used in our comorbidity index, and this should improve coding consistency.

The Dr Foster Unit is affiliated with the Centre for Patient Safety and Service Quality at Imperial College Healthcare NHS Trust, which is funded by the National Institute of Health Research. We are grateful for support from the NIHR Biomedical Research Centre funding scheme. We also thank Liz Robb and Nick Flatt for their helpful comments.

Contributors: AB and PA conceived the study. AB performed all analyses and wrote the first draft. All authors contributed in the revision of the manuscript. AB is the guarantor.

Competing interests: All authors have completed the unified competing interest form at www.icmje.org/coi_disclosure.pdf (available on request from the corresponding author) and declare no support from any organisation for the submitted work; The Dr Foster Unit at Imperial is principally funded via a research grant by Dr Foster Intelligence, an independent healthcare information company and joint venture with the Information Centre of the NHS. The unit also receives funding for HSMR work, particularly the US HSMRs, from the Rx Foundation in Boston. Dr Foster Intelligence publishes HSMRs and provides them to the NHS. All authors are members of the steering committee or technical committee of the NHS HSMR working group.

Provenance and peer review: Not commissioned; externally peer reviewed.

1   Lilford R, Pronovost P. Using hospital mortality rates to judge hospital performance: a bad idea that just won't go away. *BMJ* 2010;340:955-7.
2   Black N. Assessing the quality of hospitals. Hospital standardised mortality ratios should be abandoned. *BMJ* 2010;340:933-4.
3   Mohammed MA, Deeks JJ, Girling A, Rudge G, Carmalt M, Stevens AJ, et al. Evidence of methodological bias in hospital standardised mortality ratios: retrospective database study of English hospitals. *BMJ* 2009;338:b780.
4   Jarman B, Gault S, Alves B, Hider A, Dolan S, Cook A, et al. Explaining differences in English hospital death rates using routinely collected data. *BMJ* 1999;318:1515-20.
5   National Audit Office. A safer place for patients: learning to improve patient safety. NAO, 2005.
6   Bottle A, Aylin P. Intelligent information: a national system for monitoring clinical performance. *Health Serv Res* 2008;43:10-31.
7   Jarman B, Bottle A, Aylin P, Browne M. Monitoring changes in hospital standardised mortality ratios. *BMJ* 2005;330:329.
8   Wright J, Dugdale B, Hammond I, Jarman B, Neary M, Newton D, et al. Learning from death: a hospital mortality reduction programme. *J R Soc Med* 2006;99:303-8.
9   Lilford R, Mohammed MA, Spiegelhalter DJ, Thomson R. Use and misuse of process and outcome data in managing performance of acute medical care: avoiding institutional stigma. *Lancet* 2004;363:1147-54.
10 Hayward RA, Hofer TP. Estimating hospital deaths due to medical errors: preventability is in the eye of the reviewer. *JAMA* 2001;286:415-20.
11 Kahn JM, Kramer AA, Rubenfeld GD. Transferring critically ill patients out of hospital improves the standardized mortality ratio. *Chest* 2007;131:68-75.
12 Nicholl J. Case-mix adjustment in non-randomised observational evaluations: the constant risk fallacy. *J Epidemiol Community Health* 2007;61:1010-3.
13 Pine M, Jordan HS, Elixhauser A, Fry DE, Hoaglin DC, Jones B, et al. Modifying ICD-9-CM coding of secondary diagnoses to improve risk-adjustment of inpatient mortality rates. *Med Decis Making* 2009;29:69-81.
14 Office for National Statistics Statistical Bulletin: Deaths and Births in England and Wales 2009. www.statistics.gov.uk/pdfdir/bdths0510.pdf.
15 Jarman B, Pieter D, van der Veen AA, Kool RB, Aylin P, Bottle A, et al. The hospital standardised mortality ratio: a powerful tool for Dutch hospitals to assess their quality of care? *Qual Safety Health Care* (in press).
16 Robb E, Jarman B, Suntharalingam G, Higgens C, Tennant R, Elcock K. Using care bundles to reduce in-hospital mortality: quantitative survey. *BMJ* 2010;340:C1234.
17 Spiegelhalter DJ. Handling over-dispersion of performance indicators. *Qual Safety Health Care* 2005:14;347-51.
18 Audit Commission. Information and data quality in the NHS. 2004. www.audit-commission.gov.uk/nationalstudies/health/other/Pages/informationanddataqualityinthenhs.aspx.
19 Campbell S, Campbell M, Grimshaw J, Walker A. A systematic review of discharge coding accuracy. *J Pub Health Med* 2001;23:205-11.
20 Charlson ME, Pompei P, Ales KL, MacKenzie CR. A new method of classifying prognostic comorbidity in longitudinal studies: development and validation. *J Chron Dis* 1987;40:373-3.
21 Healthcare Commission. Investigation into Mid Staffordshire NHS Foundation Trust. 2009. www.cqc.org.uk/_db/_documents/Investigation_into_Mid_Staffordshire_NHS_Foundation_Trust.pdf.

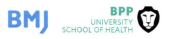

Importance of accurately identifying disease in studies using electronic health records

Douglas G Manuel, senior scientist[1 2 3 4 5], Laura C Rosella, fellow[4 5 6],
Thérèse A Stukel, senior scientist[4 6]

Ottawa Hospital Research Institute, 1053 Carling Ave, Ottawa, Ontario, Canada K1Y 4E9

Statistics Canada, Ottawa

Departments of Family Medicine and Epidemiology and Community Medicine, University of Ottawa

Institute for Clinical Evaluative Sciences, Toronto, Ontario

Dalla Lana School of Public Health, University of Toronto, Toronto

Ontario Agency for Health Protection and Promotion, Toronto, Ontario

Correspondence to: D G Manuel
dmanuel@ohri.ca

Cite this as: BMJ 2010;341:c4226

DOI: 10.1136/bmj.c4226

http://www.bmj.com/content/341/bmj.c4226

ABSTRACT

Use of routinely collected electronic health data to identify people for epidemiology studies and performance reports can lead to serious bias

Disease registries and similar databases have facilitated epidemiological studies that contribute to our understanding of the natural course of disease and the value of medical and surgical interventions.[1] These data have also allowed us to study the performance of health care, including patient safety and quality of care.[2 3] However, there is an increasing possibility of inaccurate results arising from a shift in the type of data used to identify people with chronic diseases. In the past, registries for cancer and other diseases were laboriously created using active reporting from individual clinical records. But increasingly, disease databases are now generated from routinely collected electronic data and applying a set of disease identification criteria en masse. For uncommon diseases, small errors in classifying people can result in a large number of incorrect entries in a database, leading to biased results and classification errors that propagate through calculations in ways that are difficult to intuitively appreciate.

How disease classification errors affect study conclusions

Routinely collected electronic data are increasingly used to identify patients with chronic diseases such as diabetes, heart disease, cancer, and arthritis, for research.[1 4] Databases that contain information on patients with a wide range of diseases are even more widely used. The United Kingdom's General Practice Research Database, for example, has been used for more than 700 studies of over 150 conditions (table 1),[5 6] and hospital discharge databases are widely used in many countries for research and performance studies.

However, few of these studies assess whether their findings may be biased by misclassification of patients in the database. We believe that the conclusions of many studies may change if their results were adjusted for bias or if there were no misclassification errors.

To illustrate our case, we estimated the potential bias in two published studies that use the Ontario Diabetes Database.[7 8] The concerns about misclassification error are described in other areas of health care, such as diagnostic accuracy studies, where methods to reduce error and reporting guidelines to disclose potential bias have been developed.[9] We applied the same principles and methods to examine bias in the use of routinely collected data to identify disease.

Estimating bias

The Ontario Diabetes Database is a well developed database generated using only routinely collected administrative data. Both studies that we examined generated study populations directly from this database, and both studies quoted a separate development study as validation that disease identification in the database was high quality (table 2).[10]

We calculated the potential percentage of misclassified people in the two study samples using a straightforward correction method described in different epidemiology settings (see bmj.com).[11 12 13] Like several other approaches to assess misclassification and bias, this method centres around estimating the predictive accuracy of disease identification in terms of "false positives"—people who do not have a disease and are incorrectly enrolled in the disease database or study—and "false negatives"—people who do have the disease but are missing from the disease database.[14 15 16] The amount that a study is biased can be estimated after misclassification is described. For example, performance studies for diabetes care will report the proportion of patients who receive care as recommended in clinical practice guidelines (such as regular haemoglobin A1c testing). Incorrectly including people without diabetes in a study of diabetes care will bias performance towards poor care because people who do not have diabetes do not need to have regular testing. In this way, false positives and classification error will almost always bias performance reporting towards poor care.

Table 3 shows the findings from the validation study[10] for the Ontario Diabetes Database and our estimate of false positives and false negatives in the study populations for each of two examples.

The first study reported an annual rate of haemoglobin A1c tests and concluded that the level of testing was unacceptably low in 2005.[7] The study reported that 58% of 36 945 patients with physician diagnosed diabetes received a haemoglobin A1c test. These results have been widely cited. The Health Council of Canada, for one, used these and other findings to conclude that care for people with diabetes in Canada is possibly the worst of any country in the Organisation for Economic Cooperation and Development.[17] Applying a sensitivity of 86.1% and specificity of 97.1% from the database validation study, we estimate that 38 186 of 63 699 participants were correctly classified as having diabetes (positive predictive value 59.9%). The remaining 25 513 patients were false positives, misclassified as having diabetes and not in need of regular haemoglobin A1c

SUMMARY POINTS

- Routinely collected electronic health data are increasingly used to identify people with chronic conditions for research
- Classification error can occur during the disease identification process
- Even when the identification process has very good sensitivity and specificity, misclassification can considerably bias study findings
- Studies using routinely collected data should assess the potential for classification error and adjust for bias

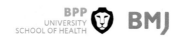

Table 1 Examples of routinely collected data used to identify people with chronic diseases

Name	Country	Description	Quality assurance	Disease ascertainment development and validation approaches	Assessment or adjustment for bias or generalisability
General Practice Research Database	United Kingdom	Primary care database of patient records comprising about 6% of the UK population. Used for over 700 studies for more than 100 conditions. Read codes are used to identify people with diseases	Standardised protocol for data entry, training for database entry, quality audits, etc	Disease diagnoses are typically validated by requesting that participating doctors verify diagnosis or provide detailed medical records. This approach is used to estimate positive predictive value but most studies do not/cannot assess sensitivity	Studies sometimes describe potential sources of bias. No identified examples of analytical assessment of bias or generalisability
Hospital discharge/ separation databases	Widespread use in many countries	Summary of hospital stay that is primarily used for "administrative" purposes such as hospital payment. Widely used to identify populations with specific diseases to monitor hospital performance and other studies. Hospital data are increasingly linked to additional population data to improve disease identification and provide additional healthcare information	Several approaches during data abstraction (data coded by specifically trained medical records staff, with a well developed quality framework and procedures) and before general use (re-abstraction studies)	Rigour of development and validation studies varies widely, including using a reference standard. Many studies do not perform specific validation studies	Studies occasionally discuss potential sources of bias from misclassification error
Diabetes databases/ registries	Canada, Scotland, and others	Generated from hospital discharge records and physician billing claims (Canada) and other databases such as those of laboratory tests (Scotland, Denmark)	Extensive for some data (see above for hospital discharge data). No/little quality assurance for other data (eg, physician billing data)	Diabetes identification algorithms developed and validated using a reference standard from clinical chart reviews	Studies occasionally discuss potential sources of bias from misclassification error

Table 2 Estimates of misclassified respondents in two published studies using sensitivity and specificity from development study

	Reported prevalence of diabetes (%)	Study base	True positives	False positives	True negatives	False negatives	Positive predictive value (%)	Negative predictive value (%)
Development study[4]	11.7	3 317	335	85	2 843	54	79.8	98.1
Haemoglobin A1c testing coverage study[7]	6.9	923 174	38 186	25 513	853 319	6 155	59.9	99.2
Trend in diabetes prevalence study[8]	8.9	9 276 945	577 579	249 840	8 356 424	93 102	69.8	98.9

The sensitivity and specificity from the development study were used to estimate the true and false positives and true and false negatives in the example studies, using the prevalence of diabetes in the example studies. See bmj.com for detailed calculations.

Table 3 Estimates of misclassified respondents in two published studies using sensitivity and specificity from development study

	Reported prevalence of diabetes (%)	Study base	True positives	False positives	True negatives	False negatives	Positive predictive value (%)	Negative predictive value (%)
Development study[10]	11.7	3 317	335	85	2 843	54	79.8	98.1
Study of haemoglobin A1c testing coverage[7]	6.9	923 174	38 186	25 513	853 319	6 155	59.9	99.2
Study of trend in diabetes prevalence[8]	8.9	9 276 945	577 579	249 840	8 356 424	93 102	69.8	98.9

The sensitivity and specificity from the development study were used to estimate the true and false positives and true and false negatives in the example studies, using the prevalence of diabetes in the example studies. See bmj.com for detailed calculations.

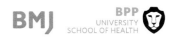

testing. Using this information (see bmj.com), we calculated an unbiased estimate of haemoglobin A1c testing among diabetes patients of 97% (36 945/38 186).

The second study reported trends in the incidence and prevalence of diabetes[8] and concluded that more adult Ontarians were diagnosed with diabetes in 2005 (8.9% or 827 419 people) than the global rate predicted for 2030.[18] The Ontario government extrapolated findings from the study to state that diabetes prevalence will increase by an additional 30% by 2010.[19] This prevalence calculation is widely quoted and is being used to support a considerably expanded diabetes strategy.[19] However, applying the database validation study, we estimate that the unbiased prevalence of diabetes in 2005 was 19% lower than the original study found (7.2% versus 8.9%). Of the 827 419 people enrolled in the Ontario Diabetes Database, we calculated that 249 840 were wrongly classified as having been diagnosed with diabetes (positive predictive value 69.8%), and that 93 102 people had diabetes diagnosed by their physician but were not enrolled in the database (false negatives).

Why does this problem happen?

It is important to recognise a subtle but critical distinction between disease databases that individually verify diagnoses from those that do not. It is one matter to identify patients with a positive confirmation test such as a cancer pathology report, manually verify the report, and then use this information to create a disease registry. It is another matter to access an entire population's electronic records and apply identification criteria to automatically classify people who have a disease and exclude those who do not. Routinely collected electronic data offer the advantage of identifying many diseases in large populations at low cost. However, mass application of identification criteria is more prone to error than the traditional, more expensive, approach of individually or manually verifying disease diagnoses for each person.

When individual verification is not done, disease databases should at least attempt to gauge the accuracy of the identification process in a representative sample. Unfortunately, this step is commonly omitted. Instead, diagnoses are identified using the corresponding codes within health services data such as international classification of disease (ICD) codes from hospital admission discharge summaries or Read codes from primary care data.[20] [21] This approach assumes that the diseases are accurately and completely recorded in the databases, which in turn assumes that well implemented quality control procedures are in place at the point of data entry.[21]

The purpose of development and validation studies is to test these assumptions. These studies run different identification algorithms against a reference population whose disease status has been individually validated (box). Identification algorithms are constructed and tested using various diagnosis codes along with procedures and services in different combinations and intensities. Identification algorithms are then compared using tests of discrimination (sensitivity, specificity, likelihood ratios) and predictive accuracy (positive and negative predictive values).[22] Other approaches for developing and validating identification methods are available.[23] [24] [25] Because studies of identification accuracy (assessing the accuracy of tests to identify people already diagnosed with a disease) are similar to those studying diagnostic accuracy (assessing the accuracy of tests to diagnose people who may have a

disease), the approaches to development, validation, and reporting are largely applicable to both types of studies.[9]

Errors can also occur when information is abstracted from a database for a study. With increased computing power and wider availability of health data it is straightforward to apply identification criteria to an entire population, including populations beyond those represented in a development study (if one exists). Rather than formally creating a database for a specific study, it is common simply to apply the identification criteria to create a study population. For example, a hospital may assess its performance by examining the quality of care for people with an acute myocardial infarction in terms of time to thrombolytic therapy or 30 day survival by identifying people with a discharge diagnosis coded for acute myocardial infarction.[26] However, if the ICD-9 code for myocardial infarction is incorrectly used, the quality measure may be biased.

Studies using electronically collected data can be grouped into three types:
- Study denominator is drawn from the database—for example, examining healthcare performance for people with a particular condition
- Study base is entire population and the numerator is people with a disease—for example, examining the incidence and prevalence of a disease in a population
- Outcome of interest is people who develop a condition—for example, study of drug side effects such as admission for hyperkalaemia (identified from hospital discharge data) in patients prescribed spironolactone.[27]

Classification errors will potentially bias different study types in different ways. Performance reports are biased only from false positive entries, whereas estimates of disease incidence are affected by both false positive and false negative entries.

Assessment of bias

Bias from misclassification should be assessed for each use of data from electronic health record systems. Unless a diagnosis is individually verified there will inevitably be some classification error, and the resulting bias is difficult to intuitively gauge because both the amount and direction of bias are affected by the study design and by various properties of disease identification including prevalence, sensitivity, and specificity. The amount of bias may be large, even when the disease identification criteria seem to be accurate or there are well instituted data quality control procedures.

There are two general approaches that are used to estimate bias. The first approach applies the level of identification accuracy from development studies to a new study. We used this approach when we estimated bias in the two published diabetes studies. The second approach validates the identification in a new study, correcting for bias as needed.

Calculating bias is not always straightforward. First, development or validation studies are required, and they should report sensitivity and specificity or similar measures of disease identification accuracy. Many studies have not validated their method of disease identification. For example, more than two thirds of peer reviewed studies using the General Practice Research Database did not perform a validation study and most of those that did calculated only specificity and positive predictive values.[5] Even well performed validation studies carry generalisability concerns. In our examples, the validation study used a diagnosis

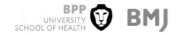

STEPS FOR CREATING AND USING A DISEASE DATABASE WHEN DISEASE STATUS IS NOT INDIVIDUALLY VERIFIED

- *Development studies*—Develop disease identification criteria by assessing the identification (or diagnostic) accuracy of different ascertainment approaches or algorithms against a reference standard of people with individually verified disease status
- *Create disease database*—Systematically apply the case identification criteria to an entire population's health data. Enrol people in the database if they satisfy case identification criteria. Regularly update the process when new data become available. Assign an enrolment (incident) date. Studies may not formally create a disease database; instead, the disease identification criteria are applied to the health data of all study participants
- *Assess for bias due to classification error*—For each use of the disease databases or disease identification algorithm, assess the potential for misclassification to bias the study results. Estimate the number of people who may be false positives and false negatives, and examine how this affects the study results
- *Validation studies*—(Re)validate the disease identification criteria in new study populations with a reference standard

of diabetes in general practice records as the reference standard. This reference standard is imperfect because, among other reasons, some patients may not have had their diagnosis in their general practice recorded because their diabetes was diagnosed and cared for exclusively by specialists. Furthermore, it may be inappropriate to assume that sensitivity and specificity from a validation study hold firm for studies with different population characteristics. Methods are available to overcome these concerns, including performing sensitivity testing using different reference standards or levels of identification accuracy (calculating bias by varying sensitivity and specificity).[9] We recommend the development and use of multi-attribute identification algorithms to estimate the probability of disease diagnoses (value of 0 to 1), rather than assigning disease status to a person (value of 0 or 1).[28]

Conclusion

As our two examples show, even in well performed studies with well developed identification criteria, there is considerable opportunity for misclassification to bias results—so much so that studies can arrive at incorrect conclusions. Most of the time, it is straightforward to calculate the amount of potential bias and adjust the findings accordingly. Our findings are applicable beyond diabetes, particularly when disease prevalence is below about 10% and the specificity of identification is less than perfect (say, less than 98%).

The problem is further magnified because once a disease database is generated, many different investigators may use it for a wide range of studies or reports, propagating classification errors in their wake. However, data users cannot estimate bias when the accuracy of identification is unknown, and people who generate the databases or apply identification algorithms to routinely collected data should clearly describe the accuracy of their classification process. Researchers using such data should also publish an estimate of the percentage of false positives and negatives and the effect of misclassified people on the study's findings. Readers of reports can reasonably ask if classification error potentially challenges the studies'

findings, and they should expect to see calculations that estimate the amount of bias.

It would be wrong to conclude that routinely collected data are poorly suited to study people with chronic conditions. Routinely collected data are improving and increasingly include more clinical information that can be used to individually verify disease or develop more accurate identification algorithms. Nevertheless, careful development and validation can help ensure that disease identification is accurate, bias can be measured, and results accordingly adjusted.

Contributors: All authors contributed to the development of the paper. DGM led the writing. LCR and TAS provided edits. DGM is the guarantor of the paper and analyses.

Competing interests: All authors have completed the unified competing interest form at www.icmje.org/coi_disclosure.pdf (available on request from the corresponding author) and declare support for this article was provided by the Population Health Improvement Research Network; DGM holds a chair in applied public health from the Canadian Institute for Health Research and the Public Health Agency of Canada; no other relationships or activities that could appear to have influenced the submitted work. The opinions, results, and conclusions reported in this paper are not necessarily those of the funding or employment sources.

Provenance and peer review: Not commissioned; externally peer reviewed.

1   Newton J, Garnes H. Disease registers in England. Institute of Health Sciences, University of Oxford, 2002.
2   Hurtado M, Swift E, Corrigan J. Envisioning the national health care quality report. National Academy Press, 2001.
3   Powell AE, Davies HT, Thomson RG. Using routine comparative data to assess the quality of health care: understanding and avoiding common pitfalls. Qual Saf Health Care 2003;12:122-8.
4   Joshy G, Simmons D. Diabetes information systems: a rapidly emerging support for diabetes surveillance and care. Diabetes Technol Ther 2006;8:587-97.
5   Herrett E, Thomas SL, Schoonen WM, Smeeth L, Hall AJ. Validation and validity of diagnoses in the General Practice Research Database: a systematic review. Br J Clin Pharmacol 2010;69:4-14.
6   General Practice Research Database. www.gprd.com.
7   Woodward G, van Walraven C, Hux JE. Utilization and outcomes of HbA1c testing: a population-based study. CMAJ 2006;174:327-9.
8   Lipscombe LL, Hux JE. Trends in diabetes prevalence, incidence, and mortality in Ontario, Canada 1995-2005: a population-based study. Lancet 2007;369:750-6.
9   Bossuyt PM, Reitsma JB, Bruns DE, Gatsonis CA, Glasziou PP, Irwig LM, et al. The STARD statement for reporting studies of diagnostic accuracy: explanation and elaboration. Ann Intern Med 2003;138:W1-12.
10 Hux JE, Ivis F, Flintoft V, Bica A. Diabetes in Ontario: determination of prevalence and incidence using a validated administrative data algorithm. Diabetes Care 2002;25:512-6.
11 Kelsey J, Thompson W, Evans A. Methods in observational epidemiology. 2nd ed. Oxford University Press, 1996.
12 Rogan WJ, Gladen B. Estimating prevalence from the results of a screening test. Am J Epidemiol 1978;107:71-6.
13 Couris CM, Polazzi S, Olive F, Remontet L, Bossard N, Gomez F, et al. Breast cancer incidence using administrative data: correction with sensitivity and specificity. J Clin Epidemiol 2009;62:660-6.
14 Lix L, Yogendran M, Burchill C, Metge C, McKeen N, Moore D, et al. Defining and validating chronic diseases: an administrative data approach. Manitoba Centre for Health Policy, 2006.
15 Mullooly JP. Misclassification model for person-time analysis of automated medical care databases. Am J Epidemiol 1996;144:782-92.
16 White E. The effect of misclassification of disease status in follow-up-studies—implications for selecting disease classification criteria. Am J Epidemiol 1986;124:816-25.
17 Health Council of Canada. Why health care renewal matters: lessons from diabetes. 2007. www.healthcouncilcanada.ca/docs/rpts/2007/HCC_DiabetesRpt.pdf.
18 Wild S, Roglic G, Green A, Sicree R, King H. Global prevalence of diabetes: estimates for the year 2000 and projections for 2030. Diabetes Care 2004;27:1047-53.
19 Ontario Ministry of Health and Longterm Care. Diabetes strategy—backgrounder. Ontario Ministry of Health and Longterm Care, 2008.
20 World Health Organization. International statistical classification of diseases and related health problems: 10th revision. WHO, 1992.
21 Schulz EB, Barrett JW, Price C. Read code quality assurance. J Am Med Inform Assoc 1998;5:337-46.
22 Habbema JDF, Eijkemans R, Krijnen P, Knottnerus JA. Analysis of data on the accuracy of diagnostic tests. In: Knottnerus JA, ed. The evidence base of clinical diagnosis. BMJ Publishing, 2002:117-44.

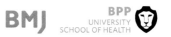

23 Lix LM, Yogendran MS, Leslie WD, Shaw SY, Baumgartner R, Bowman
    C, et al. Using multiple data features improved the validity of
    osteoporosis case ascertainment from administrative databases. *J Clin
    Epidemiol* 2008;61:1250-60.

24 Sturmer T, Thurigen D, Spiegelman D, Blettner M, Brenner H. The
    performance of methods for correcting measurement error in case-
    control studies. *Epidemiology* 2002;13:507-16.

25 Mower WR. Evaluating bias and variability in diagnostic test reports.
    Ann Emerg Med 1999;33:85-91.

26 Tu JV, Khalid L, Donovan LR, Ko DT. Indicators of quality of care for
    patients with acute myocardial infarction. *CMAJ* 2008;179:909-15.

27 Juurlink DN, Mamdani MM, Lee DS, Kopp A, Austin PC, Laupacis A,
    et al. Rates of hyperkalemia after publication of the Randomized
    Aldactone Evaluation Study. *N Engl J Med* 2004;351:543-51.

28 Van Walraven C, Austin PC, Manuel D, Knoll G, Jennings A, Forster AJ.
    The usefulness of administrative databases for identifying disease
    cohorts is increased with a multivariate model. *J Clin Epidemiol*
    2010;63:1000-10.

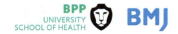

Verification problems in diagnostic accuracy studies: consequences and solutions

Joris A H de Groot, clinical epidemiologist[1], Patrick M M Bossuyt, professor of clinical epidemiology[2], Johannes B Reitsma, associate professor of clinical epidemiology[2], Anne W S Rutjes, senior researcher[3], Nandini Dendukuri, assistant professor clinical epidemiology and biostatistics[4], Kristel J M Janssen, clinical epidemiologist[1], Karel G M Moons, professor of clinical epidemiology[1]

[1]Julius Center for Health Sciences and Primary care, UMC Utrecht, PO Box 85500, 3508GA Utrecht, Netherlands

[2]Department of Clinical Epidemiology, Biostatistics and Bioinformatics, Academic Medical Center Amsterdam, 1100 DE Amsterdam, Netherlands

[3]Division of Clinical Epidemiology and Biostatistics, Institute of Social and Preventive Medicine-University of Bern, 3012 Bern, Switzerland

[4]Royal Victoria Hospital, Quebec, Canada H3A 1A1

Correspondence to: J A H de Groot
j.degroot-17@umcutrecht.nl

Cite this as: BMJ 2011;343:d4770

DOI: 10.1136/bmj.d4770

http://www.bmj.com/content/343/bmj.d4770

The accuracy of a diagnostic test or combination of tests (such as in a diagnostic model) is the ability to correctly identify patients with or without the target disease. In studies of diagnostic accuracy, the results of the test or model under study are verified by comparing them with results of a reference standard, applied to the same patients, to verify disease status (see first panel in figure).[1] Measures such as predictive values, post-test probabilities, ROC (receiver operating characteristics) curves, sensitivity, specificity, likelihood ratios, and odds ratios express how well the results of an index test agree with the outcome of the reference standard.[2] Biased and exaggerated estimates of diagnostic accuracy can lead to inefficiencies in diagnostic testing in practice, unnecessary costs, and physicians making incorrect treatment decisions.

The reference standard ideally provides error-free classification of the disease outcome presence or absence. In some cases, it is not possible to verify the definitive presence or absence of disease in all patients with the (single) reference standard, which may result in bias. In this paper, we describe the most important types of disease verification problems using examples from published diagnostic accuracy studies. We also propose solutions to alleviate the associated biases.

Partial verification

Often not all study subjects who undergo the index test receive the reference standard, leading to missing data on disease outcome (see middle panel in figure). The bias associated with such situations of partial verification is known as partial verification bias, work-up bias, or referral bias.[3] [4] [5]

Clinical examples of partial verification

Various mechanisms can lead to partial verification (see examples in table 1).

When the condition of interest produces lesions that need biopsy and subsequent histological verification (as in many cancers), it is impossible to verify negative index test results ("where to biopsy?"). An example is F-18 fluorodeoxyglucose positron emission tomography (FDG-PET) to detect possible distant metastases before planning curative surgery in patients with carcinoma of the oesophagus: only the hotspots detected by PET can be sampled by biopsy and verified histologically.[6]

Ethical reasons can also play a role in withholding a reference standard. Angiography is still considered the best method for detecting pulmonary embolisms, but, because of its invasiveness and risk of serious complications, it is now considered unethical to perform this reference standard in low risk patients, such as those with a low clinical probability and negative D-dimer result.[10]

Sometimes the reference standard may be temporarily unavailable, or patients and doctors may decide to refrain from disease verification. In a study evaluating the accuracy of digital rectal examination and prostate specific antigen (PSA) for the early detection of prostate cancer, 145 out of 1000 men fulfilled the criterion for verification by the reference standard (transrectal ultrasound combined with biopsy). However, 54 of these men did not undergo the reference standard, for unknown reasons.[7] In another study the accuracy of dobutamine-atropine stress echocardiography for the diagnosis of coronary artery disease was assessed, with coronary angiography as the reference.[8] Only a small proportion of patients received this reference standard because the clinicians' decision to refer to angiography depended on the patient's history and test results.

Potential for bias

The above examples show that partial disease verification, and thus missing disease outcome status in some of the patients, is often not completely at random or non-selective. It is usually based on results of the index test under study or other observed patient variables or test results. If so, the missing outcome status is selectively missing, as the reason for disease verification is associated with other information. For example, patients with a positive index test result or with a high clinical suspicion based on other variables (that is, high probability before the index test) are often more likely to be verified by the reference test than patients with

SUMMARY POINTS

- In studies of diagnostic accuracy studies, ideally all patients undergoing the index test are verified by the reference standard
- This is not always possible, and incomplete or improper disease verification is one of the major sources of bias in diagnostic accuracy studies
- Partial verification bias occurs when not all patients are verified by the reference standard; instead, disease verification is related to other, previous (index) test results or patient characteristics. Multiple imputation methods can be used to correct for the partial verification bias
- An alternative reference test may be used for those cases where verification with the preferred reference test is not possible. This can result in differential verification bias if the results of both reference tests are treated as equal and interchangeable, when they are really of different quality or define the target condition differently. Instead, the estimated accuracy of the diagnostic index test should be reported separately for each reference test

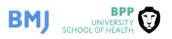

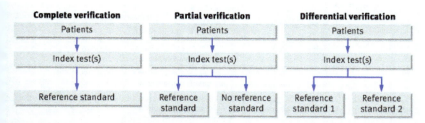

Complete verification	Partial verification	Differential verification
Patients	Patients	Patients
Index test(s)	Index test(s)	Index test(s)
Reference standard	Reference standard / No reference standard	Reference standard 1 / Reference standard 2

Diagnostic accuracy studies with (a) complete verification by the same reference standard, (b) partial verification, or (c) differential verification

negative test results or a low probability before the index test. Simply leaving such selectively unverified patients out of the analysis will leave a non-random (selective) part of the original group for analysis and thus generate biased estimates of the accuracy of the index test under study.

The direction and size of this bias will depend on how selective the reason for non-verification is, the number of patients whose results are not verified, and the ratio between the number of patients with positive and negative index test results that remain unverified.[5] The bias always occurs in the estimates of the sensitivity and specificity of the diagnostic index test or model under study, and often also in the predictive value. When the reason for partially missing outcomes is based only on the results of the index test, the predictive values of this index test will indeed be unbiased (see below). If, however, the reason for referral for reference testing is not only due to the index test results but also to other patient information, the predictive values of the index test will be affected.[15]

Corrections for partial verification bias

One of the early methods to correct for partial verification bias was developed by Begg and Greenes.[16] Briefly, this method uses only the pattern of disease and non-disease verified by the reference standard among the patients with a positive or negative result of the (single) index test under study. This pattern is then used to calculate the expected number of diseased and non-diseased among the non-verified patients with a positive or negative index test result to obtain an inflated 2×2 table as if all patients were verified by the reference standard. This correction method assumes that the reason for referral to the reference test is only due to the result of the index test under study. Hence, conditional on these index test results, the decision to verify is in fact a random process. The method can also be extended to more than one test result, but this requires exact knowledge of the reasons and patterns behind the partial verification.[16] [17]

More recently, multiple imputation methods have been proposed to correct for partial verification problems.[18] [19] Multiple imputation can be viewed as a "statistical" workout of the intuitive "diagnostic reasoning" of the clinician. Just as a clinician in practice decides whether to refer a patient for disease verification by a (more invasive, burdensome, or costly) reference standard based on all available patient information, multiple imputation techniques also use all available information of a patient—and that of similar patients—to estimate the most likely value of the missing reference test result in non-verified patients.

Imputation methods comprise two phases—an imputation phase where each missing reference test result is estimated and imputed from all available patient information, and an analysis phase where accuracy estimates of the diagnostic index test or model are computed by standard procedures based on the now completed dataset. Several imputation variants are available, ranging from single imputation of missing reference test values to multiple imputation.[20] [21] Instead of filling in a single value for each missing value, as with single imputation, multiple imputation procedures replace each missing value with a set of plausible values to represent the uncertainty about the imputed value. These multiple imputed datasets are then analysed, one by one, again by standard procedures. The results from these analyses are combined to produce accuracy estimates of the diagnostic index test(s) or model and confidence intervals that properly reflect the uncertainty due to missing values.[20] [21]

For optimal application of multiple imputation techniques to address partial verification, it is important for researchers to collect as much detailed data as possible on study subjects that could potentially drive the (selective) referral for reference testing. The performance of the multiple imputation or other correction methods will improve with more and better information that may be involved in disease verification decisions. The flexibility of the multiple imputation method enables the incorporation of multiple pieces of observed patient information, not only the results of the index test under study, thereby increasing the likelihood of correctly imputing missing reference test values in patients in whom the disease status was selectively not verified.[17] [18] [19]

The discussed mathematical methods to correct for selectively missing verification, and thus partial verification bias, make use of observed (patient) information or variables. They assume that the reasons for missing verification depend on the observed information only. Clearly, this assumption cannot be tested with the data at hand, since non-observed information is, by definition, not available. If one expects selectively missing reference test results as a result of unobserved information, there are methods to perform additional (sensitivity) analysis to quantify to what extent the diagnostic accuracy estimates of the index test change under these situations.[22] [23]

Differential verification

Another common approach in diagnostic accuracy studies is to use an alternative, second best, reference test in those subjects for whom the first, preferred reference test cannot or will not be used (see third panel in figure). Although this seems a clinically appealing and ethical approach, bias arises when the results of the two reference tests are treated as interchangeable. Both reference tests are, almost by definition, of different quality in terms of classification of the target disease or may even define the target disease differently.[24] [25] Hence, simply combining all disease outcome data in a single analysis (table 2), as if both reference tests are yielding the same disease outcomes, does not reflect the "true" pattern of disease presence and absence. Such an estimation of disease prevalence differs from what one would have obtained if all subjects had undergone the preferred reference standard. Consequently, all estimated measures of the accuracy of the diagnostic index test or model will be biased. This is called differential verification bias.[3] [4]

When evaluating a new marker for acute appendicitis, histopathology of the appendix is the preferred reference test, but clinical follow-up is sometimes used as an alternative (for example, if histopathology is considered too invasive). Compared with histopathology, clinical follow-up is likely to have a higher implicit threshold to detect

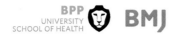

Table 1   Examples of diagnostic accuracy studies with problems in disease verification

Index test(s)	Target condition	Reference standard	Problem	Study
Partial verification				
Positron emission tomography (PET)	Distant metastases	Histology of biopsy	Only PET hotspots were (can be) biopsied	Lee 2001[6]
Digital rectal examination and prostate specific antigen	Prostate cancer	Combination of transrectal ultrasound plus biopsy	54/145 men not verified for unknown reasons	Pode 1995[7]
Dobutamine-atropine stress echocardiography	Coronary artery disease	Coronary angiography	Only a small sample of patients verified because of clinicians' decision	Elhendy 1998[8]
Hepatic scintigraphy	Liver cancer	Liver biopsy with pathology	39% of index test positives and 63% of test negatives not verified for unspecified reasons	Kline 2001[9]
D-dimer and alveolar dead space measurement	Pulmonary embolism	Pulmonary angiography	Not all patients verified for unspecified reasons	Drum 1972[10]
Differential verification				
Elbow extension test	Elbow fracture	Radiography or follow-up	Index test positives received radiography, index test negatives received follow-up	Appelboam 2008[11]
D-dimer test	Deep vein thrombosis (DVT)	Ultrasonography of the legs	Patients with negative D-dimer test or clinically low risk of DVT were verified by follow-up at 3 months	Buller 2009[12]
Patient history, physical examination, and laboratory tests	Serious bacterial infection	Cultures of blood, spinal fluid, urine, stools, or a panel diagnosis	Mixture of reference standards, as used in clinical practice	Bleeker 2001[13]
Ventilation/perfusion lung scans	Acute pulmonary embolism	Scintigraphy, pulmonary angiography, or follow-up	Mixture of reference standards, as used in clinical practice	PIOPED Investigators 1990[14]

Table 2   Effect of differential disease verification in a diagnostic accuracy study. If the preferred reference test (R) is used only to verify positive index test results while an alternative reference test (S) is used to validate index test negatives, simply combining the results ignores the fact that both reference tests have different abilities to determine disease presence or absence, and so the disease status is ambiguously defined

Index test result	Reference test results								
	Verification with test R			Verification with test S			Differential verification with either		
	+ve	−ve		+ve	−ve		+ve?	−ve?	
+ve	a	b	+	−	−	≠	a	b	
−ve	−	−		c	d		c	d	

appendicitis, so it will label more patients as non-diseased (that is, no appendicitis). Thus, these two reference tests define the target condition in a different way. Histopathology might seem the preferred reference test because it reveals even the smallest number of inflamed cells, but one could argue that the more relevant information for clinical practice is not whether the patient has inflamed cells but whether the patient will recover without intervention. This would make clinical follow-up the preferred reference, even though it would be unethical to adopt for all subjects and to withhold surgery. This does mean that accuracy estimates from a combination of histopathology and follow-up will differ systematically from what one would have obtained if all index test results had been verified by either clinical follow-up or histology.

Because accuracy estimates of the new index test ignore the use of different reference tests, they are also difficult to interpret. In situations of differential verifications such as this, the results should be corrected and reported separately for each reference standard to provide informative and unbiased measures of accuracy of the diagnostic index test or model. We illustrate this with a clinical example from the recent literature.

Clinical example

In a recent study[11] the elbow extension test (EET) was examined for its accuracy in ruling out elbow fractures. The preferred reference test was radiography. For unstated reasons (costs, efficiency, or minimising radiation exposure), radiography was planned in patients with a positive EET result whereas the patients with a negative EET received a structured follow-up assessment by telephone after 7-10 days to verify whether elbow fracture was absent (the alternative reference test). Only patients who met any of the pre-specified recall criteria were asked to return to the emergency department for radiography. The rest were considered not to have a clinically significant elbow fracture. The resulting data are shown in table 3.

The authors reported overall estimates of accuracy of the EET, ignoring the use of different reference standards (table 4, first row). Though both radiography and structured follow-up are useful verification methods, their results are not necessarily interchangeable.

The availability of 181 patients with a negative EET who were, after all, evaluated by radiography ("protocol violations" in table 3) enables us to apply the above mentioned correction methods for partial verification, under

Table 3 Distribution of patients in study of diagnostic accuracy of elbow extension test (EET) verified against radiography (for positive EET) or clinical follow-up (for negative EET)*

	Radiography			Follow-up	
	Fracture	No fracture		Fracture	No fracture
Positive EET	521	617		NA	NA
Negative EET	14†	167†		3	414

*Data from Appelboam et al, 2008.[11]

†Data available as a result of protocol violations.

Table 4 Sensitivity, specificity, and predictive values of elbow extension test* depending on whether correction was made for differential verification. All values are percentages (95% confidence intervals)

Analysis	Sensitivity	Specificity	Negative predictive value	Positive predictive value
No correction	96.8 (95.0 to 98.2)	48.5 (45.6 to 51.4)	97.2 (95.5 to 98.3)	45.8 (42.9 to 48.7)
Correction†	91.8 (88.0 to 95.7)	47.2 (44.2 to 50.2)	92.3 (88.6 to 95.9)	45.8 (42.6 to 49.0)

*Data from Appelboam et al, 2008.[11]

†Corrected for partial verification (accuracy with respect to radiography) by method of Begg and Greenes, 1983.[16]

the assumption that, conditional on the index test result, the decision to verify is a random process.

The corrected values of sensitivity and specificity clearly show the consequences of differential verification (table 4, second row). We found differences in the estimates of EET accuracy when verification bias is simply ignored and when it is adjusted for. The negative predictive value (the item of primary interest, to rule out elbow fractures), with respect to radiography alone was lower than the value reported by the authors and fell below the desired value of ≥97%. This clearly shows that two reference tests should not be viewed as one.

(For a more detailed discussion of this example and the possibilities to correct for differential verification, see de Groot et al, 2011[26])

Further corrections for differential verification bias
Recently, a Bayesian method was proposed for simultaneously adjusting for differential verification bias and for the fact that these multiple reference tests were imperfect.[26] The method produces accuracy measures both with respect to the latent disease status and with respect to the use of different reference tests. The former can be considered as a more general measure of performance of the index test with respect to a theoretically defined target condition or disease status since none of the reference tests used is considered perfect. However, the index test's accuracy measures for each of the reference standards may be considered of greater clinical relevance, as these reflect the accuracy against the reference tests that are commonly also performed in daily practice, and on which patient management decisions will often be based.

Conclusion
In diagnostic accuracy studies, all efforts should be made to verify as many test results as possible, preferably all, with the optimal reference test to avoid bias. In practice, the burden on patients, costs, or other reasons often prevent this from happening (table 1).[27]

If test outcome is verified by the reference test for only some of the patients, which is usually selective disease verification based on other observed patient information, we advise the use of the mathematical correction methods described above.[16 17 19]

There is insufficient knowledge to make general statements about what proportion of missing reference standard results might be acceptable and at which point

correction methods will become unreliable. Following various statistical guidelines,[18 19 20 21 28 29] we recommend the use of correction methods even with small rates of missing verification data. Even small proportions of missing outcomes may yield biased accuracy estimates of the index test(s) or model under study if the non-verified sample is highly selective.

What upper limits of missing reference test data can still be corrected for is even harder to say.[4] Recently Janssen et al showed that, even for large amounts of missing data, imputation leads to less biased results than simply ignoring the (selectively) non-measured subjects.[28] The authors warn that this possibility for imputation depends on how selective or different the observed and non-observed subjects are and how many results remain to build "good enough" imputation models. In any case, authors applying correction or imputation methods for addressing partial verification should provide insight in both issues—how many subjects had missing reference test values and how different were the verified and non-verified patients by comparing both groups on their observed characteristics.[29 30]

If the preferred reference test is not possible and thus missing in complete subgroups, applying a different, usually inferior, reference test will obviously produce different information about the disease status. In such cases, the results should be reported separately for each reference test to provide more clinically informative and unbiased measures of diagnostic accuracy.[3] If in these situations one still wants to quantify the accuracy of the diagnostic index test or model with regard to the same underlying target condition, one should also correct for possible imperfections of the applied reference tests.[26]

Contributors: KGMM is guarantor for the article and heads a research team aimed at improving methods for quantification of the diagnostic and prognostic value of medical tests, biomarkers, and other devices. KJMJ and JAHdG are clinical epidemiologists in his team. PMMB and JBR lead the Biomarker and Test Evaluation (BiTE) programme to develop and appraise methods for evaluating medical tests and biomarkers, and spearheaded the STARD initiative to improve the reporting of diagnostic accuracy studies. AWSR's PhD thesis was on sources of bias and variation in diagnostic accuracy studies and she currently works to update QUADAS, a tool for the quality assessment of studies of diagnostic accuracy included in systematic reviews. ND is engaged in research in the area of methods for diagnostic studies.

Funding: We acknowledge the support of the Netherlands Organization for Scientific Research (projects 9120.8004 and 918.10.615).

Competing interests: All authors have completed the ICJME unified disclosure form at www.icmje.org/coi_disclosure.pdf (available on request from the corresponding author) and declare that they have no financial or non-financial interests that may be relevant to the submitted work.

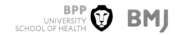

In diagnostic accuracy studies the ability of a test or combination of tests to correctly identify patients with or without the target condition is verified by applying a reference standard in all patients who have undergone the index test. Incomplete or improper disease verification is one of the major sources of bias in diagnostic accuracy studies. This study describes the various types of disease verification problems, including empirical examples, and proposes solutions to alleviate the associated biases

Provenance and peer review: Not commissioned; externally peer reviewed.

1   Knottnerus JA, Muris JW. Assessment of the accuracy of diagnostic tests: the cross-sectional study. In: Knottnerus JA, ed. *The evidence base of clinical diagnosis* . 2nd ed. BMJ Books, 2002:39-60.
2   Knottnerus JA, van Weel C. General introduction: evaluation of diagnostic procedures. In: Knottnerus JA, ed. *The evidence base of clinical diagnosis* . 2nd ed. BMJ Books, 2002:1-18.
3   Rutjes AW, Reitsma JB, Irwig LM, Bossuyt PM. Sources of bias and variation in diagnostic accuracy studies. In: Rutjes AWS, ed. *Partial and differential verification in diagnostic accuracy studies* . Rutjes, 2005:31-44.
4   Rutjes AW, Reitsma JB, Coomarasamy A, Khan KS, Bossuyt PM. Evaluation of diagnostic tests when there is no gold standard. A review of methods. *Health Technol Assess* 2007;11:iii, ix-51.
5   Reitsma JB, Rutjes AW, Khan KS, Coomarasamy A, Bossuyt PM. A review of solutions for diagnostic accuracy studies with an imperfect or missing reference standard. *J Clin Epidemiol* 2009;62:797-806.
6   Lee J, Aronchick JM, Alavi A. Accuracy of F-18 fluorodeoxyglucose positron emission tomography for the evaluation of malignancy in patients presenting with new lung abnormalities: a retrospective review. *Chest* 2001;120:1791-7.
7   Pode D, Shapiro A, Lebensart P, Meretyk S, Katz G, Barak V. Screening for prostate cancer. *Isr J Med Sci* 1995;31:125-8.
8   Elhendy A, van Domburg RT, Poldermans D, Bax JJ, Nierop PR, Geleijnse ML, et al. Safety and feasibility of dobutamine-atropine stress echocardiography for the diagnosis of coronary artery disease in diabetic patients unable to perform an exercise stress test. *Diabetes Care* 1998;21:1797-802.
9   Drum DE, Christacopoulos JS. Hepatic scintigraphy in clinical decision making. *J Nucl Med* 1972;13:908-15.
10 Kline JA, Israel EG, Michelson EA, O'Neil BJ, Plewa MC, Portelli DC. Diagnostic accuracy of a bedside D-dimer assay and alveolar dead-space measurement for rapid exclusion of pulmonary embolism: a multicenter study. *JAMA* 2001;285:761-8.
11 Appelboam A, Reuben AD, Benger JR, Beech F, Dutson J, Haig S, et al. Elbow extension test to rule out elbow fracture: multicentre, prospective validation and observational study of diagnostic accuracy in adults and children. *BMJ* 2008;337:a2428.
12 Buller HR, Ten Cate-Hoek AJ, Hoes AW, Joore MA, Moons KG, Oudega R, et al. Safely ruling out deep venous thrombosis in primary care. *Ann Intern Med* 2009;150:229-35.
13 Bleeker SE, Moons KG, rksen-Lubsen G, Grobbee DE, Moll HA. Predicting serious bacterial infection in young children with fever without apparent source. *Acta Paediatr* 2001;90:1226-32.
14 The PIOPED Investigators. Value of the ventilation/perfusion scan in acute pulmonary embolism. Results of the prospective investigation of pulmonary embolism diagnosis (PIOPED). *JAMA* 1990;263:2753-9.
15 Little RA, Rubin DB. *Statistical analysis with missing data* . Wiley, 1987.
16 Begg CB, Greenes RA. Assessment of diagnostic tests when disease verification is subject to selection bias. *Biometrics* 1983;39:207-15.
17 de Groot JA, Janssen KJ, Zwinderman AH, Bossuyt PM, Reitsma JB, Moons KG. Correcting for partial verification bias: a comparison of methods. *Ann Epidemiol* 2011;21:139-48.
18 Harel O, Zhou XH. Multiple imputation for correcting verification bias. *Stat Med* 2006;25:3769-86.
19 de Groot JA, Janssen KJ, Zwinderman AH, Moons KG, Reitsma JB. Multiple imputation to correct for partial verification bias revisited. *Stat Med* 2008;27:5880-9.
20 Donders AR, van der Heijden GJ, Stijnen T, Moons KG. Review: a gentle introduction to imputation of missing values. *J Clin Epidemiol* 2006;59:1087-91.
21 Rubin DB. *Multiple imputation for non response in surveys* . Wiley, 1987.
22 Kosinski AS, Barnhart HX. Accounting for non-ignorable verification bias in assessment of diagnostic tests. *Biometrics* 2003;59:163-71.
23 Kosinski AS, Barnhart HX. A global sensitivity analysis of performance of a medical diagnostic test when verification bias is present. *Stat Med* 2003;22:2711-21.
24 Whiting P, Rutjes AW, Reitsma JB, Glas AS, Bossuyt PM, Kleijnen J. Sources of variation and bias in studies of diagnostic accuracy: a systematic review. *Ann Intern Med* 2004;140:189-202.
25 Lijmer JG, Mol BW, Heisterkamp S, Bonsel GJ, Prins MH, van der Meulen JH, et al. Empirical evidence of design-related bias in studies of diagnostic tests. *JAMA* 1999;282:1061-6.
26 de Groot JA, Dendukuri N, Janssen KJ, Reitsma JB, Bossuyt PM, Moons KG. Adjusting for differential-verification bias in diagnostic-accuracy studies: a bayesian approach. *Epidemiology* 2011;22:234-41.
27 Oostenbrink R, Moons KG, Bleeker SE, Moll HA, Grobbee DE. Diagnostic research on routine care data: prospects and problems. *J Clin Epidemiol* 2003;56:501-6.
28 Janssen KJ, Donders AR, Harrell FE Jr, Vergouwe Y, Chen Q, Grobbee DE, et al. Missing covariate data in medical research: to impute is better than to ignore. *J Clin Epidemiol* 2010;63:721-7.
29 Mackinnon A. The use and reporting of multiple imputation in medical research—a review. *J Intern Med* 2010;268:586-93.
30 Van der Heijden GJ, Donders AR, Stijnen T, Moons KG. Imputation of missing values is superior to complete case analysis and the missing-indicator method in multivariable diagnostic research: a clinical example. *J Clin Epidemiol* 2006;59:1102-9.

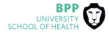

Interpretation of random effects meta-analyses

Richard D Riley, senior lecturer in medical statistics[1],
Julian P T Higgins, senior statistician[2], Jonathan J Deeks, professor of biostatistics[1]

Department of Public Health,
Epidemiology and Biostatistics,
Public Health Building, University
of Birmingham, Birmingham B15
2TT, UK

MRC Biostatistics Unit, Institute
of Public Health, Cambridge CB2
0SR, UK

Correspondence to: R D Riley
r.d.riley@bham.ac.uk

Cite this as: BMJ 2011;342:d549

DOI: 10.1136/bmj.d549

http://www.bmj.com/content/342/
bmj.d549

ABSTRACT

Summary estimates of treatment effect from random effects meta-analysis give only the average effect across all studies. Inclusion of prediction intervals, which estimate the likely effect in an individual setting, could make it easier to apply the results to clinical practice

Meta-analysis is used to synthesise quantitative information from related studies and produce results that summarise a whole body of research.[1] A typical systematic review uses meta-analytical methods to combine the study estimates of a particular effect of interest and obtain a summary estimate of effect.[2] For example, in a meta-analysis of randomised trials comparing a new treatment with placebo, researchers will collect the estimates of treatment effect for each study, as measured by a relevant statistic such as a risk ratio, and then statistically synthesise them to obtain a summary estimate of the treatment effect.

Meta-analyses use either a fixed effect or a random effects statistical model. A fixed effect meta-analysis assumes all studies are estimating the same (fixed) treatment effect, whereas a random effects meta-analysis allows for differences in the treatment effect from study to study. This choice of method affects the interpretation of the summary estimates. We examine the differences and explain why a prediction interval can provide a more complete summary of a random effects meta-analysis than is usually provided.

Difference between fixed effect and random effects meta-analyses

Figure 1 shows two hypothetical meta-analyses, in which estimates of treatment effect are computed and synthesised from 10 studies of the same antihypertensive drug. Each study provides an unbiased estimate of the standardised mean difference in change in systolic blood pressure between the treatment group and the control group. Negative estimates indicate a greater blood pressure reduction for patients in the treatment group than the control group.

The two meta-analyses give identical summary estimates of treatment effect of −0.33 with a 95% confidence interval of −0.48 to −0.18, but the first uses a fixed effect model

and the second a random effects model. In the following two sections we explain why the summary result should be interpreted differently in these two examples because of the different meta-analysis models they use.

Fixed effect meta-analysis

Use of a fixed effect meta-analysis model assumes all studies are estimating the same (common) treatment effect. In other words, there is no between study heterogeneity in the true treatment effect. The implication of this model is that the observed treatment effect estimates vary only because of chance differences created from sampling patients. Hypothetically, if all studies had an infinite sample size, there would be no differences due to chance and the differences in study estimates would completely disappear.

I^2 measures the percentage of variability in treatment effect estimates that is due to between study heterogeneity rather than chance.[3] I^2 is 0% in our fixed effect meta-analysis example, suggesting the variability in study estimates is entirely due to chance. This is visually evident by the narrow scatter of effect estimates with large overlap in their confidence intervals (fig 1, top). The summary result of −0.33 (95% confidence interval of −0.48 to −0.18) in our example thus provides the best estimate of a common treatment effect, and the confidence interval depicts the uncertainty around this estimate. As the confidence interval does not contain zero, there is strong evidence that the treatment is effective.

Random effects meta-analysis

A random-effects meta-analysis model assumes the observed estimates of treatment effect can vary across studies because of real differences in the treatment effect in each study as well as sampling variability (chance). Thus, even if all studies had an infinitely large sample size, the observed study effects would still vary because of the real differences in treatment effects. Such heterogeneity in treatment effects is caused by differences in study populations (such as age of patients), interventions received (such as dose of drug), follow-up length, and other factors.

In the random effects example in figure 1, I^2 is 71%, suggesting 71% of the variability in treatment effect estimates is due to real study differences (heterogeneity) and only 29% due to chance.[3] This is visually evident from the wide scatter of effect estimates with little overlap in their confidence intervals, in contrast to the fixed effect example (fig 1). The random effects model summary result of −0.33 (95% confidence interval −0.48 to −0.18) provides an estimate of the average treatment effect, and the confidence interval depicts the uncertainty around this estimate. As the confidence interval does not contain zero, there is strong evidence that on average the treatment effect is beneficial.

SUMMARY POINTS

- Meta-analysis combines the study estimates of a particular effect of interest, such as a treatment effect
- Fixed effect meta-analysis assumes a common treatment effect in each study and variation in observed study estimates is due only to chance
- Random effects meta-analysis assumes the true treatment effect differs from study to study and provides an estimate of the average treatment effect
- Interpretation of random effects meta-analysis is aided by a prediction interval, which provides a predicted range for the true treatment effect in an individual study

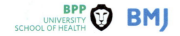

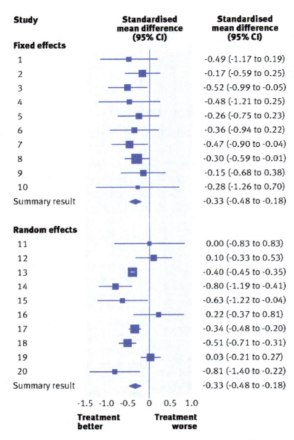

Study	Standardised mean difference (95% CI)	Standardised mean difference (95% CI)
Fixed effects		
1		-0.49 (-1.17 to 0.19)
2		-0.17 (-0.59 to 0.25)
3		-0.52 (-0.99 to -0.05)
4		-0.48 (-1.21 to 0.25)
5		-0.26 (-0.75 to 0.23)
6		-0.36 (-0.94 to 0.22)
7		-0.47 (-0.90 to -0.04)
8		-0.30 (-0.59 to -0.01)
9		-0.15 (-0.68 to 0.38)
10		-0.28 (-1.26 to 0.70)
Summary result		-0.33 (-0.48 to -0.18)
Random effects		
11		0.00 (-0.83 to 0.83)
12		0.10 (-0.33 to 0.53)
13		-0.40 (-0.45 to -0.35)
14		-0.80 (-1.19 to -0.41)
15		-0.63 (-1.22 to -0.04)
16		0.22 (-0.37 to 0.81)
17		-0.34 (-0.48 to -0.20)
18		-0.51 (-0.71 to -0.31)
19		0.03 (-0.21 to 0.27)
20		-0.81 (-1.40 to -0.22)
Summary result		-0.33 (-0.48 to -0.18)

-1.5 -1.0 -0.5 0 0.5 1.0

Treatment better   **Treatment worse**

Fig 1 Forest plots of two distinct hypothetical meta-analyses that give the same summary estimate (centre of diamond) and its 95% confidence interval (width of diamond). In the fixed effect meta-analysis (top) the summary result provided the best estimate of an assumed common treatment effect. In the random effects meta-analysis (bottom) the summary result gives the average from the distribution of treatment effects across studies

Use and interpretation of meta-analysis in practice

Unfortunately, meta-analysis results are often interpreted in the same manner regardless of whether a fixed effect

---

How to calculate a prediction interval

A random effects meta-analysis combines the study estimates of a parameter of interest (eg, a treatment effect) in order to estimate the average value (denoted by μ) and the standard deviation of the parameter (denoted by τ) across studies. The term random denotes that the μ value is not common to all studies, and that the parameter value in an individual study can vary randomly about the average value due to unexplained heterogeneity. Methods to estimate μ and τ are discussed elsewhere.[2]

After a random effects meta-analysis, a prediction interval can be calculated to give a range for the predicted parameter value in a new study. Assuming the random effects (that is, the individual study parameter values) are normally distributed with between-study standard deviation (τ), then the prediction interval is approximately[6]

$$\hat{\mu} - t_{k-2}\sqrt{\hat{\tau}^2 + SE(\hat{\mu})^2}, \quad \hat{\mu} + t_{k-2}\sqrt{\hat{\tau}^2 + SE(\hat{\mu})^2}$$

Fig 2

where $\hat{\mu}$ is the estimate of the average parameter value across studies; $SE(\hat{\mu})$ is the standard error of $\hat{\mu}$; $\hat{\tau}$ is the estimate of between study standard deviation; t_{k-2} is the $100(1-\alpha/2)$ percentile of the t distribution with $k-2$ degrees of freedom, where k is the number of studies in the meta-analysis and α is usually chosen as 0.05, to give a 5% significance level and thus 95% prediction interval. A t distribution, rather than a normal distribution, is used to help account for the uncertainty of $\hat{\tau}$. The correct number of degrees of freedom for this t distribution is complex, and we use a value of $k-2$ largely for pragmatic reasons.

As an example computation, for the fibromyalgia syndrome meta-analysis (fig 3) the effect of interest is the standardised mean difference in pain (for the antidepressant group minus the control group) and $\hat{\mu} = -0.425$, $SE(\hat{\mu}) = 0.063$, $\hat{\tau} = 0.18$, and a $t_{k-2}^{\alpha} = t_{20}^{0.05} = 2.086$, leading to a 95% prediction interval of -0.83 to -0.02.

Finally, it is important to work on a scale that helps meet the normal assumption for the random effects. In particular, when the parameter under investigation is a ratio measure (such as a relative risk or odds ratio), then $\hat{\mu}$, $\hat{\tau}$ and the subsequent prediction interval are best derived on the natural log scale and the results subsequently exponentiated back to the original scale.

---

or random effects model is used. We reviewed 44 Cochrane reviews that each reported a random effects meta-analysis and found that none correctly interpreted the summary result as an estimate of the average effect rather than the common effect.[4] Furthermore, only one indicated why the summary result from a random effects meta-analysis was clinically meaningful,[5] arguing that, although real study differences (heterogeneity) in treatment effects existed (because of different doses), the studies were reasonably clinically comparable as the same drug was used and patient characteristics were similar.

Another problem is that a fixed effect meta-analysis model is often used even when heterogeneity is present. We examined 31 Cochrane reviews that did not use a random effects model and found that 26 had potentially moderate or large heterogeneity between studies ($I^2 > 25\%$ as a guide[3]) yet still used a fixed effect model, without justifying why.[4] Ignoring heterogeneity leads to an overly precise summary result (that is, the confidence interval is too narrow) and may wrongly imply that a common treatment effect exists when actually there are real differences in treatment effectiveness across studies.

Benefits of using prediction intervals

After a random effects meta-analysis, researchers usually focus on the average treatment effect estimate and its confidence interval. However, it is important also to consider the potential effect of treatment when it is applied within an individual study setting, as this may be different from the average effect. This can be achieved by calculating a prediction interval (fig 2).[6]

Intervals akin to prediction intervals are commonly used in other areas of medicine. For example, when considering the blood pressure of an individual or the birthweight of an infant, we not only compare it with the average value but also with a reference range (prediction interval) for blood pressure or birthweight across the population. In the meta-analysis setting, our measures are treatment effects, and we work at the study level (rather than the individual level) with a population of study effects. We therefore can report the range of effects across study settings, providing a more complete picture for clinical practice. For instance, consider the random effects analysis in figure 1 again, for which the 95% prediction interval is -0.76 to 0.09. Although most of this interval is below zero, indicating the treatment will be beneficial in most settings, the interval overlaps zero and so in some settings the treatment may actually be ineffective. This finding was masked when we focused only on the average effect and its confidence interval.

A prediction interval can be provided at the bottom of a forest plot (fig 3). It is centred at the summary estimate, and its width accounts for the uncertainty of the summary estimate, the estimate of between study standard deviation in the true treatment effects (often denoted by the Greek letter τ), and the uncertainty in the between study standard deviation estimate itself.[6] It can be calculated when the meta-analysis contains at least three studies, although the interval may be very wide with so few studies. A prediction interval will be most appropriate when the studies included in the meta-analysis have a low risk of bias.[7] Otherwise, it will encompass heterogeneity in treatment effects caused by these biases, in addition to that caused by genuine clinical differences.

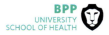

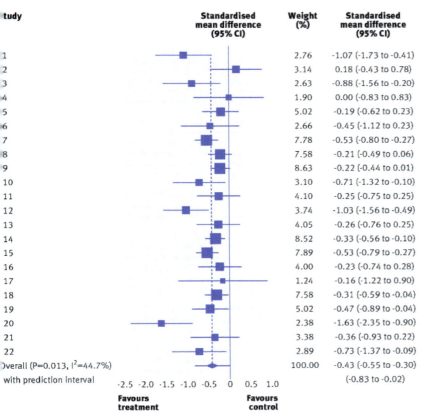

Fig 3 Random effects meta-analysis of 22 studies that examine the effect of antidepressants on reducing pain in patients with fibromyalgia syndrome[8]

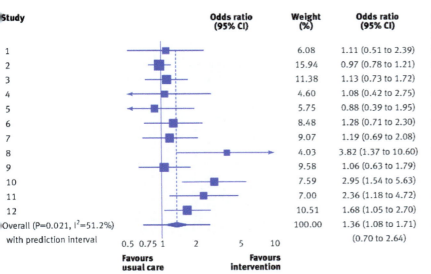

Fig 4 Random effects meta-analysis of 12 trials that examine the effect of inpatient rehabilitation designed for geriatric patients versus usual care on improving functional outcome[9]

Examples

Antidepressants for reducing pain in fibromyalgia syndrome

Hauser and colleagues report a meta-analysis of randomised trials to determine the efficacy of antidepressants for fibromyalgia syndrome, a chronic pain disorder associated with multiple debilitating symptoms.[8] Twenty two estimates of the standardised mean difference in pain (for the antidepressant group minus the control group) were available from the included trials (fig 3), with negative values indicating a benefit for antidepressants. Studies used different classes of antidepressants, and other clinical and methodological differences also existed, resulting

in large between study heterogeneity in treatment effect (I^2=45%; between study standard deviation estimate=0.18). The authors therefore used a random effects meta-analysis and obtained a summary result of −0.43 (95% confidence interval −0.55 to −0.30), concluding that "antidepressant medications are associated with improvements in pain."

The summary result here relates to the average effect of antidepressants across the trials. As the confidence interval is below zero, it provides strong evidence that on average antidepressants are beneficial; however, it does not indicate whether antidepressants are always beneficial. The authors acknowledge the heterogeneity of treatment effects but conclude that "although study effect sizes differed, results were mostly consistent." This can be quantified more formally by a 95% prediction interval, which we calculated as −0.83 to −0.02 (fig 2). This interval is entirely below zero and shows that antidepressants will be beneficial when applied in at least 95% of the individual study settings, an important finding for clinical practice.

Inpatient rehabilitation in geriatric patients

Bachmann and colleagues did a random effects meta-analysis of 12 randomised trials to summarise the effect of inpatient rehabilitation compared with usual care on functional outcome in geriatric patients (fig 4).[9] The summary odds ratio estimate is 1.36 (1.07 to 1.71), which indicates that the average effect of the intervention is to make the odds of functional improvement 1.36 times higher than usual care. As the confidence interval is above one, it provides strong evidence that the average intervention effect is beneficial.

However, there is large between study heterogeneity in intervention effect (I^2=51%; between study standard deviation estimate=0.27), possibly because of differences in the type of intervention used (such as general or orthopaedic rehabilitation) and length of follow-up, among other factors. Responding to the heterogeneity, the authors state: "Pooled effects should be interpreted with caution because the true differences in effects between studies might be due to uncharacterised or unexplained underlying factors or the variability of outcome measures on functional status."[9] This cautionary note can be quantified by presenting a 95% prediction interval, which we calculate as 0.70 to 2.64. This interval contains values below 1 and so, although on average the intervention seems effective, it may not always be beneficial in an individual setting. Further research is needed to identify causes of the heterogeneity, in particular the subtypes of geriatric rehabilitation programmes that work best and the subgroups of patients that benefit most.

Discussion

Between study heterogeneity in treatment effects is a common problem for meta-analysts. Although it is desirable to identify the causes of heterogeneity (by using meta-regression or subgroup analyses, for example),[10] this is often not practically possible.[11] [12] For instance, there may be too few studies to examine heterogeneity reliably; no prespecified idea of what factors might cause heterogeneity; or a lack of necessary information (such as no individual participant data[13]). Even when factors causing heterogeneity are identified, unexplained heterogeneity may remain. Thus random effects meta-analysis, which accounts for unexplained heterogeneity, will continue to be prominent in the medical literature. Including a prediction interval, which indicates the possible treatment effect in an individual

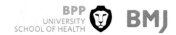

setting, will make these analyses more useful in clinical practice and decision making.[14] Although our examples focused on the synthesis of randomised trials, prediction intervals can also be used in other meta-analysis settings such as studies of diagnostic test accuracy[15] and prognostic biomarkers.[16]

We thank David Spiegelhalter and Simon Thompson for their comments and acknowledge their role in developing the concept of a prediction interval from random effects meta-analysis (see Higgins et al[6]). We thank the reviewers and editors for their helpful comments, which have greatly improved the content and clarity of the paper.

Contributors: All authors have undertaken applied and methodological research in the meta-analysis field over many years and work closely with the Cochrane Collaboration. JPTH and RDR conceived the paper. RDR performed the review of 44 Cochrane reviews that used random effects meta-analysis. JPTH (with colleagues Simon Thompson and David Spiegelhalter) identified the need for a prediction interval and subsequently derived how to calculate it. RDR and JJD performed the analyses for the two examples. RDR wrote the first draft and produced the figures and tables. All authors contributed to revising the paper accordingly. RDR is the guarantor.

Competing interests: All authors have completed the unified competing interest form at www.icmje.org/coi_disclosure.pdf (available on request from the corresponding author) and declare no support from any organisation for the submitted work; no financial relationships with any organisation that might have an interest in the submitted work in the previous three years; RDR and JJD are statistics editors for the *BMJ*.

Provenance and peer review: Not commissioned; externally peer reviewed.

1   Egger M, Davey Smith G. Meta-analysis: Potentials and promise. *BMJ* 1997;315:1371-4.

2   Sutton AJ, Abrams KR, Jones DR, Sheldon TA, Song F. *Methods for Meta-analysis in medical research* . John Wiley, 2000.

3   Higgins JP, Thompson SG, Deeks JJ, Altman DG. Measuring inconsistency in meta-analyses. *BMJ* 2003;327:557-60.

4   Riley RD, Gates SG, Neilson J, Alfirevic Z. Statistical methods can be improved within Cochrane pregnancy and childbirth reviews. *J Clin Epidemiol* 2010 Nov 24. [Epub ahead of print].

5   King J, Flenady V, Cole S, Thornton S. Cyclo-oxygenase (COX) inhibitors for treating preterm labour. *Cochrane Database Syst Rev* 2005;2:CD001992.

6   Higgins JPT, Thompson SG, Spiegelhalter DJ. A re-evaluation of random effects meta-analysis. *J R Stat Soc Ser A* 2009;172:137-59.

7   Higgins JPT, Green S, eds. *Cochrane handbook for systematic reviews of interventions* . John Wiley, 2008.

8   Häuser W, Bernardy K, Üceyler N, Sommer S. Treatment of fibromyalgia syndrome with antidepressants: a meta-analysis. *JAMA* 2009;301:198-209.

9   Bachmann S, Finger C, Huss A, Egger M, Stuck AE, Clough-Gorr KM. Inpatient rehabilitation specifically designed for geriatric patients: systematic review and meta-analysis of randomised controlled trials. *BMJ* 2010;340:c1718.

10 Thompson SG. Why sources of heterogeneity in meta-analysis should be investigated. *BMJ* 1994;309:1351-5.

11 Thompson SG, Higgins JPT. How should meta-regression analyses be undertaken and interpreted? *Stat Med* 2002;21:1559-74.

12 Higgins J, Thompson S, Deeks J, Altman D. Statistical heterogeneity in systematic reviews of clinical trials: a critical appraisal of guidelines and practice. *J Health Serv Res Policy* 2002;7:51-61.

13 Riley RD, Lambert PC, Abo-Zaid G. Meta-analysis of individual participant data: conduct, rationale and reporting. *BMJ* 2010;340:c221.

14 Ades AE, Lu G, Higgins JPT. The interpretation of random-effects meta-analysis in decision models. *Med Decis Making* 2005;25:646-54.

15 Reitsma JB, Glas AS, Rutjes AW, Scholten RJ, Bossuyt PM, Zwinderman AH. Bivariate analysis of sensitivity and specificity produces informative summary measures in diagnostic reviews. *J Clin Epidemiol* 2005;58:982-90.

16 Riley RD, Sauerbrei W, Altman DG. Prognostic markers in cancer: the evolution of evidence from single studies to meta-analysis, and beyond. *Br J Cancer* 2009;100:1219-29.

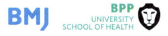

Differential dropout and bias in randomised controlled trials: when it matters and when it may not

Melanie L Bell, senior research fellow[1], Michael G Kenward, professor[2], Diane L Fairclough, professor[3], Nicholas J Horton, professor[4]

Psycho-Oncology Co-operative Research Group (PoCoG), University of Sydney, Sydney Australia

Department of Medical Statistics, London School of Hygiene and Tropical Medicine, London, UK

Department of Preventive Medicine and Biometry, University of Colorado at Denver, Denver, CO, USA

Department of Mathematics and Statistics, Smith College, Northampton, MA, USA

Correspondence to: M L Bell melanie.bell@sydney.edu.au

Cite this as: BMJ 2013;346:e8668

DOI: 10.1136/bmj.e8668

http://www.bmj.com/content/346/bmj.e8668

ABSTRACT

Dropout in randomised controlled trials is common and threatens the validity of results, as completers may differ from people who drop out. Differing dropout rates between treatment arms is sometimes called differential dropout or attrition. Although differential dropout can bias results, it does not always do so. Similarly, equal dropout may or may not lead to biased results. Depending on the type of missingness and the analysis used, one can get a biased estimate of the treatment effect with equal dropout rates and an unbiased estimate with unequal dropout rates. We reinforce this point with data from a randomised controlled trial in patients with renal cancer and a simulation study.

Introduction

Dropout in longitudinal randomised controlled trials is common and a potential source of bias in terms of evidence based medicine. A review of 71 randomised controlled trials in four top medical journals showed dropout rates of 20% or more in 18% of the trials.[1] Similar rates were found in a review of quality of life outcomes.[2] In specialist journals, the rates are likely to be higher.

When dropout rates differ between treatment arms, so that fewer patients are followed up in one arm than the other, it is sometimes called "differential dropout" or "differential attrition." Despite extensive literature on incomplete data methods for randomised controlled trials, guidance from the CONSORT reports, and the National Research Council's recent report on missing data,[3] many applied researchers have misconceptions about how to handle dropout.[1 2 4] Two common misunderstandings about differential dropout need to be debunked:

- Myth 1—if dropout rates in longitudinal clinical trials are similar between study arms, bias is not a concern.
- Myth 2—if dropout rates are dissimilar between study arms, the results will necessarily be biased.

Although differential dropout can bias results, equal dropout rates between study arms does not imply that results will be unbiased (myth 1). The inverse is true as well: unequal dropout rates do not mean the results are biased (myth 2). Whether dropout rates between the arms

are differential or not can be a red herring; the two key factors are the type of missingness and the statistical analysis. Our aims were to show that for continuous outcome data biased estimates of treatment effects can be obtained when no differential dropout occurs (refute myth 1); unbiased estimates of treatment effects can be obtained when differential dropout occurs (refute myth 2); and when missingness is non-random, the degree of bias depends, in part, on the actual mechanism of dropout. We begin with an example from a real randomised controlled trial and then show the generalisability of our assertions with a computer simulation study (see glossary).

Example

A phase III randomised controlled trial was carried out to compare two treatments in patients with advanced renal cell carcinoma (details discussed elsewhere[6]). This disease is aggressive, and the treatment is toxic; patients discontinue treatment (one form of dropout) owing to toxicity, disease progression, and death.

Quality of life and symptom sub-studies are commonly carried out in clinical trials, as patient reported outcomes are increasingly recognised as important for understanding patients' experience during treatment and providing support for or against experimental treatments.[7] The renal cell trial used a quality of life questionnaire that included questions on physical and functional wellbeing, as well as disease specific questions. One aim was to determine whether the two treatments affected these aspects of quality of life differently. One hundred and ninety seven patients were assessed at four time points: baseline and two, eight, and 17 weeks.

The term "dropout" also refers to the situation in which all outcome data are missing after a certain point. In the renal cell trial, the dropout rates for quality of life were 64% for the control arm and 70% for the experimental arm. To investigate the myths, we averaged 50 multiply imputed datasets to create one complete dataset, in which no outcome data were missing, thereby enabling calculation of a "true" treatment effect. We then deleted observations to create datasets with equal and unequal dropout rates to investigate bias in the estimated treatment effect and its relation to the analytical approach. Details are in the web appendix.

Key concepts

Types of missing data

To investigate the effect of dropout in the example, we need to understand the different types of missing data and how they relate to bias. Rubin defined a taxonomy of missingness,[8] shown in the glossary, which underpins the

SUMMARY POINTS

- Equal dropout rates between treatment arms in a randomised controlled trial do not imply that estimates of treatment effect are unbiased
- Similarly, unequal dropout rates do not imply that estimates are biased
- Bias depends on the type of missingness, the analysis method, and the effect that is being estimated
- Likelihood based methods such as mixed models can be used to estimate unbiased treatment effects, under assumptions regarding the missingness mechanism(s)

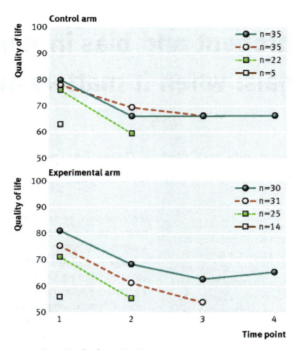

Fig Quality of life (QoL) stratified by treatment arm and dropout time. Possible range of QoL=0-100, with higher values indicating better QoL. If data were missing completely at random (MCAR), the within arm trajectories would be indistinguishable. As patients with lower baseline QoL are more likely drop out, these data are not MCAR

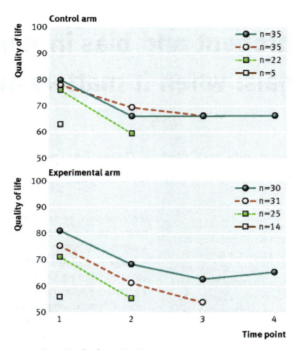

choice of appropriate analytical approach in a trial with dropout. If patients withdraw from a study for a reason unrelated to their disease or treatment (for example, because they have moved overseas) their data are probably missing completely at random, because systematic differences between them and the patients who remained in the study are unlikely. If patients withdraw from the study for reasons related to their disease or treatment (such as progression or toxicity) the missing data are either missing at random or missing not at random; their quality of life measures would have been, on average, worse than those of patients who remained in the study. One can distinguish between missing at random and missing completely at random by testing, for example, whether baseline quality of life or progression rates differ between dropouts and completers or by using a graphical approach.[4] The figure shows quality of life plotted against time for the renal cell trial, stratified by dropout time. As the trajectories differ substantially by dropout time, the data are not missing completely at random; patients with lower baseline quality of life were more likely to drop out, particularly in the experimental arm. Distinguishing between missing at random and missing not at random from the data under analysis is generally impossible.[6][9]

Statistical analysis: what works and what does not work

Bias in the estimate of treatment effect caused by dropout can also depend on the analytical approach used. When data are missing completely at random or missing at random, likelihood based mixed models (see glossary) can yield unbiased estimates of treatment effect.[6][10][11] The mixed model for repeated measures is appropriate if participants are assessed at common time points, as is usual in clinical trials. This model allows the outcome to potentially differ by group and time.[5][12] Implementation in a variety of software packages (SAS, Stata, SPSS, and R code are shown in the appendix) is straightforward. If no dropouts occur, the estimate of the difference between treatment and control

arms from this mixed model will yield identical results to the simple calculation of a difference in means. Even if dropout differs between the treatment groups, if the data are missing completely at random or missing at random and an appropriate mixed model is used then estimates of the treatment effect will, on average, be unbiased. This is because information from patients with complete data is used to implicitly impute the missing values. (Other methods, such as multiple imputation, Bayesian, and weighted approaches also can give unbiased estimation,[9][13] but these are more computationally intensive, may offer no advantage over the likelihood based approach, and are beyond the scope of this paper.) Table 1 shows the lack of bias with mixed models in the renal cell trial.

Unfortunately, data from randomised controlled trials are not typically analysed using methods that are valid under missing at random, which can in many circumstances lead to biased estimates.[1][2][4] More commonly, simpler methods

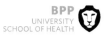

Table 1 Treatment effect estimates and statistical significance at time 4: difference in quality of life between control and experimental arms (QoLcontrol−QoLexperimental) in renal cell trial

Analysis	Dataset and dropout rates (control %:experimental %)							
	Real data (64:70)		Equal dropout (41:44)		Unequal dropout (25:51)		Unequal dropout (51:25)	
	Estimate	P value	Estimate (% bias*)	P value	Estimate (% bias*)	P value	Estimate (% bias*)	P value
True difference	?		7.2	0.002	7.2	0.002	7.2	0.002
Mixed model	8.1	0.03	7.2 (0)	0.005	7.2 (0)	0.008	8.5 (18)	<0.001
Complete case†	0.4	0.9	4.5 (−38)	0.1	2.0 (−72)	0.5	12.5 (74)	<0.001
Mean imputation‡	5.0	0.008	5.9 (−18)	0.003	3.4 (−53)	0.1	9.0 (25)	<0.001
Last observation carried forward§	6.3	0.01	5.1 (−29)	0.05	5.9 (−18)	0.03	9.9 (38)	<0.001

Complete dataset was created by averaging 50 multiply imputed datasets, then patients were dropped out using missing at random process (see web appendix for more detail); true estimate from this complete dataset is 7.2 (see web appendix for more detail).

*100×(estimate−true)/true, where estimate=difference in mean quality of life at final time point.

†No imputation used.

‡Missing values replaced with mean of patient's previously observed values.

§Missing values replaced with patient's last observed value.

such as complete case analysis and single imputation are used, and these are valid only under strong and typically unrealistic assumptions. These methods have been shown to be biased if data are not missing completely at random.[6] [9] [11] Complete case analysis includes only participants with complete data, which can cause bias if those who drop out are sicker. Popular single imputation methods are last observation carried forward and mean imputation. With last observation carried forward, patients with declining health and quality of life who drop out will have their missing quality of life values replaced by their last observed values, which is likely to overestimate quality of life and yield biased estimates. Last observation carried forward, because of its unlikely assumptions about trajectories over time, is generally biased even when data are missing completely at random.[3] [9] [11] The common misuse of these methods has potentially serious consequences.[14] In the renal cell trial, these methods were associated with bias of up to a 74% overestimate and 72% underestimate of the treatment effect for the complete dataset (table 1). (Note that we cannot know what the bias is for the non-augmented real dataset.) This bias translates to a standardised effect size of 0.4 (0.4 of the baseline standard deviation). In some cases, the statistical significance changed as well, which may have implications for decision making.

When data are missing not at random, no method of obtaining unbiased estimates exists that does not incorporate the mechanism of non-random missingness, which is nearly always unknown. Some evidence, however, shows that the use of a method that is valid under missing at random can provide some reduction in bias.[11] This is the main reason that experts recommend methods such as mixed modelling as the primary analysis followed by sensitivity analyses,[15] [16] in which the stability of estimates is examined when assumptions about missingness are varied.[3] [6] [9] [11]

Returning to the myths, we see from table 1 that biased estimates can result from equal dropout, particularly if complete case analysis is used, suggesting that myth 1 may be false. Of the methods shown, the mixed model gave almost unbiased treatment estimates, even when the dropout rates were different, suggesting that myth 2 may also be false. To confirm this, we did a simulation study.

Simulation study

The simulation study involved creation of 10000 datasets representing a two arm randomised controlled trial for quality of life, with 200 participants, over three time points, in which the true treatment effect was known. We deleted data to make equal and unequal dropout scenarios. We created different types of missingness and different "directions" of dropout (patients in the treatment group dropped out when they had good outcomes, and patients in the control group dropped out when they had poor outcomes). We used two common patterns for quality of life over time: a linear decline and a temporary change. We analysed each of these datasets by computing the difference in mean quality of life at the final time point between the treatment and control groups by using complete case analysis, single imputation, and a mixed model. Details are given in the appendix.

Myth 1—Table 2 (second and fourth columns) shows that equal dropout rates do not guarantee unbiased results. In the equal dropout simulation, the single imputation approaches all yielded biased estimates of the treatment effect, for every type of dropout, even missing completely at random. Last observation carried forward, for example, underestimated the treatment effect by 22% for missing completely at random for both the same and different direction mechanisms. For missing at random, last observation carried forward underestimated by 24% for the same direction mechanism but overestimated by 6% for the different direction mechanism.

Myth 2—Table 2 (third and fifth columns) shows that unequal dropout rates do not imply biased results. The mixed model yielded unbiased estimates for all missing completely at random and missing at random scenarios, regardless of equal or unequal dropout rates and differing mechanisms (directions) for dropout.

Dropout mechanism—Our third aim was to show that the magnitude of the bias depends, in part, on the dropout mechanism. The bias when using the simple methods was larger for the differing directions dropout mechanism, compared with the same direction, when data were missing at random and for all analyses, including the mixed model, for missing not at random data.

The complete case approach gave unbiased treatment estimates for the situation of equal dropout rates with the same direction of dropout. For most other situations, it gave biased results, with as much as 80% underestimation. Most of the bias took the form of underestimation, but this was not uniform, as cases of overestimation also occurred, showing that the bias that occurs when complete case and single imputation techniques are used is not predictable.

Results for the temporary change pattern of quality of life were very similar and are shown in the web appendix. The bias does not change with sample size; we did the same

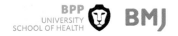

Table 2 Comparison of simple methods and mixed modelling for linear decline pattern

Missingness and analysis	Percentage bias*				
	Same direction†			Different direction†	
	Equal dropout (30%)	Unequal dropout (20% treatment, 40% control)		Equal dropout (30%)	Unequal dropout (20% treatment, 40% control)
No missing data:					
Complete case	0	0		0	0
Mixed model	0	0		0	0
Missing completely at random:					
Complete case‡	−1	0		0	0
Mean imputation§	−27	−46		−27	−47
Last observation carried forward¶	−22	−40		−22	−41
Mixed model	0	0		0	0
Missing at random:					
Complete case‡	0	26		−60	−61
Mean imputation§	−28	−17		−6	−24
Last observation carried forward¶	−24	−19		6	−10
Mixed model	1	0		0	0
Missing not at random:					
Complete case‡	0	35		−80	−82
Mean imputation§	−28	−5		−44	−61
Last observation carried forward¶	−25	−2		−41	−57
Mixed model	0	−18		−40	−41

*100×(estimate−true)/true, where estimate=difference in mean quality of life (QoL) at final time point.

†Different direction=patients in treatment group dropped out when they had high QoL, patients in control group dropped out when they had poor QoL; same direction=patients in both group dropped out when QoL scores were low.

‡No imputation used.

§Missing values replaced with mean of patient's previously observed values.

¶Missing values replaced with patient's last observed value.

simulations with 2000 datasets, and the results were very similar to those shown in table 2.

Discussion

We have shown that the two myths described in the introduction are indeed myths: equal dropout rates can still yield biased estimates of treatment effects, and studies with unequal dropout rates can be analysed to produce unbiased results. Likelihood based analyses, such as the mixed model presented here, represent one approach for valid analysis when the dropout mechanism is data missing completely at random or missing at random. A non-random mechanism will typically lead to bias under any analysis that does not incorporate this (usually unknown) mechanism. Because of this, if missing not at random is suspected a sensitivity analyses should be done.[3 6 9 11] We have discussed these concepts in the context of quality of life in oncology trials, but the results are generalisable to any randomised controlled trial with continuous outcomes and dropout.

Unfortunately, the consideration of differential dropout in the literature has omitted a discussion of key elements. In a review of randomised controlled trials of palliative care, Thomas et al stated that they "recorded an attrition analysis as performed only if the authors reported an analysis assessing if the intervention and control arms were differentially affected by attrition."[17] Heneghan et al, in considering differential attrition in randomised controlled trials in diabetes, created a "relative attrition statistic."[18] Neither of these papers discusses type of missingness or analyses used for estimation of treatment effect.

The CONSORT statement says: "There should be concern when the frequency or the causes of dropping out differ between the intervention groups."[19] Although this is certainly true, it may be misinterpreted as researchers focus on frequency instead of cause and are lulled into complacency about unbiased estimation when dropout rates are equal between trial arms. We do not wish to give the misleading impression that unequal dropout rates between arms in a clinical trial is not a problem, but we wish to stress that it does not always cause bias. An important reason to consider differential dropout is the acceptability and uptake of the intervention. Different adverse effect profiles between the arms, for example, could cause differential dropout. We recommend, as do others in the missing data field, that a sensible analytical approach for data with dropout begins with an assumption of missing at random, includes careful examination and documentation of the missingness mechanism(s), and includes sensitivity analyses if missing not at random data are suspected.[3 6 9 11 15] With appropriate analyses, such as use of mixed models, bias can be eliminated or reduced.

Data presented are derived (and used with permission) from a trial conducted by Memorial Sloan-Kettering Cancer Center and Eastern Cooperative Oncology Group funded by the National Cancer Institute grant CA-05826.

Contributors: MLB had the original idea, did the analyses, and wrote the first draft. DLF aided in design. All authors revised the manuscript and approved the final version.

Competing interests: All authors have completed the ICMJE uniform disclosure form at www.icmje.org/coi_disclosure.pdf (available on request from the corresponding author) and declare: no support from any organisation for the submitted work; no financial relationships with any organisations that might have an interest in the submitted work in the previous three years; no other relationships or activities that could appear to have influenced the submitted work.

Provenance and peer review: Not commissioned; externally peer reviewed.

1   Wood AM, White IR, Thompson SG. Are missing outcome data adequately handled? A review of published randomized controlled trials in major medical journals. *Clin Trials* 2004;1:368-76.

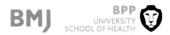

2 Fielding S, Maclennan G, Cook JA, Ramsay CR. A review of RCTs in four medical journals to assess the use of imputation to overcome missing data in quality of life outcomes. *Trials* 2008;9:51.

3 Panel on Handling Missing Data in Clinical Trials, National Research Council. The prevention and treatment of missing data in clinical trials. National Academies Press, 2010.

4 Joly F, Vardy J, Pintilie M, Tannock IF. Quality of life and/or symptom control in randomized clinical trials for patients with advanced cancer. *Ann Oncol* 2007;18:1935-42.

5 Fitzmaurice GM, Laird NM, Ware JH. Applied longitudinal analysis. 2nd ed. Wiley, 2011.

6 Fairclough DF. Design and analysis of quality of life studies in clincial trials. 2nd ed. Chapman & Hall/CRC, 2010.

7 Au HJ, Ringash J, Brundage M, Palmer M, Richardson H, Meyer RM, for the NCIC CTG Quality of Life Committee. Added value of health-related quality of life measurement in cancer clinical trials: the experience of the NCIC CTG. *Expert Rev Pharmacoecon Outcomes Res* 2010;10:119-28.

8 Rubin DB. Inference and missing data. *Biometrika* 1976;63:581-92.

9 Carpenter J, Kenward M. Missing data in randomised controlled trials—a practical guide. National Institute for Health Research, 2008.

10 Carpenter JR, Kenward MG, Vansteelandt S. A comparison of multiple imputation and doubly robust estimation for analyses with missing data. *J R Stat Soc Series A Statistics in Society* 2006;169:571-84.

11 Molenberghs G, Thijs H, Jansen I, Beunckens C, Kenward MG, Mallinckrodt C, et al. Analyzing incomplete longitudinal clinical trial data. *Biostatistics* 2004;5:445-64.

12 Mallinckrodt CH, Clark WS, Carroll RJ, Molenberghs G. Assessing response profiles from incomplete longitudinal clinical trial data under regulatory considerations. *J Biopharm Stat* 2003;13:179-90.

13 Robins JM, Rotnitzky A, Zhao LP. Analysis of semiparametric regression models for repeated outcomes in the presence of missing data. *J Am Stat Assoc* 1995;90:106-21.

14 Molnar FJ, Man-Son-Hing M, Hutton B, Fergusson DA. Have last-observation-carried-forward analyses caused us to favour more toxic dementia therapies over less toxic alternatives? A systematic review. *Open Med* 2009;3:e31-50.

15 Carpenter J, Roger J, Kenward M. Analysis of longitudinal trials with protocol deviations: a framework for relevant, accessible assumptions and inference via multiple imputation. *J Biopharm Stat* [forthcoming].

16 White IR, Horton NJ, Carpenter J, Pocock SJ. Strategy for intention to treat analysis in randomised trials with missing outcome data. *BMJ* 2011;342:d40.

17 Thomas RE, Wilson D, Sheps S. A literature review of randomized controlled trials of the organization of care at the end of life. *Can J Aging* 2006;25:271-93.

18 Heneghan C, Perera R, Ward AA, Fitzmaurice D, Meats E, Glasziou P. Assessing differential attrition in clinical trials: self-monitoring of oral anticoagulation and type II diabetes. *BMC Med Res Methodol* 2007;7:18.

19 Moher D, Hopewell S, Schulz KF, Montori V, Gøtzsche PC, Devereaux PJ, et al. CONSORT 2010 explanation and elaboration: updated guidelines for reporting parallel group randomised trials. *BMJ* 2010;340:c869.

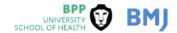

Rethinking pragmatic randomised controlled trials: introducing the "cohort multiple randomised controlled trial" design

Clare Relton, research fellow[1] [3], David Torgerson, director of clinical trials unit[2], Alicia O'Cathain, professor of health services research[1], Jon Nicholl, director of the Medical Care Research Unit[1]

[1]School for Health and Related Research, University of Sheffield, Sheffield

[2]Department of Health Sciences, University of York, Heslington, York

[3]School of Healthcare, University of Leeds, Leeds

Correspondence to: C Relton
c.relton@sheffield.ac.uk

Cite this as: BMJ 2010;340:c1066

DOI: 10.1136/bmj.c1066

http://www.bmj.com/content/340/bmj.c1066

ABSTRACT

Pragmatic trials are important for informing routine clinical practice, but current designs have shortcomings. Clare Relton and colleagues outline the new "cohort multiple randomised controlled trial" design, which could help address the problems associated with existing approaches

Introduction

Randomised controlled trials are generally held to be the "gold standard" for establishing how well an intervention works. Trials that aim to determine the efficacy of a treatment by using a double blind, placebo controlled design (that is, explanatory trials) are, however, sometimes criticised. For example, although the design of explanatory trials results in strong internal validity—we can depend upon the results of a given trial—such trials may have limited external validity: we can't be confident that we can apply the results to routine clinical practice. Pragmatic trials,[1] [2] which aim to inform healthcare decision making in practice, have been offered as a solution in that they retain the rigour of randomisation (thus eliminate selection bias) but retain the characteristics of normal clinical practice.

The implementation and interpretation of both pragmatic and explanatory randomised controlled trials are associated with significant problems. This article describes a trial design that helps address these problems—the "cohort multiple randomised controlled trial" approach.

Problems with randomised controlled trials

Existing clinical trial designs can have shortcomings in four areas: recruitment; ethics; patient preferences; and treatment comparisons.

SUMMARY POINTS

- The "cohort multiple randomised controlled trial" (cmRCT) design tackles some of the problems associated with pragmatic trial designs, such as recruitment
- The cmRCT design has several innovative features: a large observational cohort of patients is recruited and used as a multiple trials facility; each randomised controlled trial uses random selection of some participants (not random allocation of all); and "patient centred" information and consent is applied
- The cmRCT design is best suited to: open trials where "treatment as usual" is compared with the offer of treatment; easily measured and collected outcomes; conditions where many trials will be conducted; and trials of desirable or expensive interventions
- Further research is required to address a range of analysis, implementation, and ethical questions related to the cmRCT design

Recruitment

The majority of randomised controlled trials have difficulty recruiting sufficient numbers of patients. For example, one investigation found that less than a third of 114 multicentre, publicly funded UK trials recruited their original target number of patients within the time originally specified.[3] Failure to recruit to target may have implications for the power and generalisability of trial results.

Moreover, many clinical trials exclude hard to reach groups and ethnic minorities,[4] resulting in disparities between the "with need" (reference) population and the trial population.[5] [6] Measures of real world effectiveness are vital for analyses of benefit, harm, and cost effectiveness. If the reference population is not adequately represented in a trial and effectiveness is variable, then such analyses cannot accurately inform real world decisions.

Ethics

The most common reason given by patients (and clinicians) for not participating in clinical trials is "concerns with information and consent."[7] In routine real world health care, patients are rarely told of treatments that their clinicians cannot with certainty provide,[8] nor are patients told their treatment will be decided by chance. On the other hand, in clinical trials providing this type of "full" information before randomisation is regarded as an ethical requirement.

Patient preferences

Standard "open" (unblinded) pragmatic trials often compare an intervention with treatment as usual. Where the "standard care" on offer is available outside the trial, however, the only incentive for the patient to participate (apart from altruism) is to receive the new intervention. If a patient is allocated to treatment as usual, he or she may withdraw from the trial (attrition bias) or exhibit disappointment bias when reporting outcomes.[9]

Treatment comparisons

A common research scenario is addressing a clinical problem with many potential treatments. Yet often each potential treatment is trialled, one at a time, in different populations by different research teams. This approach yields many trials of different interventions, with heterogeneous trial populations and often short term and heterogeneous outcomes—a situation that is both financially and scientifically inefficient on three counts.

Firstly, lack of collection of long term outcomes hinders the measurement of infrequent adverse events and outcomes

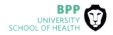

that occur far in the future. Secondly, systematic reviews of studies on a particular topic often conclude that "there was heterogeneity in populations and outcomes"; thus greater homogeneity in trial outcomes and populations is required to be able to synthesise the results of trials effectively. Thirdly, heterogeneity of trial populations and outcomes presents difficulties when making indirect comparisons between interventions; for example, the effectiveness of treatments A versus C, where only trials of treatments A versus B and B versus C exist. Indirect comparisons—where two interventions are compared through their relative effect versus a common comparator—can succeed, but sometimes result in significant discrepancies compared with the results of head to head randomised trials.[10] Many competing interventions have thus not been compared, or have been compared inaccurately, which is a waste of valuable information and money.

Previous solutions

Three alternative trial designs have attempted to address the recruitment and patient preferences issues inherent in existing clinical trial designs: the patient preference,[11] comprehensive cohort,[12 13] and randomised consent (Zelen) designs.[14]

Both the patient preference design and the comprehensive cohort design make some allowance for patient preferences regarding random allocation or type of treatment by collecting data from both randomised and non-randomised patients, thus increasing the overall number of patients recruited but not the numbers randomised. Both these designs have the limitation that if large numbers of patients express a preference, there might be insufficient "indifferent" patients available to be randomised. Designs where patients are asked their preferences and randomised irrespective of these will not necessarily solve problems of attrition or failure to recruit participants with a very strong preference.[15]

In randomised consent (Zelen) designs, consent is sought after randomisation. However, these designs are subject to ethical criticisms, such as the lack of information regarding all trial treatment options to all patients, and scientific criticism, because of the dilution of effect owing to "cross-over" of patients to the non-randomised treatment. Despite these criticisms, reviews report the existence of more than 60 randomised consent designs with ethics committee approval.[16 17 18]

The "cohort multiple randomised controlled trial" design

To address some of the shortcomings of existing trial designs we propose a new approach primarily for pragmatic randomised controlled trials—the "cohort multiple randomised controlled trial" (cmRCT) design (figure).

The key features of this design are:

(I)   Recruitment of a large observational cohort of patients with the condition of interest
(II) Regular measurement of outcomes for the whole cohort
(III) Capacity for multiple randomised controlled trials over time
      For each randomised controlled trial:
(IV) Identification of all eligible patients in the whole cohort (NA)
(V)   Random selection of some patients (nA) from all eligible patients in the cohort, who are then offered the trial intervention
(VI) Comparison of the outcomes in randomly selected patients (nA) with the outcomes in eligible patients not

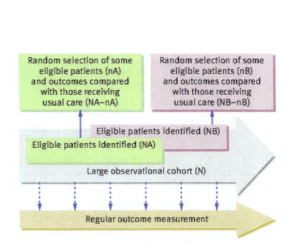

Fig The "cohort multiple randomised controlled trial" design. Firstly, a large observational cohort of patients with the condition of interest is recruited (N) and their outcomes regularly measured. Then for each randomised controlled trial, information from the cohort is used to identify all eligible patients (NA). Some eligible patients (nA) are randomly selected and offered the trial intervention. The outcomes of these randomly selected patients (nA) are then compared with the outcomes of eligible patients not randomly selected; that is, those receiving usual care (NA − nA). This process can be repeated for further randomised controlled trials (for example, NB)

randomly selected; that is, those receiving usual care (NA − nA)
(VII)"Patient centred" informed consent; that is, the process of obtaining patient information and consent aims to replicate that in real world routine health care.

The recruitment and regular follow-up of a large cohort of patients (features I and II) are characteristic of longitudinal observational studies. In the cmRCT design, however, all patients in the cohort consent at the outset to provide data to be used to look at the benefit of treatments for the condition of interest. Feature III, the capacity for multiple randomised controlled trials over time using patients from the same cohort, is unique to the cmRCT design. Random selection of some eligible cohort patients (feature V), the comparison of their outcomes with the outcomes in eligible patients not randomly selected (feature VI), and the similarity of the patient centred informed consent approach to real life situations (feature VII) offer solutions to the ethical criticisms of randomised consent (Zelen) designs.

Randomisation: random selection of some
Feature V and VI offer an alternative process for randomisation in clinical trials. The purpose of randomisation in experimental research is to generate two or more groups whose selection and treatment have not been influenced by anyone or anything other than chance and where all known or unknown prognostic factors are distributed evenly at baseline. Generating two groups whose membership is a result of chance can be achieved by either random allocation of all participants or random selection of some, because each approach produces the same effect. The random selection of nA patients from all patients (NA) in our example has the same effect as the random allocation of NA into two groups, nA and nB, because it is solely owing to chance whether any one patient is selected into nA. For the purposes of a randomised controlled trial, random

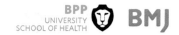

selection from NA into nA provides two groups where all known or unknown prognostic factors are distributed at baseline purely by chance: nA and (NA − nA).

Randomisation is generally conceived as "random allocation of all" and as something that is "done" to all patients, and thus requires their prior consent. With randomisation conceived of as "random selection of some," however, then nothing is "done" to all patients and prior consent of all patients is not required.

Information and consent: "patient centred"

The final feature of the cmRCT design (feature VII) is the adoption of a "patient centred" approach to informed consent, in which the process of obtaining patient information and consent aims to replicate that in real world routine health care rather than conform to the needs of trial design. All cohort patients consent to provide observational data at the outset; however, consent to "try" a particular intervention is sought only from those offered that intervention, thus replicating the patient centred information and consent procedures that exist in routine health care, where clinicians provide patients with the information they need, at the time they need it.

The rationale for this approach is twofold. Firstly, the primary motive for patients to enter clinical trials is not altruism, but their own direct benefit as patients.[19] Clinical trial informed consent procedures should, therefore, put the needs of the patient at the centre; that is, patients should not be told about treatments that they might not then receive, nor should they be told that their treatment will be allocated by chance. Secondly, the greater the similarity between patients' experiences in trials and their experiences in routine health care, then the greater the generalisability of the trial results to patients in routine health care.

Benefits of the approach

The cmRCT design will, we believe, help to address some of the shortcomings that prevent many pragmatic randomised controlled trials fulfilling their potential of giving robust evidence that clinicians can apply to their usual clinical populations.

Compared with randomised controlled trials, longitudinal observational studies can recruit a greater quantity and more representative sample of patients. Moreover, compared with doing individual pragmatic trials, using an observational cohort has important additional benefits:

A   A facility for multiple randomised controlled trials
B   Long term outcomes as standard
C   Ongoing information as to the natural history of the condition and to treatment as usual
D   Increased comparability between each trial conducted within the cohort
E   Increased efficiency, particularly for expensive or high risk interventions

The cmRCT approach enables more reliable direct and indirect comparisons than is possible with trials conducted using current randomised controlled trial designs because all treatments have the same "treatment as usual" comparator and use the same core outcomes.

Furthermore, researchers using standard randomised controlled trial designs often struggle to recruit and consequently have to randomly allocate all patients to either group in equal proportions to maximise statistical power within their total sample. The large numbers of patients recruited to the cohort in the cmRCT approach increases the statistical power of any randomised controlled trials and enables unequal randomisation. For example, a small number of patients could be randomly selected to be offered an expensive treatment and compared with a large number of unselected patients. Unequal randomisation thus improves the efficiency of trials of high cost interventions compared with equal allocation. These factors strengthen the inferences in the trial, lower treatment costs compared with standard designs (that is, once the cohort is established, it potentially allows for rapid and cheap recruitment of patients for any randomised controlled trials), and allows significant cost savings for trials of expensive treatments. Furthermore, data on treatment refusers provides information on the acceptability of the treatment and thus the generalisability of the trial results.

Role of the cmRCT design

There are certain circumstances, populations, clinical conditions, and treatments where the cmRCT design is more, or less, suitable than current strategies (box). The approach is best suited to the examination of long term conditions for which many pragmatic clinical trials will likely be conducted in the future. The design is also suitable for both primary and secondary care settings, and for conditions with easily reported patient outcomes.

The cmRCT design cannot be used for trials that have a placebo comparator because such trials could not use feature VI (comparison to treatment as usual) or feature VII (patient centred informed consent) as patients are never told that they may receive placebo in routine health care. However, features I to V could be used for placebo trials and benefits A to E would still accrue.

Challenges of the design

A potential problem with our approach is that significant numbers of patients may refuse to receive the intervention being trialled. An intention to treat analysis will, therefore, dilute any treatment effects. There are two ways of dealing with this problem. Firstly, we could use the statistical method complier average causal effect (CACE) analysis,[20] which provides unbiased estimates of the treatment effect for patients who comply with the protocol (albeit usually with loss of power), unlike per protocol or on treatment analysis.

Secondly, we could try to avoid some potential non-compliance by presenting cohort patients with a list of possible interventions at enrolment and asking which they would consider agreeing to use if offered. This process identifies the potential compliers in advance and consequently reduces dilution effects; however, care must be taken to avoid false expectation of future treatment and the loss of feature VII, patient centred information and consent.

In researching interventions already available in routine health care, it will be necessary to identify and monitor which patients use or have used these.

Furthermore, discrete trials are currently supported by private and public funding infrastructures and institutional frameworks, to the tune of £100000 per trial. Existing infrastructures and frameworks might struggle to determine a funding approach for cmRCTs.

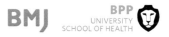

USING THE COHORT MULTIPLE RANDOMISED CONTROLLED TRIAL DESIGN

Most suited to:

Settings
- Open trials with "treatment as usual" as the comparator
- Studies that aim to inform healthcare decisions in routine practice (pragmatic trials)
- Research questions that address easily measured and collected outcomes

Populations
- Stable populations
- Easily identified populations

Clinical conditions
- Clinical conditions for which many trials will be conducted; for example, obesity, diabetes, chronic pain
- Chronic conditions
- Conditions for which previous trials have struggled with recruitment

Treatments
- Treatments highly desired by patients
- Expensive treatments

Least suited to:

Settings
- Closed trial designs with masking or a placebo arm
- Studies that aim to further knowledge as to how and why a treatment works (efficacy trials)
- Research questions that address hard to measure and hard to collect outcomes

Population
- Populations with high attrition
- Unstable patient populations
- Difficult to identify populations

Clinical conditions
- Acute or short term conditions

Treatments
- Treatments not highly desired by patients

Examples of the cmRCT design

Campbell and colleagues[18] recently adapted the randomised consent (Zelen) method and developed an approach in which patients consented to an observational study and were then all randomly allocated to either intervention or control in a randomised controlled trial. Although this method shares several features with the cmRCT design (features I, II, IV, and VII), it does not have the capacity for multiple randomised controlled trials (feature III) or use random selection of some instead of random allocation of all (features V and VI).

We have obtained ethical approval for and have conducted a pilot study of the cmRCT design.[21] In this pilot, a large observational cohort of 856 women aged 45-64 was recruited and their outcomes measured. A total of 72 women reported frequent or severe menopausal hot flushes, or both. Of these 72 women, 48 were eligible for the trial treatment (NA) and 24 were randomly selected to be offered the treatment (nA). The outcomes of the randomly selected patients were then compared with the outcomes of those eligible patients not randomly selected (NA − nA) using both intention to treat analysis and CACE analysis.[20]

Patients were not told about the treatments that they were not randomly selected to be offered.

The clinical outcomes of this pilot will be reported separately. However, a post hoc evaluation of the design found that the design was acceptable to patients, clinicians, and the NHS Research ethics committee. The concept of multiple trials within a single cohort of patients (feature III) has not yet been tested.

The cmRCT design is currently being used to address questions in the management of obesity (http://clahrc-sy.nihr.ac.uk/theme-obesity.html). The 20 year study is projected to recruit a cohort of 20 000 adults aged 16 years or more, and multiple trials will be embedded within this cohort. To maximise the long term benefits of this study, it is planned that the cohort will be "open" and will be replenished with new recruits (16 and 17 year olds) every two years.

Summary

The cmRCT design appears to be a workable and useful approach to pragmatic research questions that aim to inform healthcare decisions within routine practice. The design is best suited to circumstances that require open (rather than blinded) trials where "treatment as usual" is compared with the offer of study treatment, and to questions with outcomes that can be easily measured in the whole cohort (for example, patient reported outcomes). Clinical conditions where many clinical trials will be conducted and trials of desirable or expensive interventions are also well suited to the cmRCT approach.

There are challenges to the cmRCT design. Further research is required to address a range of analysis and implementation questions related to the design and the ethics of patient centred informed consent for pragmatic randomised controlled trials.

In his Harveian oration at the Royal College of Physicians, London, Professor Michael Rawlins, chair of the National Institute for Health and Clinical Excellence, called for "investigators to continue to develop and improve their methodologies in order to help decision makers appraise the evidence."[22] We hope that the cmRCT design goes some way towards addressing the problems associated with existing approaches. If these problems are addressed, then perhaps the most important problem of all will be resolved—the non-implementation of the results of clinical research.

Contributors: JN and CR had the original idea for the article. This article arose from CR's doctoral research, which was supervised by JN and AO at the School for Health and Related Research at the University of Sheffield. CR wrote the article and prepared the initial and subsequent draft. JN reviewed and commented on every draft. AO and DT commented on later drafts. AO, DT, CR, and JN agreed the final draft. CR is guarantor for the article. JN and CR jointly conceived the cmRCT design.

Funding: A pre-doctoral training fellowship award from the Department of Health's National Coordinating Centre for Research Capacity Development funded CR's doctoral research and the pilot of the cmRCT design. All work has been independent from the funders in every way.

Competing interests: All authors have completed the Unified Competing Interest form at www.icmje.org/coi_disclosure.pdf (available on request from the corresponding author) and declare that (1) CR, AOC, and JN have received financial support from the University of Sheffield and DT has received financial support from the University of York for the submitted work; (2) CR, AOC, JN, and DT have no relationships with any companies that might have an interest in the submitted work in the previous three years; (3) their spouses, partners, or children have no financial relationships that may be relevant to the submitted work; and (4) no author has any non-financial interests that may be relevant to the submitted work.

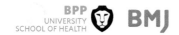

Ethical approval: The protocol of the cmRCT pilot study was approved by the South Sheffield NHS Research Ethics Committee (ref 06/Q2305/181). NHS Scientific Review Approval was also obtained (consortium ref: ZF89).

Provenance and peer review: Not commissioned; externally peer reviewed.

1 Schwartz D, Lellouch J. Explanatory and pragmatic attitudes in therapeutical trials. *J Chronic Dis* 1967;20:637-48.
2 Thorpe KE, Zwarenstein M, Oxman AD, Treweek S, Furberg CD, Altman DG, et al. A pragmatic-explanatory continuum indicator summary (PRECIS): a tool to help trial designers. *J Clin Epidemiol* 2009;62:464-75.
3 McDonald AM, Knight RC, Campbell MK, Entwistle VA, Grant AM, Cook JA, et al. What influences recruitment to randomised controlled trials? A review of trials funded by two UK funding agencies. *Trials* 2006;7:9.
4 Mason S, Hussain-Gambles M, Leese B, Atkin K, Brown J. Representation of South Asian people in randomised clinical trials: analysis of trials' data. *BMJ* 2003;326:1244-5.
5 Bartlett C, Doyal L, Ebrahim S, Ebrahim S, Davey P, Bachmann M, et al. The causes and effects of socio-demographic exclusion from clinical trials. *Health Technol Assess* 2005;9:38.
6 Britton A, McKee M, Black N, McPherson K, Sanderson C, Bain C. Choosing between randomised and non randomised studies: a systematic review. *Health Technol Assess* 1998;2:13.
7 Ross S, Grant A, Counsell C, Gillespie W, Russell I, Prescott R. Barriers to participation in randomised controlled trials: a systematic review. *J Clin Epidemiol* 1999;52:1143-56.
8 Firth J. Should you tell patients about beneficial treatments that they cannot have? *BMJ* 2007;334:826.
9 Torgerson DJ, Torgerson CJ. *Designing randomised trials in health, education and the social sciences: an introduction*. Palgrave Macmillan, 2008.
10 Song F, Altman DG, Glenny AM, Deeks JJ. Validity of indirect comparison for estimating efficacy of competing interventions: empirical evidence from published meta-analyses. *BMJ* 2003;326:472-7.
11 Brewin CR, Bradley C. Patient preferences and randomised clinical trials. *BMJ* 1989;299:313-5.
12 Francis T Jr, Korns RF, Voight RB, Boisen M, Hemphill FM, Napier JA, et al. An evaluation of the 1954 poliomyelitis vaccine trials. *Am J Public Health* 1954;45:1-63.
13 Olschewski M, Scheurlen H. Comprehensive cohort study: an alternative to randomised consent design in a breast preservation trial. *Methods Inf Med* 1985;24:131-4.
14 Zelen M. A new design for randomized clinical trials. *N Engl J Med* 1979;300:1242-5.
15 Preference Collaborative Review Group. Patients' preferences within randomised trials: systematic review and patient level meta-analysis. *BMJ* 2008;337:a1864-6.
16 Adamson J, Cockayne S, Puffer S, Torgerson DJ. Review of randomised trials using the post-randomised consent (Zelen's) design. *Contemp Clin Trials* 2006;27:305-19.
17 Schellings R, Kessels AG, ter Riet G, Knottnerus JA, Sturmans F. Randomized consent designs in randomized controlled trials: systematic literature search. *Contemp Clin Trials* 2006;27:330-2.
18 Campbell R, Peters T, Grant C, Quilty B, Dieppe P. Adapting the randomised consent (Zelen) design for trials of behavioural interventions for chronic disease: a feasibility study. *J Health Serv Res Policy* 2005;10:220-5.
19 Healthtalkonline. Clinical trials—deciding whether to take part: risks and benefits. Reasons for wanting to take part—personal benefit. 2008. www.healthtalkonline.org/medical_research/clinical_trials/Topic/3635/topicList.
20 Hewitt CE, Torgerson DJ, Miles JVN. Is there another way to take account of noncompliance in randomized controlled trials? *Can Med Assoc J* 2006;175:347.
21 Relton C. *A new design for pragmatic RCTs: a "patient cohort" RCT of treatment by a homeopath for menopausal hot flushes*. [PhD thesis] ISRCTN 0287542. University of Sheffield, 2009.
22 Rawlins M. Harveian oration 2008. www.rcplondon.ac.uk/pubs/brochure.aspx?e=262.

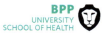

Correlation in restricted ranges of data

J Martin Bland, professor of health statistics[1],
Douglas G Altman, professor of statistics in medicine[2]

Department of Health Sciences, University of York, York YO10 5DD

Centre for Statistics in Medicine, University of Oxford, Oxford OX2 6UD

Correspondence to: Professor M Bland martin.bland@york.ac.uk

Cite this as: BMJ 2011;342:d556

DOI: http://dx.doi.org/10.1136/bmj.d556

http://www.bmj.com/content/342/bmj.d556

In a study of 150 adult diabetic patients there was a strong correlation between abdominal circumference and body mass index (BMI) (r = 0.85).[1] The authors went on to report that the correlation differed in different BMI categories as shown in the table.

The authors' interpretation of these data was that in patients with low or high BMI values (BMI <25 kg/m² and BMI >35 kg/m²) the correlation was strong, but in those with BMI values between 25 and 35 kg/m² the correlation was weak or missing. They concluded that measuring abdominal circumference is of particular importance in subjects with the most frequent BMI category (25 to 35 kg/m²).

When we restrict the range of one of the variables, a correlation coefficient will be reduced. For example, fig 1 shows some BMI and abdominal circumference measurements from a different population. Although these people are from a rather thinner population, the correlation coefficient is very similar, r = 0.82 (P<0.0001). When we divide the sample into the same four restricted ranges of BMI at 20, 25, and 30 kg/m², the correlation coefficient in each interval is smaller than the correlation coefficient for the whole sample. This phenomenon is to be expected; it is a result of restricting the range of data, not any particular property of BMI and abdominal circumference.

One interpretation of the correlation coefficient r is that r² is the proportion of the variation in abdominal circumference explained or predicted by the variation in BMI. If we restrict the range of BMI values we reduce the variation in BMI,

which will explain less variation in abdominal circumference, and r will fall. If we further reduce the variation in BMI until all remaining patients have the same BMI, then we cannot explain any variation in abdominal circumference and the correlation must be zero. (By contrast within any of the sections of fig 1 the fitted regression line would be the same, apart from random variation.)

For another example, fig 2 shows the weights and heights of the same sample, with different symbols for men and women. Clearly, the lower end of the height range for men is higher than the lower end of the range for women, but the upper ends of the ranges are very similar. The men's heights (SD 6.0 cm) are less variable than those of the women (SD 8.9 cm) or the heights of both sexes combined (also SD 8.9 cm). The correlation coefficients for women and for both men and women are very similar and considerably larger than that for men alone.

The same phenomenon can arise when the sample is restricted using another variable related to the ones being studies. For example, the correlation between weight and height of schoolchildren will increase as the age range is increased. But a spurious correlation may also be seen in such a situation, for example between shoe size and spelling ability.[2] Such an example illustrates the well worn phrase that an observed association does not imply causation.

Correlation coefficients are a property of the variables and also the population in which they are measured. If we look at a restricted population, we should not conclude that there is little or no relation between the variables because the correlation coefficient is small. But given a clear relation in the whole group, we see no point in looking within categories of one of the variables. In any case, regression is generally the preferred approach to considering the relation between two continuous variables.

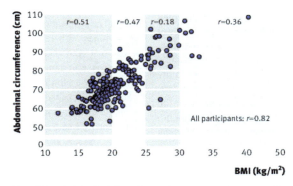

Fig 1 BMI and abdominal circumference in 202 men and women, with correlation coefficients in four restricted ranges and overall

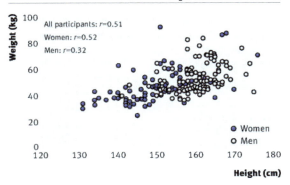

Fig 2 Weight and height in 202 men and women, with correlation coefficients

BMI group	r
<25	0.62
25 to 30	0.50
30 to 35	−0.09
>35	0.86
All patients	0.85

Correlation between abdominal circumference and body mass indeed (BMI) in 1450 adult patients with diabetes

Acknowledgements: The data are taken from a student elective project by Dr Malcolm Savage.

Contributors: JMB and DGA jointly wrote and agreed the text, JMB did the statistical analysis.

Competing interests: All authors have completed the Unified Competing Interest form at www.icmje.org/coi_disclosure.pdf (available on request from the corresponding author) and declare: no support from any organisation for the submitted work; no financial relationships with any organisations that might have an interest in the submitted work in the previous 3 years; no other relationships or activities that could appear to have influenced the submitted work.

1   Nádas J, Putz Z, Kolev G, Nagy S, Jermendy G. Intraobserver and interobserver variability of measuring waist circumference. Med Sci Monit 2008;14:CR15-8.
2   Goodwin LD, Leech NL. Understanding correlation: factors that affect the size of r. J Exp Educ 2006;74:251-66.

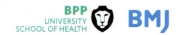

Is a subgroup effect believable? Updating criteria to evaluate the credibility of subgroup analyses

Xin Sun, research fellow[1] [2], Matthias Briel, senior researcher[1] [3], Stephen D Walter, professor[1], Gordon H Guyatt, professor[1] [4]

[1]Department of Clinical Epidemiology and Biostatistics, McMaster University, Hamilton, ON, Canada

[2]Center for Clinical Epidemiology and Evidence-Based Medicine, West China Hospital, Sichuan University, Chengdu, China

[3]Basel Institute for Clinical Epidemiology and Biostatistics, University Hospital Basel, Basel, Switzerland

[4]Department of Medicine, McMaster University, Hamilton, Canada

Correspondence to: Gordon H Guyatt, 1200 Main Street West, Rm 2C12, Hamilton, Ontario, Canada, L8N 3Z5
guyatt@mcmaster.ca

Cite this as: *BMJ* 2010;340:c117

DOI: 10.1136/bmj.c117

http://www.bmj.com/content/340/bmj.c117

ABSTRACT

How can we tell the difference between spurious and real subgroup effects? This article identifies new criteria and proposes a checklist for judging the credibility of subgroup analyses

Introduction

Subgroup analyses in randomised controlled trials (RCTs) or in meta-analyses of RCTs examine whether treatment effects vary according to patient group, way of giving an intervention, or approach to measuring an outcome. Subgroup analyses are common and often associated with claims of difference of treatment effects between subgroups—termed "subgroup effect", "effect modification", or "interaction between a subgroup variable and treatment".[1] [2] [3] A difference in effect between subgroups, if true, is likely to have important implications for clinical practice and policy making. Many subgroup claims are, however, subsequently shown to be false.[4] Thus, investigators, clinicians, and policy makers face the challenge of whether or not to believe apparent differences in effect.

Debates about subgroup effects may be framed in terms of absolute acceptance or rejection. For instance, in an intense academic debate,[5] [6] [7] [8] [9] [10] [11] one camp maintained that effects of propranolol on death differed in two groups of study centres, whereas the other remained highly sceptical. This "yes" versus "no" polarised approach is undesirable and destructive, mainly because it ignores the uncertainty that is inevitably part of such judgments. An approach that is more productive and more realistic is to place the likelihood that a subgroup effect is real on a continuum from "highly plausible" to "extremely unlikely", possibly by using a visual analogue scale. The question is then a decision of where on this continuum a putative subgroup effect lies.

In 1991, Yusuf et al[12] discussed principles of analysing and interpreting subgroup effects, and stated that qualitative interactions (that is, when treatment is beneficial in one subgroup but harmful in another) are rare. They advocated a priori specification of subgroup hypotheses, completion of a small number of subgroup analyses, and use of an interaction test for analysing subgroup effects. In the subsequent year, Oxman and Guyatt[13] suggested seven criteria to guide inferences about the credibility of subgroup analyses. The greater the extent to which these criteria are met, the more plausible the putative subgroup effect is.

Since 1992, these seven criteria have been widely used to assess hypothesised subgroup effects,[14] [15] [16] [17] [18] [19] [20] [21] [22] [2] and have undergone only minimal cosmetic revisions.[4] After years of use of the 1992 criteria, we had begun to perceive limitations. These limitations became vivid when deciding on the credibility of a subgroup hypothesis of a large multicentre randomised trial.[24] On the basis of this experience, a review of published methodological articles addressing subgroup analyses, and consultation with clinicians and epidemiologist colleagues, we identified four new criteria that could further aid differentiation between spurious and real subgroup effects. We now believe that failure to consider these criteria could result in misleading inferences about subgroup hypotheses. In this article, we describe these new criteria, use real-world examples to show how they influence the strength of inference of subgroup hypotheses, and discuss their implications. Finally, we propose a re-structured checklist of items addressing study design, analysis, and context.

Relative versus absolute effect in subgroup analyses

A crucial issue in subgroup analyses is that the effects should be examined with relative rather than absolute measures. By contrast with relative effects, which in most situations remain constant across varying baseline risks, absolute risk reductions will typically vary with baseline risk.

For example, consider the effect of statin therapy on major coronary events (that is, non-fatal myocardial infarction and coronary heart disease death) in patients with varying coronary risks. A 45 year old non-smoking woman without a family history of heart disease and without diabetes presents with a raised serum cholesterol (>5.2 mmol/L and a blood pressure of 130/85 mm Hg. Her risk of major coronary events in the next decade is 5%. Compare this woman to a 65 year old smoking male with a family history of heart diseases and diabetes, presenting with a raised serum cholesterol (> 6.2 mmol/L), and blood pressure of 160/90 mm Hg. His risk of major coronary events is 50%.

A meta-analysis showed that statin therapy could reduce the relative risk of major coronary events by 29.2%.[25] This relative effect was consistent across subgroups, including the determinants of coronary risk discussed in the previous paragraph. Because of the constant reduction in relative risk across subgroups (that is, we are confident that there is no subgroup effect for the relative effect measure), we can infer a reduction in absolute risk of major coronary events by 1.5% (from 5% to 3.5%) in the first patient and 14.6% (from 50% to 35.4%) in the second patient. If we were considering absolute risk reduction, an evident subgroup

SUMMARY POINTS

- Seven existing criteria help clinicians assess the credibility of putative subgroup effects on a continuum from "highly plausible" to "extremely unlikely"
- We suggest four additional criteria: subgroup definition on the basis of baseline characteristics, independence of the subgroup effect, a priori specification of the direction of the subgroup effect, and consistency across related outcomes
- We propose a re-structured checklist of items addressing study design, analysis, and context

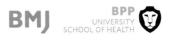

effect would exist (low risk patients, such as our female patient, have an absolute risk reduction of 1.5%, whereas high risk patients, such as our male patient, an absolute risk reduction of 14.6%).

This example shows how subgroup effects are often present when using the absolute risk reduction, but rarely present when using a relative effect measure. Indeed, in the presence of known prognostic factors that allow definition of groups at varying risk, if no subgroup effect is associated with these factors for relative measures of effect, a subgroup effect for absolute measures must exist. Our subsequent discussion, therefore, focuses exclusively on putative subgroup differences in relative effects.

The original seven criteria for subgroup analyses

The box shows the seven 1992 criteria,[13] in a re-structured checklist addressing design, analysis, and context of subgroup analyses in this paper. Inferences about subgroup effects are stronger, if, at the design stage, the comparison is made within rather than between studies, the subgroup hypothesis is specified a priori, and a small number of hypotheses are tested; if, in the analysis, the test for interaction between treatment and a subgroup variable (for example, age, sex, disease severity) suggests that chance is an unlikely explanation for apparent differences; and if, on the basis of the context, the difference in effect between subgroup categories is large and consistent across studies, and indirect evidence exists to support the difference (biological rationale).

New criteria to judge the credibility of subgroup effects

1 Is the subgroup variable a characteristic measured at baseline or after randomisation?

Subgroups can be defined according to characteristics measured at baseline or after randomisation. Subgroups defined according to post-randomisation characteristics might be influenced by tested interventions; that is, the apparent difference of treatment effect between subgroups can be explained by the intervention itself, or by differing prognostic characteristics in sub-groups that emerge after randomisation, rather than by the subgroup characteristic itself. Thus, the credibility of subgroup hypotheses based on post-randomisation characteristics is severely compromised, and can be rejected simply on this criterion.

For instance, in a randomised trial of 1200 critically ill patients,[26] intensive insulin therapy, compared with conventional therapy, did not significantly reduce all-cause hospital mortality (37.3% v 40.0%, P=0.33). In 767 patients who stayed in the intensive care unit (ICU) for at least 3 days, the intensive insulin therapy group had a lower all-cause hospital mortality (43.0% v 52.5%, P=0.009), whereas in 433 patients who stayed in the ICU for less than three days, intensive therapy seemed to increase all-cause hospital mortality (26.5% v 18.9%, P=0.05). Because the subgroups were not selected on the basis of characteristics at baseline, the most likely explanation of the results is not that insulin therapy is harmful in those destined to stay in ICU for less than 3 days and beneficial in those destined to stay for more than three days, but rather that an effect of treatment was to create prognostic imbalance between groups in those who ultimately stayed less than three days or at least three days. Such post-randomisation subgroup

analyses have very low credibility—in most cases, they can be readily dismissed.

2 Was the *direction* of the subgroup effect specified a priori? Even if specified *a priori*, a putative subgroup effect is unlikely to be compelling if the investigator has little idea of the direction of the effect. A subgroup effect consistent with the *pre*-specified direction will increase the credibility of a subgroup analysis; failure to specify the direction—or worse yet, getting the direction wrong—weakens the case for a real underlying subgroup effect.

Users should look for explicit statements of a priori specification of subgroup hypothesis and subgroup direction in the primary study reports. In view of emerging evidence of differences between protocols and study reports,[27] statements about what was included in registered or publicly available protocols finalised before the study or systematic review are desirable.

For instance, Russell et al[28] compared the effect of vasopressin versus norepinephrine infusion on 28-day mortality in a randomised trial of 778 patients with septic shock. As the primary subgroup analysis, the authors hypothesised a priori that the benefit of vasopressin over norepinephrine would be larger in patients with more severe septic shock. It turned out, however, that the benefit of vasopressin seemed to be greater in the patients with less severe septic shock (RR 1.04 in more severe v 0.74 in less severe septic shock, interaction P=0.10). The investigators' failure to correctly identify the direction of the subgroup effect appreciably weakens any inference that vasopressin is superior to norepinephrine in the less severely ill patients.

3 Is the significant subgroup effect independent?

When examining subgroup hypotheses, one must address the likelihood that the differences in effects can be explained by chance. The statistical approach that addresses this issue is called a test for interaction (the interaction meaning that the treatment effect differs across subgroup categories). The null hypothesis of the test for interaction is that no difference exists in the underlying true effect between subgroup categories. The lower the P value, the less likely it is that chance explains the apparent subgroup effect. Inevitably, the choice of a threshold for the P value involves subjective judgment. Rather than use of a threshold, a preferable way of assessing the P value is that as it gets smaller, the subgroup hypothesis becomes increasingly credible: we can be sceptical of any hypothesis with a P value of greater than 0.1, begin to consider the hypothesis if the P value is between 0.1 and 0.01, and take the hypothesis seriously when P values reach 0.001 or less.

When testing multiple hypotheses in a single study, the analyses might yield more than one apparently significant interaction. These significant interactions might, however, be associated with each other, and thus explained by a common factor. For instance, in a meta-analysis examining the effect of aspirin on the prevention of cardiovascular events, aspirin reduced the risk of stroke in women, whereas it had no apparent effect in men.[29] However, the men were generally younger than the women, suggesting that age, rather than sex, might explain the interaction.[30]

Expressing this in general terms, in a particular analysis, treatment effects apparently differ according to patients'

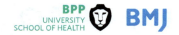

CRITERIA TO ASSESS THE CREDIBILITY OF SUBGROUP ANALYSES

Design

- Is the subgroup variable a characteristic measured at baseline or after randomisation?*
- Is the effect suggested by comparisons within rather than between studies?
- Was the hypothesis specified a priori?
- Was the direction of the subgroup effect specified a priori*
- Was the subgroup effect one of a small number of hypothesised effects tested?

Analysis

- Does the interaction test suggest a low likelihood that chance explains the apparent subgroup effect?
- Is the significant subgroup effect independent?*

Context

- Is the size of the subgroup effect large?
- Is the interaction consistent across studies?
- Is the interaction consistent across closely related outcomes within the study?*
- Is there indirect evidence that supports the hypothesised interaction (biological rationale)?

*New criteria.

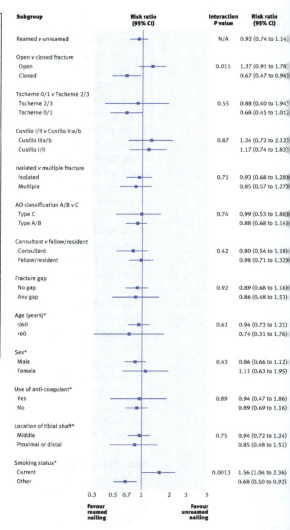

Fig 1 Effect of reamed v unreamed nailing on re-operation in patients with fracture: a priori and post-hoc subgroup analyses. First point estimate and confidence interval indicates main effect. Subsequent pairs of point estimates and confidence intervals indicate effect of reamed v unreamed nailing on re-operation in categories of 12 subgroup variables. *Subgroup analyses done post hoc. Subgroup analysis by Tscherne type included patients with closed facture only, and analysis by Gustilo type included open fracture only. In our analysis of significant and non-significant interactions, these two interactions were not included in regression model, resulting in ten interaction terms included in model.

status on variables A and B. A and B are statistically associated with each other. The difference of effects between patients in different categories with respect to A might, therefore, be explained by B (that is, the apparent effects of A on the size of treatment effect are due to confounding with B).

Another example comes from a trial of reamed versus unreamed nailing of tibial fractures.[24] Reamed and unreamed nailing produced no significant difference in the rate of re-operation (RR 0.92, 95% CI 0.74 to 1.14, fig 1). Analysis of seven a priori hypotheses suggested that reamed nailing had a lower re-operation rate in closed fractures (RR 0.64, 95% CI 0.47 to 0.96) while resulted in a higher re-operation rate in open fractures (RR 1.27, 95% CI 0.91 to 1.78, interaction P= 0.011, fig 1). We subsequently used the trial data to explore five additional hypotheses, one of which suggested that reamed nailing was superior in current smokers (RR 0.68, 95% CI 0.50 to 0.92) and unreamed nailing better in others (that is, ex-smokers and lifetime non-smokers) (RR 1.56, 95% CI 1.04 to 2.36, interaction P=0.001, fig 1).

We wondered if the apparently significant difference in treatment effect between smokers and non-smokers could be explained by fracture type (open v closed). In other words, one possibility was that the reason for the apparent smoking effect was that smokers tended to have open fractures and others tended to have closed fractures. In this case, the apparent association between preferred procedure (reamed or unreamed nailing) and smoking status might actually be due to confounding between smoking and fracture type (open and closed). To check for the independence of the interaction effect of smoking with procedure (reamed v unreamed), we included the interaction terms of treatment with smoking and treatment with fracture type in the same regression model. The analysis showed that the smoking interaction remained significant (P value changed from 0.001 to 0.006) after adjusting for the interaction of fracture type with treatment. This suggests that the apparent smoking interaction cannot be explained by an association between smoking status and open versus closed fractures.

An additional check for independence of the association could include all significant and non-significant interactions

in the regression model. Persisting significance of interaction terms strengthens the subgroup effect inference. In our analysis, this additional regression including both significant and non-significant hypothesised interactions (that is, the ten interactions between patient characteristics with treatment in fig 1) showed a persistent smoking interaction (P=0.008), thus providing further support for the independence of the smoking subgroup effect. A note of caution: adjustment for significant and non-significant interaction terms might be compromised by a limited sample size and small number of events,[31] providing a further rationale for pre-specifying a limited number of important interactions.

4 Is the interaction consistent across closely related outcomes within the study?

If a subgroup effect is real, it is likely to manifest itself across all closely related outcomes. For example, in a randomised trial of 1692 patients with refractory non-small-

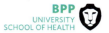

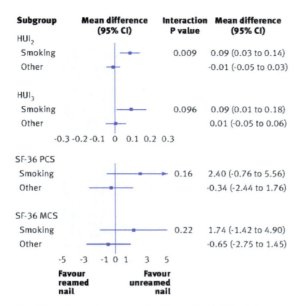

Fig 2 Effect of reamed v unreamed nailing on Health Utility Index (HUI, 2a) and Short Form-36 (SF-36, 2b) in subgroups of smoking and other tibial fracture patients. PCS=physical component summary. MCS=mental component summary.

cell lung cancer, Thatcher et al[32] compared the effect of gefitinib versus placebo on survival. The primary analysis showed a trend for a survival benefit with gefitinib over placebo (hazard ratio (HR) 0.89, 95% CI 0.77 to 1.02, P=0.087). Tests of a priori hypotheses indicated differential effects on survival in non-smokers (HR 0.67, 95% CI 0.49 to 0.92) and smokers (HR 0.92, 95% CI 0.79 to 1.06; interaction P=0.07). Secondary analyses on time to treatment failure showed similar differences of effects in non-smokers (HR 0.55, 95% CI 0.42 to 0.72) versus smokers (HR 0.89, 95% CI 0.78 to 1.01, interaction P=0.0015). The consistency of the subgroup effect across outcomes enhances its credibility.

In the trial of reamed versus unreamed nailing of tibial fractures,[24] unreamed nailing apparently reduced re-operations in current smokers while reamed nailing reduced re-operations in other patients (ex-smokers and lifetime non-smokers) (fig 1). To examine whether the difference existed in other outcomes, we tested the interactions between treatment and smoking status on quality of life measured by the Health Utility Index and short form-36 (fig 2). Results consistently suggested the superiority of unreamed nailing over reamed nailing in current smoking patients, and no or a small difference between unreamed and reamed nailing in other patients. This result strengthens the inference about an interaction with type of nailing and smoking status.

Discussion

Clinical and policy decision making always involves uncertainty. It is unlikely that a subgroup claim will meet either all or none of our criteria—in almost all instances, a subgroup claim will meet some but not all the criteria. Treating the likelihood that a subgroup effect is real as a continuum reflects the nature of the uncertainty. Judgment about its credibility will depend on how strongly clinicians and policy makers believe the subgroup effect is real. In other words, they will judge considering each criterion: the greater the extent to which criteria are met, the more likely the subgroup effect is real. When summarising the strength of the subgroup inferences, one can imagine—and possibly

apply—a visual analogue scale with anchors of "highly plausible" and "extremely unlikely".

For clinical practice and policy decision making, differences in prognosis, and the differences in absolute risk reduction that are associated with differences in prognosis, are far more important than relative subgroup effects for two reasons. First, identifiable and substantial differences in prognosis are fairly common, and one can be confident that potentially important differences in absolute effect across prognostic subgroups will occur. True subgroup differences in relative effects are, by contrast, fairly uncommon. Second, even if true differences in the effects of treatment across subgroups exist, those differences might not be large enough to mandate differences in management across those subgroups. This might be the case, for instance, if treatment is beneficial in all patients, but the size of treatment effect differs between subgroups. Assuming constant relative risk reductions, and using baseline risk to calculate absolute risk reductions for patient groups associated with validated differentiating prognostic characteristics, provides an optimum approach to trading off desirable and undesirable treatment results.[33]

We re-structured the checklist of items including the seven original and the four new criteria (table 1). This checklist is organised according to the design, analysis, and context of subgroup analysis.

The importance of these criteria varies, but the relative weight that should be applied to each criterion remains uncertain. If a credible weighting scheme could be established it might improve the efficiency and accuracy of judgments. One approach would be to develop a formal measurement instrument, allocating a specific weight to each criterion, and to validate the instrument by applying it to subgroup analyses that have been established to be real or spurious.

Contributors: All authors conceptualised the ideas in the manuscript and read and approved the manuscript. XS developed the first draft and incorporated comments from authors for successive drafts. GHG is the guarantor.

Funding: XS is supported by a grant from the National Natural Science Foundation of China (grant No. 70703025). MB is supported by Santésuisse and the Gottfried and Julia Bangerter-Rhyner Foundation.

Competing interests: None declared.

Provenance and peer review: Not commissioned; externally peer reviewed.

1　Assmann SF, Pocock SJ, Enos LE, Kasten LE. Subgroup analysis and other (mis)uses of baseline data in clinical trials. *Lancet* 2000;355:1064-9.
2　Bhandari M, Devereaux PJ, Li P, Mah D, Lim K, Schunemann HJ, et al. Misuse of baseline comparison tests and subgroup analyses in surgical trials. *Clin Orthop Relat Res* 2006;447:247-51.
3　Wang R, Lagakos SW, Ware JH, Hunter DJ, Drazen JM. Statistics in medicine— reporting of subgroup analyses in clinical trials. *N Engl J Med* 2007;357:2189-94.
4　Guyatt G, Wyer PC, Ioannidis J. When to believe a subgroup analysis. In: Guyatt G, Rennie D, Meade MO, Cook DJ, eds. *User's guide to the medical literature: a manual for evidence-based clinical practice* . 2nd ed. AMA, 2008: 571-83.
5　Horwitz RI, Singer BH, Makuch RW, Viscoli CM. Can treatment that is helpful on average be harmful to some patients? A study of the conflicting information needs of clinical inquiry and drug regulation. *J Clin Epidemiol* 1996;49:395-400.
6　Altman DG. Within trial variation—a false trail? *J Clin Epidemiol* 1998;51:301-3.
7　Feinstein AR. The problem of cogent subgroups: a clinicostatistical tragedy. *J Clin Epidemiol* 1998;51:297-9.
8　Horwitz RI, Singer BH, Makuch RW, Viscoli CM. On reaching the tunnel at the end of the light. *J Clin Epidemiol* 1997;50:753-5.
9　Horwitz RI, Singer BH, Makuch RW, Viscoli CM. Clinical versus statistical considerations in the design and analysis of clinical research. *J Clin Epidemiol* 1998;51:305-7.
10　Senn S, Harrell F. On wisdom after the event. *J Clin Epidemiol* 1997;50:749-51.

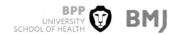

11   Smith GD, Egger M. Incommunicable knowledge? Interpreting and applying the results of clinical trials and meta-analyses. *J Clin Epidemiol* 1998;51:289-95.

12   Yusuf S, Wittes J, Probstfield J, Tyroler HA. Analysis and interpretation of treatment effects in subgroups of patients in randomized clinical trials. *JAMA* 1991;266:93-8.

13   Oxman AD, Guyatt GH. A consumer's guide to subgroup analyses. *Ann Intern Med* 1992;116:78-84.

14   Akl EA, Terrenato I, Barba M, Sperati F, Sempos EV, Muti P, et al. Low-molecular-weight heparin vs unfractionated heparin for perioperative thromboprophylaxis in patients with cancer: a systematic review and meta-analysis. *Arch Intern Med* 2008;168:1261-9.

15   Billingham LJ, Cullen MH. The benefits of chemotherapy in patient subgroups with unresectable non-small-cell lung cancer. *Ann Oncol* 2001;12:1671-5.

16   Bundy DG, Berkoff MC, Ito KE, Rosenthal MS, Weinberger M. Interpreting subgroup analyses: is a school-based asthma treatment program's effect modified by secondhand smoke exposure? *Arch Pediatr Adolesc Med* 2004;158:469-71.

17   Cranney A, Tugwell P, Wells G, Guyatt G. Meta-analyses of therapies for postmenopausal osteoporosis *I. Systematic reviews of randomized trials in osteoporosis: introduction and methodology. *Endocr Rev* 2002;23:496-507.

18   Freemantle N. Interpreting the results of secondary end points and subgroup analyses in clinical trials: should we lock the crazy aunt in the attic? *BMJ* 2001;322:989-91.

19   Hatala R, Keitz S, Wyer P, Guyatt G, for the Evidence-Based Medicine Teaching Tips Working Group. Tips for learners of evidence-based medicine. 4. Assessing heterogeneity of primary studies in systematic reviews and whether to combine their results. *CMAJ* 2005;172:661-5.

20   Heckman GA, McKelvie RS. Necessary cautions when considering digoxin in heart failure. *CMAJ* 2007;176:644-5.

21   Kirpalani H, Barks J, Thorlund K, Guyatt G. Cooling for neonatal hypoxic ischemic encephalopathy: do we have the answer? *Pediatrics* 2007;120:1126-30.

22   Jaeschke R, O'Byrne PM, Mejza F, Nair P, Lesniak W, Brozek J, et al. The safety of long-acting beta-agonists among patients with asthma using inhaled corticosteroids: systematic review and metaanalysis. *Am J Respir Crit Care Med* 2008;178:1009-16.

23   Szczurko O, Cooley K, Busse JW, Seely D, Bernhardt B, Guyatt GH, et al. Naturopathic care for chronic low back pain: a randomized trial. *PLoS One* 2007;2:e919.

24   Bhandari M, Guyatt G, Tornetta P 3rd, Schemitsch EH, Swiontkowski M, Sanders D, et al. Randomized trial of reamed and unreamed intramedullary nailing of tibial shaft fractures. *J Bone Joint Surg Am* 2008;90:2567-78.

25   Thavendiranathan P, Bagai A, Brookhart MA, Choudhry NK. Primary prevention of cardiovascular diseases with statin therapy: a meta-analysis of randomized controlled trials. *Arch Intern Med* 2006;166:2307-13.

26   Van den Berghe G, Wilmer A, Hermans G, Meersseman W, Wouters PJ, Milants I, et al. Intensive insulin therapy in the medical ICU. *N Engl J Med* 2006;354:449-61.

27   Chan A-W. Bias, spin, and misreporting: time for full access to trial protocols and results. *PLoS Med* 2008;5:e230.

28   Russell JA, Walley KR, Singer J, Gordon AC, Hebert PC, Cooper DJ, et al. Vasopressin versus norepinephrine infusion in patients with septic shock. *N Engl J Med* 2008;358:877-87.

29   Berger JS, Roncaglioni MC, Avanzini F, Pangrazzi I, Tognoni G, Brown DL. Aspirin for the primary prevention of cardiovascular events in women and men: a sex-specific meta-analysis of randomized controlled trials. *JAMA* 2006;295:306-13.

30   Ridker PM, Cook NR, Buring JE. Use of aspirin as primary prevention of cardiovascular events. *JAMA* 2006;296:391.

31   Babyak MA. What you see may not be what you get: a brief, nontechnical introduction to overfitting in regression-type models. *Psychosom Med* 2004;66:411-21.

32   Thatcher N, Chang A, Parikh P, Rodrigues Pereira J, Ciuleanu T, von Pawel J, et al. Gefitinib plus best supportive care in previously treated patients with refractory advanced non-small-cell lung cancer: results from a randomised, placebo-controlled, multicentre study (Iressa Survival Evaluation in Lung Cancer). *Lancet* 2005;366:1527-37.

33   Dans AL, Dans LF, Guyatt G. Applying results to individual patients. In: Guyatt G, Rennie D, Meade MO, Cook DJ, eds. User's guide to the medical literature: a manual for evidence-based clinical practice. 2nd ed. AMA, 2008: 273-89.

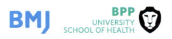

Target practice: choosing target conditions for test accuracy studies that are relevant to clinical practice

S J Lord, research fellow[1][2], L P Staub, PhD candidate[1], P M M Bossuyt, professor of clinical epidemiology[3], L M Irwig, professor of epidemiology[2]

[1]National Health and Medical Research Council Clinical Trials Centre, University of Sydney, 92-94 Parramatta Road, Locked Bag 77, Camperdown NSW 2050, Australia

[2]Screening and Test Evaluation Program, School of Public Health, University of Sydney

[3]Department of Clinical Epidemiology and Biostatistics, Academic Medical Centre, University of Amsterdam, Amsterdam, Netherlands

Correspondence to: S J Lord sally. lord@ctc.usyd.edu.au

Cite this as: BMJ 2011;343:d4684

DOI: 10.1136/bmj.d4684

http://www.bmj.com/content/343/bmj.d4684

ABSTRACT

Clinicians should seek information about how well a new test detects disease that will benefit from clinical intervention rather than simply the presence of any disease

Test accuracy varies depending on how the presence of disease is defined. For example, the sensitivity of computed tomographic (CT) colonography to detect colorectal neoplasia has been estimated at 96% for detecting invasive cancer, 86% for medium to large polyps, but as low as 45% when polyps of all sizes are included in the definition of disease.[1] To interpret these results, we need to decide whether all polyps, or what type of polyps, are important to detect.

In this paper, we explain how this principle applies when reading studies of test accuracy. When a disease threshold or set of criteria is available to define a clinically meaningful subset of disease, estimates of test accuracy for detecting the entire spectrum of disease will not apply to this subset. Therefore, clinicians need to look for estimates of test accuracy for detecting classifications of disease that are useful in clinical practice. The clinical value of a test cannot be interpreted from estimates of test accuracy if the disease definition is not clearly stated or if its clinical importance is ambiguous or unknown.

Defining disease for test accuracy studies

The diagnostic accuracy of a test measures how well it distinguishes between the presence and absence of disease. This is traditionally expressed as the sensitivity and specificity of the test. Test sensitivity is the proportion of patients with disease who are correctly identified. Test specificity is the proportion of patients without disease who are correctly identified.

To estimate sensitivity and specificity, accuracy studies require an explicit definition of disease as a dichotomous "present or absent" outcome and a reference standard that can be used to verify the true disease status (box). Typically, the definition of disease is based on the best available information about the pathological or molecular basis of disease. For example, trisomy 21 is defined by the presence of an additional chromosome 21. Here, the diagnostic threshold is reasonably clear: everyone with this characteristic is classified as having the syndrome; those without are excluded. Accuracy studies of screening tests for trisomy 21, such as ultrasound assessment of fetal nuchal translucency, measure how well the tests can correctly classify individuals according to this binary definition of disease using chromosome studies as the reference standard.

However, clinical disease is often not binary: there is no clear fixed threshold to distinguish between the presence and absence of disease. Furthermore, cases vary in severity and clinical consequences and are rarely managed as a single condition. Since test accuracy varies depending on what spectrum of disease is examined, its accuracy in detecting all disease may not reflect accuracy in detecting clinically relevant cases at one end of this spectrum.

The figure shows the common scenario where a disease has a broad spectrum of pathological presentations, ranging from mild to severe based on histology, extent, or location. For example, the presence of carotid artery stenosis can refer to all stenotic lesions, from mild plaques to fully occluded arteries. At a clinical level, disease is usually further classified based on evidence about differences in patient prognosis or treatment outcomes for subgroups of disease. These subgroups are used to guide decisions about management such as a choice between monitoring and treatment for clinically important cases.

The figure distinguishes between clinically important disease (disease associated with symptoms or a high risk of future clinical events) and disease that will benefit from treatment (disease for which the benefits of a specified treatment exceed the harms). Clinical studies are needed to define the threshold or boundaries for these subgroups. For some diseases these clinical definitions will overlap. For genital *Chlamydia trachomatis* infection, for example, all cases of disease are clinically important and recommended for treatment. For other diseases, different subgroups can be defined.

The target condition

When measuring test accuracy, the target condition is the classification of disease you wish to detect. To define the target condition we must think about the clinical decisions the test will be used to guide and determine the most appropriate threshold or criteria to dichotomise the presence or absence of disease for these decisions. The principle of defining the target condition to represent a clinically relevant classification of disease is not new[2] and is well recognised for some diseases, such as colorectal neoplasia and carotid artery stenosis.

SUMMARY POINTS

- Studies of test accuracy traditionally measure how well the test distinguishes between the presence and absence of disease
- Such studies may underestimate or overestimate a test's clinical value if a narrower spectrum of disease is relevant for diagnosis and management decisions
- Accuracy studies should use clinically relevant disease as the target condition
- Definition of the target condition should be based on evidence from prognostic studies and treatment trials

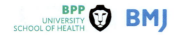

EXAMPLE OF INTERPRETATION OF TEST SENSITIVITY AND SPECIFICITY: COMPUTED TOMOGRAPHIC COLONOGRAPHY TO DETECT COLORECTAL NEOPLASIA IN A SCREENING POPULATION

Target

- To identify polyps that need further investigation by colonoscopy and biopsy. This requires a threshold for disease to be specified—eg, one or more polyps ≥10 mm (research shows high risk of advanced adenoma and progression to cancer for this subgroup)

Accuracy of computed tomographic colonography[1]

- *93% sensitivity*—of 100 patients with polyps ≥10 mm, 93 will be correctly identified as requiring colonoscopy and biopsy and seven will be misclassified as having normal or clinically unimportant results and will miss out on appropriate investigation and management
- *97% specificity*— Of 100 patients with no polyps ≥10 mm, 97 will be correctly classified as having normal or clinically unimportant results and three will be misclassified as having polyps and receive unnecessary further investigation

---

When test results will be used to rule in or rule out disease from further investigation or management, we need to consider whether all cases of disease are clinically important and, if not, what is the threshold for identifying cases that are clinically important. This is essentially a prognostic question and is best answered by studies that report patient outcomes for subgroups of disease using different disease thresholds. Clinically important carotid artery stenosis, for example, is commonly defined as ≥50% narrowing of the artery diameter, based on evidence from prognostic studies about the risk of stroke for patients with this severity of disease compared with those with mild stenosis or no disease.[3]

When test results will be used to select treatment, the target condition is best defined by treatment trials. For example, trial evidence suggests clear benefits from surgery exceeding harms only for those with 70-99% stenosis.[4] Thus the target condition for test accuracy can be based on these trial defined boundaries.

Although the target condition and reference standard are sometimes regarded as interchangeable terms, there is an important distinction between them: the target condition represents the classification of disease required to investigate a particular clinical problem (such as important carotid artery stenosis), whereas the reference standard represents the best available method to detect this condition (such as angiography). If more than one target condition is important, test accuracy can be measured separately for each.

The choice of target condition is related to but separate from other factors that limit the application of test research into practice, including the importance of measuring test accuracy in patient groups similar to those who will have the test in practice and reporting separate accuracy estimates for different patient subgroups.[5][6]

Why target condition should be clinically defined

When the target condition matches the best available evidence based classification of disease for diagnosis or treatment decisions, the clinical consequences of a true and false positive and negative test result can be clearly appreciated: test sensitivity represents the proportion of patients with the condition who will receive appropriate management; and test specificity represents the proportion of patients without the condition who will avoid further

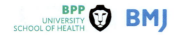

Fig Defining the target condition to represent a clinically relevant spectrum of disease

unnecessary tests or treatment. In contrast, if the definition of the target condition is not clearly defined, or its clinical importance is ambiguous, estimates of sensitivity and specificity may underestimate or overestimate the clinical value of the test. Consider human papillomavirus (HPV) testing to screen for precancerous cervical abnormalities. Here the target is high grade cervical intraepithelial neoplasia rather than all HPV infections, many of which do not warrant further investigation. HPV test sensitivity for detecting high grade intraepithelial neoplasia can be directly interpreted in clinical terms; test sensitivity for detecting all HPV infection cannot.[7]

The target condition should always be based on the best available evidence about the threshold or criteria for the intervention that the test will be used to guide. For CT colonography screening for colorectal cancer and pre-malignant polyps, the critical decision is whether to refer for colonoscopy. The risk of advanced adenoma is low for tiny polyps and increases with polyp size.[8] This evidence has been used to support a referral threshold for polyps ≥10 mm or, at most, ≥6 mm. Thus the most clinically relevant target for measuring test accuracy is having at least one polyp over the threshold size regardless of (unknown) histology.[1]

Unfortunately, poor reporting of the definition of the target condition and its relevance for clinical decisions is widespread in accuracy studies, even for conditions where clinically meaningful subgroups are well defined. In their systematic review of CT colonography for detecting colorectal polyps, Halligan et al found that only half of the accuracy studies (12/24) reported sufficient data to construct a two by two table to calculate per patient sensitivity and specificity according to polyp size.[1] In Wardlaw et al's review of imaging tests for carotid artery stenosis, 41 studies met current standards for reporting accuracy results. Of these, 30 (73%) did not provide data using standard criteria for defining clinically important (50-99%) stenosis, 12 (29%) did not provide data for 70-99% stenosis, and 7 (17%) provided data for neither of these subgroups.[9]

These reviews also show the potential magnitude of bias if test accuracy for detecting a broad disease spectrum is used as a proxy for a more narrowly defined clinically important subgroup (CT colonography test sensitivity: 93% for detecting polyps ≥10mm; 86% for polyps ≥6mm, and as low as 45% for all polyps); or if test accuracy for detecting one segment of the disease spectrum is applied to another segment (Doppler ultrasound sensitivity 89% for detecting 70-99% carotid artery stenosis; 36% for 50-69% stenosis[9]).

For conditions where the threshold for clinically important disease has not yet been defined, interpreting

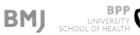

test accuracy is even more challenging. For example, studies have shown that CT pulmonary angiography is more sensitive than ventilation-perfusion (V/Q) scanning for detecting pulmonary emboli. These studies commonly include all emboli, regardless of location and size, in the definition of disease. However, the clinical importance of small subsegmental pulmonary emboli is uncertain.[10] If some of the extra cases detected by angiography represent this end of the disease spectrum, the improved sensitivity may not translate into improved patient outcomes. Ignoring this uncertainty when interpreting test accuracy results will overestimate the clinical value of angiography.[10] [11] The problems of new diagnostic technologies that are capable of detecting early or milder disease that is of uncertain clinical importance have been well documented in other areas, including cardiovascular and infectious diseases,[12] [13] spinal disorders,[14] and various cancers.[15] [16]

Clinical implications

Current guidelines for reporting and appraising studies of test accuracy do not include guidance about choosing the most relevant target condition.[17] [18] To make evidence based judgments about the clinical value of a test, clinicians need to be clear about what they are seeking to detect. When reading test accuracy studies, they should look for information about what target condition was chosen and why. Studies should include an explicit statement about the clinical consequences of correctly detecting or excluding this target and interpret the results in these terms. If the target condition is not clearly defined or does not match your reason for testing, seek more relevant evidence.

Reports of a new test having higher sensitivity for detecting potentially serious disease are compelling, but interpretation is not straightforward if the new test shifts the threshold for detecting disease. To recognise these situations, readers should consider whether the extra information provided by a more sensitive test will lead to a broader definition of disease than existing tests. If so, the clinical value of the new test will depend on whether the prognosis or response to treatment of the extra cases detected is likely to be similar to that of cases detected by existing tests. When the value is uncertain, authors should be explicit about the lack of evidence. For example, examining the clinical value of adding magnetic resonance imaging (MRI) to CT to rule out spinal injuries in obtunded patients, Schoenfeld et al reported that there are "little objective data correlating many of the identifiable MRI soft tissue abnormalities with the clinical assessment of instability."[14]

Research implications

Collaboration between clinicians and researchers is essential to define the clinical role of the test and choose the most appropriate target condition. This dialogue should focus on identifying the major clinical decisions the test will be used to guide and locating the best available evidence to determine the optimal disease threshold or criteria for making this decision.

Clinically defined target conditions will sometimes be substantially different from the traditional pathological definitions of disease. For example, a recent study of imaging strategies for acute abdominal pain used a target condition of patients requiring treatment within 24 hours rather than a traditional pathological diagnosis of appendicitis or other

disease, resulting in more clinically relevant estimates of accuracy.[19]

The target condition is likely to change as new tests and treatments are introduced that shift the threshold for clinically important disease and the threshold at which treatment benefits exceed harms. Therefore, we encourage researchers to report test results using different disease thresholds in a multidimensional table. This will allow readers to select accuracy estimates that are most relevant to how they will use the test. Ideally, study data would also be stored in a publicly accessible format that could be re-examined when new indications for tests and treatments arise.

Attempts to define the target condition will often point to the need for clinical studies that better define optimal thresholds for diagnosis and intervention. Consider quantitative polymerase chain reaction testing for cytomegalovirus in patients who have received transplants; these tests are highly sensitive for detecting copies of viral DNA in peripheral blood, but the optimal criteria for starting (expensive) treatment for this devastating disease has not yet been established.[13]

We recognise that even when trial evidence is available to develop standard disease criteria for treatment decisions, in practice the treatment threshold is not fixed. Clinical decisions about treatment thresholds may vary for different patient groups and according to clinician experience, clinician and patient preferences, and resources. Even so, we believe the development of standard evidence based disease classifications is essential to ensure accuracy estimates are meaningful to practice and to promote consistency between studies that will allow better comparisons between tests and over time.

We thank Eveline Staub, Michael Solomon, and Reginald S A Lord for their comments on drafts of this manuscript. We also thank Angela Webster and Benjamin Jonker for providing examples.

Funding: This work was supported through an Australian National Health and Medical Research Council Project Grant (No 571044) and Program Grant (No 402764).

Contributors: PB suggested the target condition as the topic for this paper, and SL and LS drafted the paper. LI led discussions to help develop and structure the ideas presented. The paper builds on earlier work from LI and PB about improving the applicability of test accuracy estimates. All authors made substantial contributions to improve the paper and approved the final version. SL is guarantor.

Competing interests: All authors have completed the ICJME unified disclosure form at www.icmje.org/coi_disclosure.pdf (available on request from the corresponding author) and declare support from the Australian National Health and Medical Research Council Project Grant (No 571044) and Program Grant (No 402764)for the submitted work; no financial relationships with any organisations that might have an interest in the submitted work in the previous three years, and no other relationships or activities that could appear to have influenced the submitted work.

Provenance and peer review: Not commissioned; externally peer reviewed.

1 Halligan S, Altman DG, Taylor SA, Mallett S, Deeks JJ, Bartram CI, et al. CT colonography in the detection of colorectal polyps and cancer: systematic review, meta-analysis, and proposed minimum data set for study level reporting. *Radiology* 2005;237:893-904.

2 Irwig L, Bossuyt P, Glasziou P, Gatsonis C, Lijmer J. Designing studies to ensure that estimates of test accuracy are transferable. *BMJ* 2002;324:669-71.

3 Autret A, Saudeau D, Betrand PH, Pourcelot L, Marchal C, De Boisvilliers S. Stroke risk in patients with carotid stenosis. *Lancet* 1987;i:888-90.

4 Rothwell PM, Eliasziw M, Gutnikov SA, Fox AJ, Taylor DW, Mayberg MR, et al. Analysis of pooled data from the randomised controlled trials of endarterectomy for symptomatic carotid stenosis. *Lancet* 2003;361:107-16.

5 Mulherin SA, Miller WC. Spectrum bias or spectrum effect? Subgroup variation in diagnostic test evaluation. *Ann Intern Med* 2002;137:598-602.

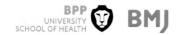

6   Whiting P, Rutjes AW, Reitsma JB, Glas AS, Bossuyt PM, Kleijnen J. Sources of variation and bias in studies of diagnostic accuracy: a systematic review. *Ann Intern Med* 2004;140:189-202.

7   Snijders PJ, van den Brule AJ, Meijer CJ. The clinical relevance of human papillomavirus testing: relationship between analytical and clinical sensitivity. *J Pathol* 2003;201:1-6.

8   Hassan C, Pickhardt PJ, Kim DH, Di GE, Zullo A, Laghi A, et al. Systematic review: distribution of advanced neoplasia according to polyp size at screening colonoscopy.. *Alimen Pharmacol Ther* 2010;31:210-7.

9   Wardlaw JM, Chappell FM, Best JJ, Wartolowska K, Berry E, NHS Research and Development Health Technology Assessment Carotid Stenosis Imaging Group. Non-invasive imaging compared with intra-arterial angiography in the diagnosis of symptomatic carotid stenosis: a meta-analysis. *Lancet* 2006;367:1503-12.

10 Anderson DR, Kahn SR, Rodger MA, Kovacs MJ, Morris T, Hirsch A, et al. Computed tomographic pulmonary angiography vs ventilation-perfusion lung scanning in patients with suspected pulmonary embolism: a randomized controlled trial. *JAMA* 2007;298:2743-53.

11 Glassroth J. Imaging of pulmonary embolism: too much of a good thing? *JAMA* 2007;298:2788-9.

12 Morrow DA. Clinical application of sensitive troponin assays. *N Engl J Med* 2009;361:913-5.

13 Szczepura A, Westmoreland D, Vinogradova Y, Fox J, Clark M. Evaluation of molecular techniques in prediction and diagnosis of cytomegalovirus disease in immunocompromised patients. *Health Technol Asses* 2006;10:1-176.

14 Schoenfeld AJ, Bono CM, McGuire KJ, Warholic N, Harris MB. Computed tomography alone versus computed tomography and magnetic resonance imaging in the identification of occult injuries to the cervical spine: a meta-analysis. *J Trauma* 113;68:109-13.

15 Esserman L, Thompson I. Solving the overdiagnosis dilemma. *J Natl Cancer Inst* 2010;102:582-3.

16 Welch HC, Black WC. Overdiagnosis in cancer. *J Natl Cancer Inst* 2010;102:605-13.

17 Bossuyt PM, Reitsma JB, Bruns DE, Gatsonis CA, Glasziou PP, Irwig LM, et al. Towards complete and accurate reporting of studies of diagnostic accuracy: the STARD initiative. *BMJ* 2003;326:41-4.

18 Whiting P, Rutjes AW, Reitsma JB, Bossuyt P, Kleijnen J. The development of QUADAS: a tool for the quality assessment of studies of diagnostic accuracy included in systematic reviews. *BMC Med Res Methodol* 2003;3:25.

19 Lameris W, van RA, van Es HW, van Heesewijk JP, van RB, Bouma WH, et al. Imaging strategies for detection of urgent conditions in patients with acute abdominal pain: diagnostic accuracy study. *BMJ* 2009;338:b2431.

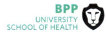

Use of serial qualitative interviews to understand patients' evolving experiences and needs

Scott A Murray, St Columba's hospice professor of primary palliative care, Marilyn Kendall, research fellow, Emma Carduff, research fellow, Allison Worth, research fellow, Fiona M Harris, research fellow, Anna Lloyd, research fellow, Debbie Cavers, research fellow, Liz Grant, senior lecturer, Aziz Sheikh, professor of primary care research and development

Primary Palliative Care Research Group, Centre for Population Health Sciences: General Practice Section, University of Edinburgh, Edinburgh EH8 9DX

Correspondence to: S A Murray scott. murray@ed.ac.uk

Cite this as: BMJ 2009;339:b3702

DOI: 10.1136/bmj.b3702

http://www.bmj.com/content/339/bmj.b3702

ABSTRACT

Interviewing patients over the course of their illness can give a much better picture of their experience than single interviews, but the approach is rarely used. **Scott Murray and colleagues** explain how to get the most from it

Longitudinal qualitative research offers considerable advantages over the more typical single "snapshot" techniques in understanding patients' changing experience of illness. Serial qualitative interviews are a convenient and efficient approach to developing an ongoing relationship between the participant and researcher, thereby facilitating discussion of sensitive and personal issues while also allowing exploration of changing needs and experiences.

Serial interview studies are widely used by social science researchers in anthropology, criminology, education, psychology, and social policy.[1][2][3][4][5][6] However, they remain underused in medicine.[7] Using our experience with the technique, we suggest when researchers might wish to use serial interviews and discuss the methods, the data generated, and how to avoid potential pitfalls.

When to use serial interviews

Serial interviews are suitable for research that aims to explore evolving and complex processes or when time is needed to develop a relationship between researcher and participants. We have used the approach to study the changing experiences and needs of people with lung and brain cancers, heart failure, severe chronic obstructive pulmonary disease, and spiritual distress, and access to care for south Asian patients at end of life (table).[8][9][10][11] Others have shown the value of this approach in, for example, understanding childhood asthma, exploring stigma related to HIV infection, reconstruction of self identity after diagnosis of chronic fatigue syndrome, complex clinician-patient interactions around requests for physician assisted suicide, and the symptom course in childhood cancer.[12][13][14][15][16]

Serial interviews can also be used to identify changes in what patients want, the most acceptable way to carry out interventions, and which outcomes are most important to patients at what times. Allowing the participant-researcher relationship to develop over time enables the generation of more private accounts and descriptions of sensitive topics that are less accessible in initial interviews. Serial interview studies can also be embedded within complex intervention studies in order to try to elucidate causal pathways. For example, we are including serial interviews in our trial of using lay outreach workers for smoking cessation in order to understand why they are (or are not) effective.

How do you conduct serial interview studies?

Recruitment

The timing of initial recruitment is important and is best driven by a sound understanding of the likely trajectory of the illness and the main issues to be explored.[17] For example, we recruited patients with lung cancer at the point of diagnosis; those with heart failure at the time of their admission to hospital—when supportive and palliative care needs become particularly relevant; and patients with glioma before formal diagnosis in order to capture their experiences from this distressing time onwards. However, when prognostic uncertainty is great, the timing of recruitment for initial and subsequent interviews can be difficult to determine.

Location of recruitment also needs consideration. Identification in hospital can be successful for patients with rare conditions, who can then be followed up in the community. However, different situations may require recruitment in other healthcare settings or even outside health care. Irrespective of where participants are recruited from, working closely with all professionals involved is crucial to ensure appropriate and ongoing access to participants. In order to make the best use of resources inclusion and exclusion criteria must be well defined, including the stage of the illness.

Data generation

Variable attrition rates and illness progression will affect the timing of second and subsequent interviews. For example, we used three month intervals in people with recently diagnosed lung cancer but six monthly interviews in people with chronic obstructive pulmonary disease, which progresses less rapidly. Researchers should identify expected transitions or key points in the course of an illness and return to speak with participants at those stages. We

SUMMARY POINTS

- Serial interviewing studies can give important insights into patients' changing experiences of illness
- The increased contact with participants allows a deeper relationship to develop, facilitating discussion of sensitive issues
- Theoretical and methodological concerns can be overcome with careful planning
- Although the method is time consuming, the benefits are well worth achieving

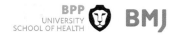

Details of six serial in-depth interview studies

Aim of study	Participants	Recruited by	Timing of initial interview	Approximate interval of interviews (months)	Length of study (months)
To compare the illness trajectories, needs, and service use of patients with cancer and those with advanced non-malignant disease[8]	20 patients with inoperable lung cancer and 20 with advanced heart failure, plus their family and professional carers	Respiratory physicians and cardiologists	Lung cancer: at diagnosisHeart failure: at hospital discharge	3	12
To inform future service developments for people with advanced heart failure[9]	30 patients with advanced heart failure, their family, and professional carers	Cardiologists and geriatricians	Hospital admission or outpatient attendance	6	12-18
To understand the experience of being diagnosed and living with a brain tumour	26 patients with suspected malignant glioma and their family carers	Neurosurgical team	During process of diagnosis	Prediagnosis, pretreatment, post-treatment, 6 month follow-up, bereavement	12 or till death
To identify the needs and service use of patients with chronic obstructive pulmonary disease and to map a framework for an intervention study	20 patients with severe disease, their family, and professional cares	Respiratory physicians and general practitioners	Severe disease, criteria from range of tests	6	18
To understand end of life care needs of South Asian patients in Scotland and to understand barriers and facilitators to accessing services[10]	25 patients, their family, and professional carers	General practitioners, community organisations	Thought by general practitioner to be in last year of life	6	18
To describe the spiritual needs of patients approaching death and to explain how and by whom such needs could best be met[11]	20 patients and their general practitioners	General practitioners	Thought by general practitioner to be in last year of life	3	6

have also found it useful to use telephone contact to assess if an interview should be brought forward to capture a changing event. The time needed for repeat interviews must be factored into the research design timetable.

Data generation must continue long enough to describe and understand the trajectory being studied. In patients with lung cancer, for example, data collection for 12 months from diagnosis will capture most deaths, but longer will be needed in a study of frail elderly patients.

Analysis

Initial analysis of transcripts of individual interviews and field notes should take place immediately, alongside continuing data generation. This allows emerging themes and concepts to be further tested and developed in subsequent interviews. Analysis may also be done across all first, second, and subsequent interviews or data synthesised from interviews at specific key points, such as immediately preceding death.

Adequate time and resources need to be allocated to allow the various longitudinal analytical opportunities to be fully exploited. Analysing all transcripts for each person as a longitudinal single unit will provide a sense of individual experience, whereas broad thematic approaches build cross-cutting themes, but at the expense of individual contexts. The longitudinal datasets generated, being typically rich in narratives, allow innovative approaches to both transcribing and analysis. For instance, as the required coding in qualitative analysis can result in fragmentation and de-contextualisation, we have transcribed some parts of the interviews of heart failure and lung cancer patients

in stanza forms, as epic poetry. These can provide an accessible insight into the patient's experience.

What type of findings might you expect?

Issues that change over time

Serial interviews can elicit changing needs or opinions—for example, in our lung cancer study some participants went from initial enthusiasm about having chemotherapy to regret, and others from refusal to deep appreciation of hospice care in later interviews. We were also able to capture the fluctuating existential anguish of increasing physical and cognitive debility in serial interviews with glioma patients and their carers. Similarly, Baker and colleagues interviewed bone marrow transplant recipients and noted changing physical problems and anxiety levels as the treatment progressed, with a feeling of impending doom emerging in later interviews.[18] The serial interviews provided a rich insight into the multifaceted roles of patients within their families and communities and the way in which these served to preserve patients' identity over time.

Serial interviews can also show how patients' experiences can be affected by external factors such as the influence of health services on their conceptualisation of illness over time.[19][20] Furthermore, serial interviews allow fluctuating and often asynchronous patterns of physical, social, psychological, and spiritual distress to be discerned. The approach allowed us to map typical trajectories of physical decline in people with cancer and organ failure.[21] We were also able to identify typical but asynchronous trajectories of psychological, social, and spiritual distress as disease

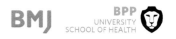

progressed in patients with advanced lung cancer.[21] [22] We were able to describe archetypal typologies of decline by following individual cases over time. This gave a much clearer picture than would have been possible by simply comparing snapshot data at different stages in the disease.

Rich and contextualised accounts

Repeating interviews allows narratives to unfold, revealing the complexity of individual situations, and helps participants and researchers to highlight deficiencies of care and make suggestions to improve services. Experiences since the last interview can be shared, with the earlier findings being developed and reflected on in the context of an evolving, participant-researcher relationship. The resulting continuous and changing account would be difficult, if not impossible, to construct from a series of snapshot interviews. Additionally, the trust fostered by repeated contact enables participants to voice sensitive or embarrassing issues and allows more private (as opposed to public) accounts to emerge.[23] We have found that repeated interviews give participants implicit permission to broach what was previously unspeakable, facilitating frank and honest discussions that might otherwise not have occurred. Detailed and contextualised accounts of sensitive illness experiences can therefore emerge.

Pitfalls and how to avoid them

Ethical issues

Ethical problems are potentially heightened in longitudinal research, including concerns around serial consent, especially if the patient is deteriorating or vulnerable.[19] [24] Intrusion, dependency, and distortion of life experience must also be avoided.[25] But we have found that patients can, and indeed want to, talk about personal and sensitive issues such as death, dying, and bereavement. Patients have said that it is sometimes easier for them to talk to a researcher rather than a clinician about these issues, and that by voicing their internal fears they have been more able afterwards to speak to their family members and friends. Serial interviews also give participants the opportunity to voice their concerns and distress and make a societal contribution through research in response to the care they have received.[26] [27]

Serial interview research can place considerable demands on researchers because it is inherently an emotionally charged process. Researchers' responsibility does not end with a final interview, and it is important to protect the wellbeing of researchers as well as participants. Accordingly, we recommend counselling and debriefing sessions for both researchers and transcribers, who should ideally have adequate maturity, experience, and access to personal or emotional support.[24] Our experiences confirm that these concerns about wellbeing can be adequately addressed and that interviewing very ill patients need not be exceptionally stressful.[28]

Attrition

As with any longitudinal research, attrition can be problematic. For example, in one study of people with glioma, none of the planned second interviews were possible because of participants' cognitive decline and lack of energy after radiotherapy.[29] Steinhauser and colleagues emphasise the importance of establishing participant-interviewer rapport from the first point of contact to try maximise retention.[30] If a firm relationship is built up between researcher and participant, few participants will be lost, except through debility or death. None theless, attrition should be factored into the design of the study. We found that by recruiting and interviewing patients and their relatives early in their illness we were able to establish relationships that facilitated interviews with relatives after patients' deaths. Grieving relatives often felt more able to take part in a bereavement interview with someone they knew and trusted, and who knew and understood their journey.

Data overload

The serial interview approach inevitably generates a large volume of interviews. The data can become difficult to manage, particularly when second and subsequent interviews have started. Effective planning is therefore essential from the outset. Furthermore, the time consuming nature of the analysis creates the danger that the process is becoming unmanageable—something that has been described as an analytical albatross.[31]

Conclusions

An understanding of the dynamic effects of disease on people's everyday lives is a prerequisite to delivering more accessible and acceptable care. People centred longitudinal research methods can make a major contribution in our understanding.[32] Serial in-depth interviews are a powerful method that resonates with the clinical aim to provide continuity of contact with patients and their families. The method is also possibly the most affordable in-depth data generation technique, and our experiences suggest that it is also likely to prove acceptable to clinicians.

Lack of awareness and concerns about some theoretical, methodological, and planning considerations currently limit use of this study design. Many of these barriers can be overcome with appropriate planning and groundwork, and although the approach is research intensive, we believe the benefits are well worth achieving. Participants consistently report serial interviews as helpful rather than harmful; researchers also find that such interviewing can be rewarding.[24]

We thank the Chief Scientist's Office of the Scottish Government, the Department of Health, London, Macmillan Cancer Support, the Economic and Social Research Council, and E Wiseman for funding the studies.

Contributors: SAM, MK, and AS conceived the paper, and all the authors wrote it and have approved the final draft. SAM is the guarantor.

Competing interests: None declared.

Provenance and peer review: Not commissioned; externally peer reviewed.

1   Kemper R, Royce A. *Chronicling cultures: Long term field research in anthropology* . Walnut Creek, CA: AltaMira, 2002.
2   Smith D, McVie S. Theory and method in the Edinburgh Study of Youth Transitions and Crime. *Br J Criminology* 2003;43:169-95.
3   White RT, Arzi HJ. Longitudinal studies: designs, validity, practicality, and value. *Res Sci Educ* 2005;35:137-49.
4   Gilligan C. *In a different voice: psychological theory and women's development* . London: Harvard University Press, 1993.
5   Corden A, Millar J. Time and change: a review of qualitative longitudinal research literature for social policy. *Soc Pol Society* 2007;6:583-92.
6   Smith N, Lister R, Middleton S. Longitudinal qualitative research. In: Becker S, Bryman A, eds. *Understanding research for social policy and practice: themes, methods and approaches* . Bristol: Policy Press, 2004.
7   Lewington S, Whitlock G, Clarke R, Sherliker P, Emberson J, Halsey J, et al. Blood cholesterol and vascular mortality by age, sex, and blood pressure: a meta-analysis of individual data from 61 prospective studies with 55,000 vascular deaths. *Lancet* 2007;370:1829-39.

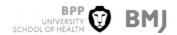

8   Murray SA, Boyd K, Kendall M, Worth A, Benton TF, Clausen H. Dying of lung cancer or cardiac failure: prospective qualitative interview study of patients and their carers in the community. *BMJ* 2002;327:929.

9   Murray SA, Worth A, Boyd K, Kendall M, Hockley J, Pratt R, et al. *Patients', carers' and professionals' experiences of diagnosis, treatment and end-of-life care in heart failure: a prospective, qualitative interview study* . London: Department of Health, British Heart Foundation, 2007.

10   Worth A, Irshad T, Bhopal R, Brown D, Lawton J, Grant E, et al. Vulnerability and access to care for South Asian Sikh and Muslim patients with life limiting illness in Scotland: prospective longitudinal qualitative study. *BMJ* 2009;338:b183.

11   Grant E, Murray SA, Kendall M, Boyd K, Tilley S, Ryan D. Spiritual issues and needs: perspectives from patients with advanced cancer and non-malignant disease. A qualitative study. *Palliat Support Care* 2004;2:371-8.

12   Peterson JW, Sterling YM. Children's perceptions of asthma: African American children use metaphors to make sense of asthma. *J Pediatr Health Care* 2009;23:93-100.

13   Buseh AG, Stevens PE. Constrained but not determined by stigma: resistance by African American women living with HIV. *Women Health* 2006;44:1-18.

14   Whitehead L. Toward a trajectory of identity reconstruction in chronic fatigue syndrome/myalgic encephalomyelitis: a longitudinal qualitative study. *Int J Nurs Stud* 2006;43:1023-31.

15   Back AL, Starks H, Hsu C, Gordon JR, Bharucha A, Pearlman RA. Clinician-patient interactions about requests for physician-assisted suicide: a patient and family view. *Arch Intern Med* 2002;162:1257-65.

16   Woodgate RL, Degner LF. Cancer symptom transition periods of children and families. *J Adv Nurs* 2004;46:358-68.

17   Lawton J, Peel E, Parry O, Douglas M. Shifting accountability: a longitudinal qualitative study of diabetes causation accounts. *Soc Sci Med* 2008;67:47-56.

18   Baker F, Zabora J, Polland A, Wingard J. Reintegration after bone marrow transplantation. *Cancer Practice* 1999;7:190-7.

19   Lawton J. Gaining and maintaining consent: ethical concerns raised in a study of dying patients. *Qual Health Res* 2001;11:693-705.

20   Lawton J, Peel E, Parry O, Araoz G, Douglas M. Lay perceptions of type 2 diabetes in Scotland: bringing health services back in. *Soc Sci Med* 2005;60:1423-35.

21   Murray SA, Kendall M, Boyd K, Sheikh A. Illness trajectories and palliative care. *BMJ* 2005;330:1007-11.

22   Murray SA, Kendall M, Grant E, Boyd K, Barclay S, Sheikh A. Patterns of social, psychological, and spiritual decline toward the end of life in lung cancer and heart failure. *J Pain Symptom Manage* 2007;34:393-402.

23   Cornwell J. *Hard-earned lives: accounts of health and illness from eas* London . London: Tavistock, 1984.

24   Kendall M, Harris F, Boyd K, Sheikh A, Murray SA, Brown D, et al. Key challenges and ways forward in researching the "good death": qualitative in-depth interview and focus group study. *BMJ* 2007;334:521-4.

25   Yates P, Stetz KM. Families' awareness of and response to dying. *Oncol Nurs Forum* 1999;26:113-20.

26   Lowes L, Paul G. Participants' experiences of being interviewed about an emotive topic. *J Adv Nurs* 2006;55:587-95.

27   Harris FM, Kendall M, Bentley A, Maguire R, Worth A, Murray S, et al. Researching experiences of terminal cancer: a systematic review of methodological issues and approaches. *Eur J Cancer Care* 2008;17:377-86.

28   Murray SA, Sheikh A. Serial interviews for patients with progressive diseases. *Lancet* 2006;368:901-2.

29   Wideheim AK, Edvardsson T, Pahlson A, Ahlstrom G. A family's perspective on living with a highly malignant brain tumor. *Cancer Nurs* 2002;25:236-44.

30   Steinhauser KE, Clipp EC, Hays JC, Olsen M, Arnold R, Christakis NA, et al. Identifying, recruiting, and retaining seriously-ill patients and their caregivers in longitudinal research. *Palliat Med* 2006;20:745-54.

31   Holland J, Thomson R, Henderson S. *Qualitative longitudinal research: a discussion paper* . Economic and Social Research Council, 2006. www.lsbu.ac.uk/families/workingpapers/familieswp21.pdf.

32   Riley J, Ross JR. Research into care at the end of life. *Lancet* 2005;365:735-7.

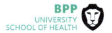

Use of multiperspective qualitative interviews to understand patients' and carers' beliefs, experiences, and needs

Marilyn Kendall, research fellow, Scott A Murray, St Columba's Hospice professor of primary palliative care, Emma Carduff, research fellow, Allison Worth, senior research fellow, Fiona Harris, research fellow, Anna Lloyd, research fellow, Debbie Cavers, research fellow, Liz Grant, senior lecturer, Kirsty Boyd, honorary clinical senior lecturer, Aziz Sheikh, professor of primary care research and development

entre for Population Health
ciences: General Practice Section,
niversity of Edinburgh, Edinburgh
H8 9DX

orrespondence to: M Kendall
1arilyn.Kendall@ed.ac.uk

ite this as: BMJ 2009;339:b4122

OI: 10.1136/bmj.b4122

ttp://www.bmj.com/content/339/
mj.b4122

ABSTRACT

A better understanding of the needs of patients and their carers can help improve services. Marilyn Kendall and colleagues describe how to conduct multiperspective studies

Linked interviews conducted with patients and their informal and professional carers can generate a richer understanding of needs and experiences than the single perspective most commonly used in qualitative studies. Interview dyads or triads, where two or three participants are interviewed as a set or case study, can explore complex complementary as well as contradictory perspectives, and there is considerable scope for using this method in a range of long term conditions.

Based on our experiences of conducting multiperspective studies and drawing on the wider literature, we summarise when researchers might find multiperspective interviews a useful approach, discuss how to use this approach, consider the data that are generated, and highlight potential pitfalls and how to avoid these.[1] [2] [3] [4] [5] This paper builds on our previous article discussing the need for longitudinal qualitative approaches.[6] Combining longitudinal and multidimensional interviews can prove particularly valuable.

When are multiperspective interviews appropriate?

Multiperspective interviews are potentially most useful when seeking to

- Understand relationships and dynamics among patients, their families, and professional carers
- Explore similarities and differences in the perceptions of patients and their family and professional carers
- Understand the individual needs of patients, carers, and professionals
- Integrate suggestions for improving services from patients, carers, and professionals.

We have used the approach mainly in the context of palliative care, where family and professional carers have an important role (table).[1] [2] [3] [4] [5] Other researchers have shown the value of a multiperspective approach in diverse clinical areas including the pattern of symptoms in childhood cancer; the couple's experience of breast cancer recurrence and prostate cancer; the complex clinician-patient interactions around requests for physician-assisted suicide; and development of a model of care giving skills for relatives of people with cancer.[7] [8] [9] [10] [11]

Dyad combinations typically include husband-wife, mother-child, and patient-carer. Triad combinations, as in a study exploring children's, parents', and professionals' views about tissue donation for research, have been used far less often.[12] In a study of patient-family dyads about information disclosure, the researchers concluded that interview triads would have given broader and deeper information.[13] More recently, another study used interviews with patients, carers, and professionals to explore views about when prognostic discussions should be instigated.[14]

How do you conduct multiperspective interview studies?

Recruitment

Our experiences have highlighted the value of a stepwise approach starting with the patient, then recruiting an informal carer, and finally health or social care professionals. Before patients give their consent, they understand that they will be invited to nominate the family members and professional carers who are most important or central to their care. The aim is to recruit those informants most likely to have relevant information for the study. Consent is obtained from each individual in turn. The aim is to complete a set of interviews over a few days or weeks, ensuring that all participants have the opportunity to reflect on whether they wish to participate and are clearly informed that they are free to withdraw at any time without adversely affecting their or their family's care and support. We found that patients were happy and able to recommend a range of key informal carers and professionals for interview. When approached in this way, the majority of carers were willing to participate.

Data generation

We usually begin by interviewing the patient alone and then the family carer in order to generate separate accounts. However, in about half the cases in our palliative care studies the patient and family carer preferred to be interviewed together. Although this can constrain the discussions, at other times patients and carers were able to prompt each other to mention or expand on specific issues or experiences. Interviewing the carer simultaneously also

SUMMARY POINTS

- Case linked interviews with patients and their carers can generate a richer understanding of needs and experiences
- Such studies can provide practical recommendations about how to deliver services
- Serial multiperspective interviewing is particularly valuable in understanding changes over the course of an illness

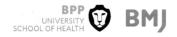

Details of multiperspective interview studies

Aims of study	Patients	Informal carers	Professional carers
To compare the illness trajectories, needs, and service use of patients with cancer and those with advanced non-malignant disease[1]	20 patients with inoperable lung cancer and 20 with advanced heart failure	Spouses, daughters, cousins, warden of sheltered accommodation	General practitioners, district nurses, community palliative care nurse, cardiologist, hospital chaplain
To inform future service developments for people with advanced heart failure[2]	30 patients with advanced heart failure	Spouses, daughters	General practitioners, heart failure nurses, geriatricians, day care staff, community nurses, hospice staff, voluntary workers
To understand the experience of being diagnosed and living with a brain tumour (2005-9)	26 patients with suspected malignant glioma	Spouses, parents, daughters, sisters	General practitioners, clinical oncologists, neurosurgeons, hospital nurses, palliative care nurses, district nurses, allied health professionals, social worker, hospital chaplains
To identify the needs and service use of patients with chronic obstructive pulmonary disease, and to map a framework for an intervention study (2006-9)	20 patients with severe disease	Spouses, daughters	General practitioners, respiratory physicians, community based and hospital based respiratory nurses, nurse from day hospice
To understand end of life care needs of South Asian patients in Scotland and to understand barriers and facilitators to accessing services[3]	25 South Asian patients	Spouses, children	General practitioners, specialist nurses, social worker, oncologist, occupational therapist, hospital manager
To describe the spiritual needs of patients approaching death and to explain how and by whom such needs could best be met[4]	20 patients with advanced malignant and non-malignant disease	Spouses, children, sisters	General practitioners, hospice staff
To explore the psychosocial impact of living with anaphylaxis on adolescents and their parents; their management of the condition; and perceptions of health care provision[5]	7 adolescents with anaphylaxis	Parents	None
To explore perceptions about anaphylaxis and its management and to formulate interventions and evaluate their acceptability to adolescents, parents, and professionals (2008-9)	26 adolescents with anaphylaxis	Parents	Allergy specialists, general practitioners, specialist nurses, school nurses, psychologists, resuscitation officers, dietitians, food and drug industry representatives, voluntary sector staff

has the advantage of allowing additional insights into the relationship. We typically interview professionals last and have found that telephone interviews, which can easily be recorded using a telephone adaptor, are the most efficient and acceptable method.

Analysis

Analysis proceeds concurrently with data generation, allowing emerging themes and concepts to be reflected on with subsequent participants. Interview transcripts and field notes from each set of patient, family, and professional carer can, however, be analysed as separate case studies and then as groups of case studies. Even a small sample will generate a variety of analytical opportunities, so qualitative software such as NVivo (www.qsrinternational.com) can be useful in organising these data.

If a longitudinal, serial dyad or triad approach is used, analysis may also be undertaken across all first interviews, then across all second and subsequent sets of interviews, or by synthesising data relating to specific key points or transitions, such as interviews with patients approaching the last days of life. By coding within as well as between cases, changes over time linked to particular patients and their associated carers and professionals can be retained and analysed in considerable depth. The context of individual patient journeys is preserved while undertaking the broader thematic analysis.[15] Creation of a matrix linking cases to the coding frame can help writing and interpretation, maximising the strengths of multiperspective data.

What type of findings might you expect?

Understanding of relationships and dynamics

Multiperspective interviews can enhance understanding of interactions such as patient-carer-doctor relationships or provide rich insights into the multifaceted roles of patients within their families and communities and the way in which these serve to maintain their identity. In one case, we conducted interviews with the patient, his wife, a specialist nurse, the church minister, his general practitioner, and an overnight nurse to develop a complex account of the experience of dying at home from lung cancer.[16]

Comparison of perceptions of patients, their family, and carers

Interviews with patient, family, and professional sometimes show concordance in their perceptions. For example, we found that an elderly man with progressive and unstable heart failure described feelings of lack of control and helplessness that were confirmed by his wife, who added that she felt like she was in prison with him. The general practitioner was experiencing similar disempowerment because he felt that he could do very little for such people.[2] In our study of the end of life care needs of South Asian patients in Scotland a participant recounted how he had suffered from discrimination and generally poor care. A linked professional confirmed that this patient's dietary needs had been unmet and his treatment been discriminatory.[3]

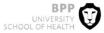

However, multiperspective data can also show differing concerns among participants. In our allergy studies, adolescents and parents gave contrasting views of the readiness of adolescents to accept responsibility for managing their condition, with parents far more anxious than adolescents about the dangers of the adolescents' ability to manage risk.[5] In a study of mothers with early breast cancer and their children, although the mothers assumed the children were unconcerned by the diagnosis, the children described themselves as being overwhelmed.[17] We found some health professionals diagnosing clinical depression at the end of life, when the patient considered the problems to be more existential or spiritual.[4]

Understanding of individual needs of participants

Interviews with multiple people can show different facets of the needs and coping strategies of participants in their role as patient, carer, or professional. Several general practitioners, as well as describing their need for better access to community nursing and social services to support dying patients at home, acknowledged that personal stresses and a lack of adequate training in communication were important barriers to effective care.[1]

Suggestions for improving services

Linked interviews not only show the complexity of individual situations and help researchers understand deficiencies in care from different perspectives, they may also contribute to formulating relevant and workable recommendations for improving services. We organised focus groups of key professionals, patients, and carers to discuss our multiperspective interview data and used the discussion to direct formulation of a framework for planning care for people with advanced heart failure.[2] [18] Interviews with bereaved carers, for example, provided in-depth accounts of their experiences that could be integrated and compared with those of the professional carers. We have also developed service recommendations by feeding back interview findings to separate groups of professional, patient, and family participants and asking them to comment on potential interventions.

Potential pitfalls and how to avoid them

Recruitment issues

Recruiting carers into a study at around the same time as the patient might seem to add complexity. Although some patients may be less willing to participate if their family carer is also to be interviewed, it can aid recruitment of vulnerable and potentially hard to access patients because the carer moves from being a protective gatekeeper to a participant.[18] Inclusion of patients who may not have an obvious family carer or friend is important, and careful exploration may identify another supportive relationship—for example, a lung cancer patient identified a sheltered housing warden.[1] We have occasionally had difficulty in recruiting busy professionals identified by patients as a key informant, and competing pressures, such as work or caring for a young family can hinder participation by family carers. Flexibility about the place and time of the interview makes refusal unusual.

Patients and carers opting to be interviewed together

Interviewing participants together is appropriate if this has been requested by participants. This can, however, have costs as well as benefits. Hearing the individual voices of

the patient and carer adequately and managing information that may be sensitive or personal in the context of a joint interview can be challenging. As most interviews take place in the patient's home, a carer wishing to add information sometimes takes the opportunity for a word alone when showing the interviewer out or, for example, by inviting the researcher to look at the garden. Patients might suggest the carer make a cup of tea, which then allows them to share information they did not want the carer to hear.

When interviews are separate some carers use the patient interview as an opportunity to go out or carry out short social activities. In our brain tumour study we found that some participants chose separate interviews when they had specific issues to discuss or were not coping or communicating well with their carers.

Joint interviews are particularly valuable when patients have cognitive impairment or communication difficulties.[19] Steinhauser has sought to overcome the difficulties of joint interviewing by providing two researchers to interview the patient and carer independently, but care must be taken not to impose separate, time consuming interviews on participants.[20]

Ethical issues

The ethical pitfalls of multiperspective research should be considered at all stages of the study. When interviewing a family or professional carer after the patient, it is often helpful to build on information from the patient interview. However, care must be taken to preserve confidentiality, particularly as carers may be curious or concerned about what has been said. Ethical issues around acting on the basis of research findings may be more acute when areas of concern—for example, about quality of care or relationships—involve or are corroborated by different interviewees. This method places emotional demands on researchers, especially if generating accounts over time, so support and debriefing from senior staff must be available.

Lack of clarity about aims and analytical strategy

Clear aims and analytical methods need to be set out and agreed at the outset because the quantity of data generated can otherwise rapidly prove overwhelming. When conducting a mixture of paired and individual interviews, both separate and joint interviews should be analysed transparently in the context in which they were generated.[21]

Conclusions

To develop personalised whole person care, we need to use patient centred research methods that can capture the multidimensional nature of the illness experience and place this understanding within a familial and health service context. Concerns about the time consuming nature of the data generation and the fact that fewer participants can be sampled have limited the use of this research method. Many of the potential barriers can be overcome with appropriate planning and groundwork. Generating data from different sources can make a major contribution to identifying people's needs and preferences.[22] Such studies elicit users' views about care in the context of their experiences and integrate these with those of professionals to provide practical recommendations about how services might be delivered more effectively.

We thank the Chief Scientist's Office of the Scottish Government, the Department of Health, London, Macmillan Cancer Support, the Economic and Social Research Council, and E Wiseman for funding the studies, and Hilary Pinnock and Michael Gallagher for permitting their studies to be highlighted.

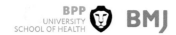

Contributors: SAM, MK, and AS conceived the paper. All the authors wrote it and have approved the final draft. MK is the guarantor.

Competing interests: None declared.

Provenance and peer review: Not commissioned; externally peer reviewed.

1   Murray SA, Boyd K, Kendall M, Worth A, Benton TF, Clausen H. Dying of lung cancer or cardiac failure: prospective qualitative interview study of patients and their carers in the community. *BMJ* 2002;325:929-32.

2   Murray SA, Worth A, Boyd K, Kendall M, Hockley J, Pratt R, et al. *Patients', carers' and professionals' experiences of diagnosis, treatment and end-of-life care in heart failure: a prospective, qualitative interview study* . London: Department of Health, British Heart Foundation, 2007.

3   Worth A, Irshad T, Bhopal R, Brown D, Lawton J, Grant E, et al. Vulnerability and access to care for South Asian Sikh and Muslim patients with life limiting illness in Scotland: prospective longitudinal qualitative study. *BMJ* 2009;338:b183.

4   Grant E, Murray SA, Kendall M, Boyd K, Tilley S, Ryan D. Spiritual issues and needs: perspectives from patients with advanced cancer and nonmalignant disease. A qualitative study. *Palliat Support Care* 2004;2:371-8.

5   Akeson N, Worth A, Sheikh A. The psychosocial impact of anaphylaxis on young people and their parents. *Clin Exp Allergy* 2007;37:1213-20.

6   Murray S, Kendall M, Carduff E, Worth A, Harris F, Lloyd A, et al. Use of serial qualitative interviews to understand patients' evolving experiences and needs. *BMJ* 2009;339:b3702.

7   Woodgate RL, Degner LF. Cancer symptom transition periods of children and families. *J Adv Nurs* 2004;46:358-68.

8   Lewis FM, Deal LW. Balancing our lives: a study of the married couple's experience with breast cancer recurrence. *Oncol Nurs Forum* 1995;22:943-53.

9   Harden JK, Northouse LL, Mood DW. Qualitative analysis of couples' experience with prostate cancer by age cohort. *Cancer Nursing* 2006;29:367-77.

10   Back AL, Starks H, Hsu C, Gordon JR, Bharucha A, Pearlman RA. Clinician-patient interactions about requests for physician-assisted suicide: a patient and family view. *Arch Intern Med* 2002;162:1257-65.

11   Schumacher KL, Beidler SM, Beeber AS, Gambino P. A transactional model of cancer family caregiving skill. *Adv Nurs Sci* 2006;29:271-86.

12   Dixon-Woods M, Cavers D, Jackson CJ, Young B, Forster J, Heney D, et al. Tissue samples as "gifts" for research: a qualitative study of families and professionals. *Med Law Int* 2008;9:131-50.

13   Kirk P, Kirk I, Kristjanson LJ. What do patients receiving palliative care for cancer and their families want to be told? A Canadian and Australian qualitative study. *BMJ* 2004;328:1343-6.

14   Clayton JM, Butow PN, Tattersall MH. When and how to initiate discussion about prognosis and end-of-life issues with terminally ill patients. *J Pain Symptom Manage* 2005;30:132-4.

15   Yin R. *Case study research: design and methods* . London: Sage, 2009.

16   Murray S, Kendall M, Boyd K, Worth A, Benton TF. Patient and carer perspectives: a man with inoperable lung cancer. *Prog Palliat Care* 2003;11:321-6.

17   Forrest G, Plumb C, Ziebland S, Stein A. Breast cancer in the family—children's perceptions of their mother's cancer and its initial treatment: qualitative study. *BMJ* 2006;332:998-1003.

18   Jaarsma T, Beattie JM, Ryder M, Rutten FH, McDonagh T, Mohacsi P, et al. Palliative care in heart failure: a position statement from the palliative care workshop of the Heart Failure Association of the European Society of Cardiology. *Eur J Heart Failure* 2009;11:433-43.

19   Pratt R. Nobody's ever asked how I felt. In: Wilkinson H, ed. *The perspectives of people with dementia: research methods and motivations*. London: Jessica Kingsley, 2002.

20   Steinhauser KE, Clipp EC, Hays JC, Olsen M, Arnold R, Christakis NA, et al. Identifying, recruiting, and retaining seriously-ill patients and their caregivers in longitudinal research. *Palliat Med* 2006;20:745-54.

21   Gysels M, Shipman C, Higginson IJ. Is the qualitative research interview an acceptable medium for research with palliative care patients and carers? *BMC Med Ethics* 2008;9:7.

22   Johnson M, Lehman R, Twycross R. *Heart failure and palliative care: a team approach* . London: Blackwell, 2006.

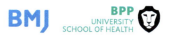

Meta-analysis of individual participant data: rationale, conduct, and reporting

Richard D Riley, senior lecturer in medical statistics[1], Paul C Lambert, senior lecturer in medical statistics[2], Ghada Abo-Zaid, postgraduate student[3]

Department of Public Health, Epidemiology and Biostatistics, University of Birmingham, Birmingham B15 2TT

[2]Centre for Biostatistics and Genetic Epidemiology, Department of Health Sciences, University of Leicester, Leicester LE1 7RH

[3]School of Mathematical Sciences, University of Birmingham, Birmingham B15 2TT

Correspondence to: R D Riley r.d.riley@bham.ac.uk

Cite this as: BMJ 2010;340:c221

DOI: 10.1136/bmj.c221

http://www.bmj.com/content/340/bmj.c221

ABSTRACT

The use of individual participant data instead of aggregate data in meta-analyses has many potential advantages, both statistically and clinically. **Richard D Riley and colleagues** describe the rationale for an individual participant data meta-analysis and outline how to conduct this type of study

Meta-analysis methods involve combining and analysing quantitative evidence from related studies to produce results based on a whole body of research. As such, meta-analyses are an integral part of evidence based medicine. Traditional methods for meta-analysis synthesise aggregate study level data obtained from study publications or study authors, such as a treatment effect estimate (for example, an odds ratio) and its associated uncertainty (for example, a standard error or confidence interval). An alternative but increasingly popular approach is meta-analysis of individual participant data, or individual patient data, in which the raw individual level data for each study are obtained and used for synthesis.[1] In this article we describe the rationale for individual participant data meta-analysis and illustrate through applied examples why this strategy offers numerous advantages, both clinically and statistically, over the aggregate data approach.[1][2] We outline when and how to initiate an individual participant data meta-analysis, the statistical issues in conducting one, how the findings should be reported, and what challenges this approach may bring.

What are individual participant data?

The term "individual participant data" relates to the data recorded for each participant in a study. In a hypertension trial, for example, the individual participant data could be the pre-treatment and post-treatment blood pressure, a treatment group indicator, and important baseline clinical characteristics such as age and sex, for each patient in

each study (table). A set of individual participant data from multiple studies often comprises thousands of patients; this is the case in the table, so for brevity we do not show all rows of data here.

This concept is in contrast to the term "aggregate data," which relates to information averaged or estimated across all individuals in a study, such as the mean treatment effect on blood pressure, the mean age, or the proportion of participants who are male. Such aggregate data are derived from the individual participant data themselves, so individual participant data can be considered the original source material.

What is an individual participant data meta-analysis?

As with any meta-analysis, an individual participant data meta-analysis aims to summarise the evidence on a particular clinical question from multiple related studies, such as whether a treatment is effective. The statistical implementation of an individual participant data meta-analysis crucially must preserve the clustering of patients within studies; it is inappropriate to simply analyse individual participant data as if they all came from a single study. Clusters can be retained during analysis by using a two step or a one step approach.[3] In the two step approach, the individual participant data are first analysed in each separate study independently by using a statistical method appropriate for the type of data being analysed; for example, a linear regression model might be fitted for continuous responses such as blood pressure, or Cox regression might be applied for time to event data such as mortality. This step produces aggregate data for each study, such as a mean treatment effect estimate and its standard error. These data are then synthesised in the second step using a suitable model for meta-analysis of aggregate data, such as one that weights studies by the inverse of the variance while assuming fixed or random (treatment) effects across studies. In the one step approach, the individual participant data from all studies are modelled simultaneously while accounting for the clustering of participants within studies. This approach again requires a model specific to the type of data being synthesised, alongside appropriate specification of the assumptions of the meta-analysis (for example, of fixed or random effects across studies).

Detailed statistical articles regarding the implementation and merits of one step and two step individual participant data meta-analysis methods are available.[4][5][6][7][8][9][10] The two approaches have been shown to give very similar results, particularly when the meta-analysis aims to estimate a single treatment effect of interest.[9][11][12] One step individual participant data meta-analyses conveniently require only a single model to be specified, but this may increase complexity for non-statisticians and requires careful separation of within study and between study variability.[9] Two step individual participant data meta-analyses are clearly more laborious, but in the second step they allow

SUMMARY POINTS

- Meta-analysis of individual participant data involves obtaining and then synthesising the raw individual level data from multiple related studies
- The application of individual participant data meta-analysis has risen dramatically from just a few articles a year in the early 1990s to an average of 49 a year since 2005
- The use of individual participant data for meta-analysis has both statistical and clinical advantages; for example, it increases the power to detect differential treatment effects across individuals in randomised trials and allows adjustment for confounding factors in observational studies
- Individual participant data meta-analyses should be protocol based, clearly reported, driven by clinical questions, and used when a meta-analysis of (published) aggregate data cannot reliably answer the clinical questions
- Statistical methods for meta-analysis of individual participant data must preserve the clustering of patients within studies. Either a one step or a two step approach should be used
- Individual participant data meta-analyses are often resource intensive but can be facilitated by the collaboration of research groups

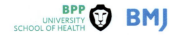

Example of individual participant data from 10 hypertension trials that assess effect of treatment versus placebo on systolic blood pressure

Study ID	Patient ID	Age (years)	Sex (1=male, 0=female)	Treatment group (1=treatment, 0=control)	Systolic blood pressure before treatment (mm Hg)	Systolic blood pressure after treatment (mm Hg)
1	1	46	1	1	137	111
1	2	35	1	0	143	133
...	...	...	...	...	...	...
1	1520	62	0	0	209	219
2	1	55	0	1	170	155
2	2	38	1	1	144	139
...	...	...	...	...	...	...
2	368	44	1	0	153	129
3	1	51	1	1	186	166
3	2	39	0	1	201	144
...	...	...	...	...	...	...
3	671	54	0	0	166	141
...	...	...	...	...	...	...
10	1	71	0	0	149	128
10	2	59	1	0	168	169
...	...	...	...	...	...	...
10	978	63	0	1	174	128

Dotted line indicates where non-displayed rows of data occur.
Hypothetical data based on Wang et al.[27]

the use of traditional, well known meta-analysis techniques such as those used by the Cochrane Collaboration[13] (for example, inverse variance fixed effect or random effects approach, or the Mantel-Haenszel method).[14] Importantly, both one step and two step approaches produce results that can inform evidence based practice, such as a pooled estimate of treatment effect across studies and how the treatment effect is modified by study level characteristics (for example, dose of treatment or study location) and patient level characteristics (for example, age or stage of disease).

Incidence of individual participant data meta-analyses over time

To assess the changes in the publication frequency of applied articles using an individual participant data meta-analysis, we performed a systematic review of the published literature. We searched Medline, Embase, and the Cochrane Library up to March 2009 using a set of search terms as described elsewhere.[15] We defined an "applied individual participant data meta-analysis" article as one describing the application and findings of a meta-analysis of individual participant data from multiple healthcare studies or multiple collaborating research groups. There was no restriction on the type of studies being synthesised. Methodological

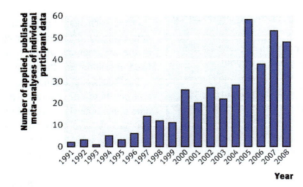

Fig 1 Number of distinct, applied meta-analyses of individual participant data published up to March 2009,* as identified by a systematic review of Medline, Embase, and the Cochrane Library. *Six articles published in 2009 were identified up to 5 March, when the review was conducted

articles, commentaries, or discussion articles regarding individual participant data meta-analysis were not included.

Our review identified 383 distinct, applied individual participant data meta-analysis articles published up to March 2009 (fig 1).[15] Only 57 articles (15%) were published before 2000, after which there was a considerable rise in the number of published articles, with an average of 49 articles published a year between 2005 and 2009. This growth is most likely the result of an increased awareness of why individual participant data meta-analyses are beneficial and the initiation of collaborations of research groups specifically to perform such studies. The 383 articles focused predominately on cancer, cardiovascular disease, and diabetes, and most assessed whether a treatment or intervention was effective, often in subgroups of patients. The assessment of risk factors for disease onset or prognostic factors for disease outcome was also popular, being the primary aim in 86 (22%) of the 383 articles, which signifies a recognition that individual participant data are particularly advantageous for time to event analyses.

When do an aggregate data meta-analysis and an individual participant data meta-analysis coincide?

In an "aggregate data meta-analysis," researchers try to replicate the two step approach to meta-analysis of individual participant data. In the first step, suitable aggregate data are extracted from the study publications or obtained directly from the study authors to allow the second step to be implemented. For example, a treatment effect estimate and its standard error are sought from each study for synthesis. If the required aggregate data can be obtained, a two step individual participant data meta-analysis and an aggregate data meta-analysis will be equivalent, provided other factors are equal (for example, number of patients, follow-up length, and so on).[8 9 12] Individual participant data are not needed if all the required aggregate data can be obtained in full from authors or the published papers themselves, which may save considerable time and resources. Researchers should note that the required aggregate data to extract will depend on the clinical questions and on the outcomes of interest and the most appropriate statistical measures to assess them. Thus liaison between clinicians and statisticians is

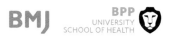

crucial to identify the aggregate data needed. Also a scoping exercise, or evidence from a previous similar review, may help establish whether such aggregate data are obtainable and reliable.

What are the advantages of a meta-analysis of individual participant data?

Meta-analysis of individual participant data has many potential advantages, both statistically and clinically, over meta-analysis of aggregate data (box 1). Aggregate data are often not available, poorly reported, derived and presented differently across studies (for example, odds ratio versus relative risk), and more likely to be reported (and in greater detail) when statistically or clinically significant, amplifying the threat of publication bias and within study selective reporting. On the contrary, having individual participant data facilitates standardisation of analyses across studies and direct derivation of the information desired, independent of significance or how it was reported. Individual participant data may also have a longer follow-up time, more participants, and more outcomes than were considered in the original study publication. This means that individual participant data meta-analyses are potentially more reliable than aggregate data meta-analyses, and the two approaches may lead to different conclusions. Four applied examples that illustrate this are shown below.[9] [16] [17] [18]

Differences in conclusions with regard to a treatment effect

Example 1: Effectiveness of laparoscopic repair at reducing persistent pain

A two step meta-analysis of individual participant data from hernia surgery trials showed that laparoscopic repair significantly reduced persistent pain compared with open repair (odds ratio 0.54, 95% CI 0.46 to 0.64).[16] In contrast, an earlier meta-analysis of published aggregate data indicated a statistically significant benefit in favour of open repair (odds ratio 2.03, 95% CI 1.03 to 4.01). This disparity occurred because the individual participant data analysis included an additional 17 trials, as few useable published aggregate data were available owing to outcome reporting bias. Furthermore, reanalysis of the individual participant data from one trial produced markedly different results to its published aggregate data.

Example 2: Effectiveness of paternal white blood cell immunisation at reducing recurrent miscarriage

The effect of paternal white blood cell immunisation on reducing recurrent miscarriage was greater in a meta-analysis of aggregate data from four published articles (live birth rate ratio (RR) 1.29, 95% CI 1.03 to 1.60) than in a two step meta-analysis of individual participant data provided by the same investigators (RR 1.17, 95% CI 0.97 to 1.37) or in a two step meta-analysis of individual participant data from four other unpublished trials (RR 1.01, 95% CI 0.74 to 1.28).[17] The effect of immunisation was statistically significant (P<0.05) only in the aggregate data meta-analysis. The different conclusions were the result of additional patients in the analysis of individual participant data and publication bias affecting the analysis of published aggregate data.

> ### BOX 1 POTENTIAL ADVANTAGES OF USING INDIVIDUAL PARTICIPANT DATA FOR A META-ANALYSIS
>
> - Consistent inclusion and exclusion criteria can be used across studies, and, if appropriate, individuals who were originally excluded can be reinstated into the analysis
> - Missing data can be observed and accounted for at the individual level
> - Results presented in the original study publications will be verified (assuming individual participant data provided can be matched to the individual participant data used in the original analyses)
> - Up to date follow-up information, potentially longer than that used in the original study publications, may be available
> - Studies that contain the same or overlapping sets of participants can be identified
> - Results for missing or poorly reported outcomes can be calculated and incorporated, thus reducing the problem of selective within study reporting
> - Results for unpublished studies can be calculated and incorporated, thus reducing the problem of publication bias
> - The statistical analysis can be standardised across studies (for example, the analysis method, how continuous variables are analysed, the time points assessed, and so on) and more appropriate or advanced methods can be applied where necessary
> - Model assumptions in each study can be assessed, such as proportional hazards in Cox regression models, and complex relationships like time dependent effects can be modelled
> - Estimates adjusted for baseline (prognostic) factors can be produced where previously only unadjusted estimates were available, which may increase statistical power and allow adjustment for potential confounding factors
> - Baseline (prognostic) factors can be adjusted for consistently across studies
> - Meta-analysis results for specific subgroups of participants can be obtained across studies (for example, those receiving a particular treatment or those with a particular biomarker level), and differential (treatment) effects can be assessed across individuals, which can help reduce between study heterogeneity
> - Prognostic models (risk scores) can be generated and validated, and multiple individual level factors can be examined in combination (for example, multiple biomarkers and genetic factors, and their interaction)
> - The correlation between multiple end points can be accounted for when each participant provides results at multiple time points, as in a meta-analysis of longitudinal data

Differences in conclusions with regard to how patient level characteristics modify treatment effect

Example 1: Effect of elevated panel reactive antibodies on the effectiveness of antilymphocyte antibody induction

An individual participant data meta-analysis of five randomised trials of antilymphocyte antibody induction therapy for renal transplant recipients showed that treatment was significantly more effective among patients with elevated (20% or more) panel reactive antibodies

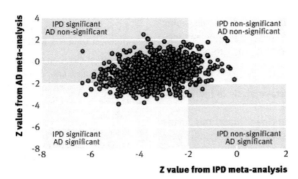

Fig 2 Comparison of the power of meta-analyses to detect a differential treatment effect across two groups of patients when individual participant data (IPD) or aggregate data (AD) are used. Adapted from Lambert et al[19]

than in those without elevated panel reactive antibodies.[18] The estimated difference in the odds of treatment failure between patients who didn't have elevated levels and those who did was -1.33 (P=0.01) on the loge scale. This important difference in treatment effect was not detected by an aggregate data meta-analysis (estimated difference in loge odds -0.014; P=0.68), because it had far less power to detect differential treatment effects across individuals than did the individual participant data analysis.

This point is illustrated in figure 2, which considers a simulated set of 1000 meta-analyses, each containing five trials where the treatment was effective for high risk patients but ineffective for low risk patients.[19] The statistical power of the meta-analysis technique used is given by the proportion of the 1000 meta-analyses that correctly detect this differential treatment effect with statistical significance (that is, the proportion that give a Z value of less than ?1.96, which equates to a P value of <0.05 and a differential treatment effect estimate in favour of high risk patients). The power is much higher when using individual participant data (90.8%) than when using aggregate data (14.8%). This difference is because individual participant data meta-analyses can model the individual risk status across (often hundreds of) patients; in contrast, aggregate data meta-analyses can only model the proportion of high risk patients across (usually a few) studies.

Example 2: Effect of gender on the effectiveness of hypertension treatment

In an aggregate data meta-analysis of 10 hypertension trials,[9] the across trials interaction between the proportion of male participants and the mean treatment effect on systolic blood pressure was estimated as 15.10 mm Hg (95% CI 8.78 to 21.41), indicating that the treatment effect was significantly less in men than in women. However, a one step individual participant data meta-analysis revealed that the within trials difference in treatment effect between men and women was actually 0.89 (95% CI 0.07 to 1.30], which is statistically but not clinically significant.[9]

This issue is shown graphically in figure 3. Each block represents a trial and the block size is inversely proportional to the standard error of the trial's treatment effect estimate. The fitted dashed lines are from the individual participant data analysis and their gradient denotes the difference in treatment effect (in mm Hg) between men and women in each trial. These lines are quite flat and suggest little difference between men and women. In contrast, the gradient of the fitted solid line across trials from the aggregate data analysis suggests a much larger treatment effect for women compared with men. The bias here in the aggregate data analysis is known as ecological bias,[18]

and is probably caused by confounding across trials. The individual participant data meta-analysis is more reliable as it directly assesses patient level information and so avoids the problem of trial level confounding.

Beyond the "grand mean"

The previous two examples importantly show that an individual participant data meta-analysis can produce more clinically relevant results than a meta-analysis of aggregate data, going beyond the "grand mean" toward individualised medicine.[20] For example, subgroups of patients with a common characteristic (such as those who are female) can be identified within individual participant data and thus a meta-analysis can be conducted specifically for that group with increased power compared with the individual studies themselves (fig 2). In contrast, the aggregate data approach is reliant on extracting summary results for each subgroup, which will often not be available. Similarly, analysis of individual participant data allows more powerful and reliable examination of treatment effects across individuals,[18] [20] as within trial information can be directly used to estimate how patients' characteristics modify treatment benefit (fig 3).[21] Multiple individual level factors can also be examined together, such as the predictive ability of combinations of biomarkers and genetic factors,[22] the results of which may facilitate stratified medicine.[23] Analyses can even be adjusted for baseline (prognostic) factors, which can increase the power of the analysis to detect a true treatment effect[24] and allows adjustment for confounding factors (a particular advantage for analyses of observational studies).

Individual participant data also enable the statistical modelling of complex relationships, such as non-linear trends and time dependent treatment effects. They even facilitate the development of prognostic models (or risk scores),[25] as a model can be constructed using individual participant data from some of the studies and then its performance validated using the individual participant data from remaining studies.[26] It is thus very clear why individual participant data are deemed the "gold standard" for meta-analysis.[1]

What are the disadvantages of a meta-analysis of individual participant data?

Meta-analysis of individual participant data is not without its disadvantages. In particular, this approach is resource intensive, because substantial time and costs are required to contact study authors, obtain their individual participant data, input and "clean" the provided individual participant data, resolve any data issues through dialog with the data providers, and generate a consistent data format across studies. For example, Ioannidis et al[22] undertook an individual participant data meta-analysis in 2002 that required 2088 hours for data management, with 1000 emails exchanged between study collaborators and the data managers. The required costs and time will clearly vary depending on the complexity of the analysis and the number of studies involved,[27] and such factors need serious consideration before embarking on an individual participant data meta-analysis or when applying for grant income. In particular, resource requirements must be considered for both the team conducting the individual participant data meta-analysis and the original study authors themselves. The latter group is often neglected, but cooperation of the original study authors is crucial to the success of the project and these individuals will often commit many hours "cleaning" and updating their data and resolving ongoing queries.

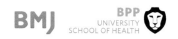

The individual participant data approach may also require advanced statistical expertise, and there may be ethical or confidentiality concerns about using patient level data. In our experience, individual participant data meta-analyses usually have the same objectives as the original studies, for which ethical approval should exist; however, this must be verified and, if in doubt, advice or approval must be sought from an ethics committee. When asking for individual participant data, researchers should stipulate that individuals' names and contact details must be erased from the data before they are supplied, so that participants can be identified only via a unique ID number interpretable solely by the original study authors.

Although a high proportion of the desired individual participant data can usually be obtained,[15] sometimes data are not available for all studies. Individual participant data might have been be lost or destroyed, or study authors may not be contactable or willing to collaborate. An individual participant data meta-analysis may then be biased if the provision of individual participant data is associated with the study results. In such a situation, it is important to examine any differences between studies that provided individual participant data and studies that did not provide individual participant data, and, if possible, consider whether the conclusions of the meta-analysis might change if those studies not providing individual participant data had been included. Meta-analysis methods for combining individual participant data with aggregate data are available for this purpose.[9 15] In many situations, however, such as the assessment of differential treatment effects across individuals,[9] aggregate data will add very little to an individual data meta-analysis and serve only to amplify why individual participant data was desired.

It is also important to recognise that the quality of individual participant data is dependent on the quality of the original studies themselves, and that the studies providing data are not necessarily of the highest quality. A meta-analysis of individual participant data from a set of poorly designed trials with many potential sources of bias is as deficient as a meta-analysis of aggregate data from these trials. Individual participant data meta-analyses should thus also include a quality assessment of the original studies and, if appropriate, make clear how the inclusion of lesser quality studies impacts on conclusions. If only low quality studies exist, it may be better to initiate a prospective individual participant data meta-analysis.

How to obtain individual participant data for a meta-analysis
Two crucial steps toward undertaking an individual participant data meta-analysis are deciding how much individual participant data are needed and obtaining the individual participant data themselves. One option is to adopt a systematic review approach, where all relevant published and unpublished studies are identified through a transparent, systematic search, and then study authors are contacted to provide the individual participant data. Authors may be more willing to agree if the clinical and methodological reasons for requiring the individual participant data are clearly outlined, preferably via a face to face meeting. It may also help to promise regular updates on the results of the individual participant data meta-analysis and provide the incentive of joint authorship on subsequent publications. Patience, politeness, and good communication are essential.

Another option is to collaborate with other research groups and agree to pool resources to answer specific clinical questions. For example, members of the receptor and biomarker group within the European Organisation for Research and Treatment of Cancer provided 18 datasets for an individual participant data meta-analysis of prognostic markers in breast cancer.[28] Such meta-analyses can also be updated prospectively as new data become available from collaborators. One concern, however, is that studies within the collaboration may not reflect the entire set of existing studies, potentially introducing bias. It is thus important for collaborations to be inclusive. For example, one individual participant data meta-analysis by the Early Breast Cancer Trialists' Collaborative Group involved over 400 named collaborators,[29] who commendably provided individual participant data for 42000 women from 78 randomised treatment comparisons.

Reporting individual participant data meta-analyses
A review of 33 applied individual participant data meta-analyses from between 1999 and 2001 noted that "clear reporting of the statistical methods used was rare" and that only a few studies actually referred to a protocol for their individual participant data project.[3] Clearly these shortcomings must be addressed. Like all good research, meta-analyses of individual participant data should be protocol driven and conducted with clear and prespecified objectives. Studies should also be clearly reported in line with the Preferred Reporting Items for Systematic Reviews and Meta-Analyses (PRISMA)[30] or Meta-analysis Of Observational Studies in Epidemiology (MOOSE)[31] guidelines for meta-analyses of randomised controlled trials and observational studies, respectively. Given that these guidelines are not specific to the individual participant data approach, in box 2 we outline some additional information that individual participant data meta-analyses should report.

An applied example of an individual participant data meta-analysis of hypertension trials
An individual participant data meta-analysis of 10 hypertension trials was conducted with the objective of estimating the effect of a treatment on systolic blood pressure.[9 32] The applied one step and two step individual participant data meta-analysis models used are described fully elsewhere.[9] Briefly, they involve fitting linear regression models that estimate the treatment effect on systolic blood pressure, having adjusted for systolic blood pressure at baseline. This "analysis of covariance" approach is the most appropriate method for analysing the change from baseline in a continuous variable[33] because it gives the most precise and least biased estimate of treatment effect. It is very difficult to undertake an analysis of covariance meta-analysis without individual participant data because individual studies analyse and report a change from baseline in a heterogeneous fashion.[34]

The one step and two step individual participant data meta-analyses gave identical results. The pooled treatment effect was estimated at -10.16 (95% CI -12.27 to -8.06), indicating that hypertension treatment reduced systolic blood pressure by, on average, 10.16 mm Hg compared with controls. There was also, however, a large between study variance of 7.13, indicating that the treatment effect varied considerably across the trials. A 95% prediction interval[35] for the underlying treatment effect in a new trial was estimated as -16.69 to -3.63. This range indicates that although there is heterogeneity among trials, in any single trial hypertension treatment is effective at reducing systolic blood pressure.

Availability of individual participant data in this example also allowed a reliable and powerful assessment of how

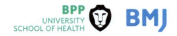

BOX 2 SUGGESTED INFORMATION TO REPORT FROM AN INDIVIDUAL PARTICIPANT DATA META-ANALYSIS, TO SUPPLEMENT THOSE REPORTING GUIDELINES OF PRISMA AND MOOSE[30 31]

- Whether there was a protocol for the individual participant data project, and where it can be found
- Whether ethics approval was necessary and (if appropriate) granted
- Why the individual participant data approach was initiated
- The process used to identify relevant studies for the meta-analysis
- How authors of relevant studies were approached for individual participant data
- How many authors (or collaborating groups) were approached for individual participant data, and the proportion that provided such data
- The number of authors who did not provide individual participant data, the reasons why, and the number of patients (and events) in the respective study
- Whether those authors who provided individual participant data gave all their data or only a proportion; if the latter, then describe what information was omitted and why
- Whether there were any qualitative or quantitative differences between those studies providing individual participant data and those studies not providing individual participant data (if appropriate)
- The number of patients within each of the original studies and, if appropriate, the number of events
- Details of any missing individual level data within the available individual participant data for each study, and how this was handled within the meta-analyses performed
- Details and reasons for including (or excluding) patients who were originally excluded (or included) by the source study investigators
- Whether a one step or a two step individual participant data meta-analysis was performed, and the statistical details thereof, including how clustering of patients within studies was accounted for
- How many patients from each study were used in each meta-analysis performed
- Whether the assumptions of the statistical models were validated (for example, proportional hazards) within each study
- Whether the individual participant data results for each study were comparable with the published results, and, if not, why not (for example, individual participant data contained updated or modified information)
- How individual participant data and non-individual participant data studies were analysed together (if appropriate).
- The robustness of the meta-analysis results following the inclusion or exclusion of non-individual participant data studies (if appropriate)

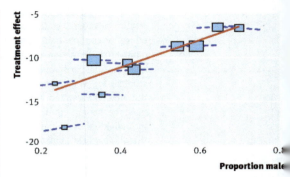

Fig 3 An example of ecological bias within an aggregate data meta-analysis

Conclusions

The decision to undertake an individual participant data meta-analysis should be driven by the clinical questions of interest and whether a meta-analysis of (published) aggregate data can reliably answer them. In many situations an individual participant data meta-analysis will offer considerable advantages, both statistically and clinically, over a meta-analysis of aggregate data, which is why individual participant data approaches are increasingly being applied.

Important challenges remain, however, not least the task of obtaining the individual participant data itself. Detailed commentaries exist regarding the often laborious and expensive process of retrieving and processing individual participant data.[22 36] Ways of addressing this difficulty include storing individual participant data in a central repository or on the internet,[37] but perhaps most crucial is the initiation of collaborations across research groups in each field. Even when individual participant data are fully available, obstacles may still remain because studies are usually collated retrospectively. Completed studies may be of poor quality (for example, poorly designed with selection biases), may not have recorded important variables, or may have used outdated treatment strategies.[38] For such reasons prospectively planned individual participant data meta-analyses have been advocated. This technique is similar to undertaking a multicentre trial, except it allows variations in the protocols of included studies. This approach maximises the power of the meta-analysis by achieving consistency in, for example, treatments received, outcomes assessed, variables collected, and how data are recorded. Prospectively planned meta-analyses are achievable[39] but currently few have been completed, so it would be encouraging to see growth in the use of this method.

We thank the two reviewers and the *BMJ* manuscript committee for their valuable comments, which have helped improve this paper.

Contributors: RDR has successfully completed an Evidence Synthesis Fellowship awarded by the Department of Health on statistical methods for individual participant data meta-analysis. He is a co-convenor of the Cochrane Prognosis Methods Group and has led workshops for the Cochrane IPD Methods Group. RDR and PCL have published numerous applied and methodological articles regarding meta-analysis, including those using individual participant data. GA-Z is currently undertaking a PhD in meta-analysis of prognosis studies using individual participant data, supervised by RDR. The aforementioned experience and knowledge of all the authors informed the content of this article, alongside the described systematic review of published individual participant data meta-analyses. RDR conceived the paper and wrote the first draft. All authors contributed to revising the paper accordingly. PCL produced the figures, and GA-Z and RDR performed the systematic review to identify published individual participant data meta-analyses. RDR is the guarantor.

Funding: None.

patient level characteristics modify the treatment effect. For example, a one step individual participant data analysis showed no clinically important difference in treatment effect between men and women. In contrast, if only aggregate data had been available, the analysis would have wrongly indicated a clinically important treatment effect difference in favour of women (fig 3).[9] A one step individual participant data analysis also revealed a non-linear effect of age on the treatment effect. Up to the age of 55 years, the treatment effect increased for each year increase in age; however, after 55 years there was no evidence of differential treatment effects according to age.[9] This finding was not detectable without individual participant data.

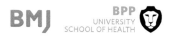

Competing interests: RDR is a statistics editor for the *BMJ*. RDR and PCL have previously published applied and methodological articles advocating the individual participant data approach to meta-analysis.

Provenance and peer review: Not commissioned; externally peer reviewed.

1   Stewart LA, Parmar MK. Meta-analysis of the literature or of individual patient data: is there a difference? *Lancet* 1993;341:418-22.
2   Oxman AD, Clarke MJ, Stewart LA. From science to practice. Meta-analyses using individual patient data are needed. *JAMA* 1995;274:845-6.
3   Simmonds MC, Higgins JPT, Stewart LA, Tierney JF, Clarke MJ, Thompson SG. Meta-analysis of individual patient data from randomized trials: a review of methods used in practice. *Clin Trials* 2005;2:209-17.
4   Turner RM, Omar RZ, Yang M, Goldstein H, Thompson SG. A multilevel model framework for meta-analysis of clinical trials with binary outcomes. *Stat Med* 2000;19:3417-32.
5   Higgins JP, Whitehead A, Turner RM, Omar RZ, Thompson SG. Meta-analysis of continuous outcome data from individual patients. *Stat Med* 2001;20:2219-41.
6   Whitehead A, Omar RZ, Higgins JP, Savaluny E, Turner RM, Thompson SG. Meta-analysis of ordinal outcomes using individual patient data. *Stat Med* 2001;20:2243-60.
7   Tudur-Smith C, Williamson PR, Marson AG. Investigating heterogeneity in an individual patient data meta-analysis of time to event outcomes. *Stat Med* 2005;24(9):1307-19.
8   Jones AP, Riley RD, Williamson PR, Whitehead A. Meta-analysis of individual patient data versus aggregate data from longitudinal clinical trials. *Clin Trials* 2009;6:16-27.
9   Riley RD, Lambert PC, Staessen JA, Wang J, Gueyffier F, Thijs L, et al. Meta-analysis of continuous outcomes combining individual patient data and aggregate data. *Stat Med* 2008;27:1870-93.
10   Riley RD, Dodd SR, Craig JV, Thompson JR, Williamson PR. Meta-analysis of diagnostic test studies using individual patient data and aggregate data. *Stat Med* 2008;27:6111-36.
11   Olkin I, Sampson A. Comparison of meta-analysis versus analysis of variance of individual patient data. *Biometrics* 1998;54:317-22.
12   Mathew T, Nordstrom K. On the equivalence of meta-analysis using literature and using individual patient data. *Biometrics* 1999;55:1221-3.
13   Higgins JPT, Green S. *Cochrane handbook for systematic reviews of interventions version 5.0.1* [updated September 2008]. The Cochrane Collaboration, 2008. www.cochrane-handbook.org.
14   Mantel N, Haenszel W. Statistical aspects of the analysis of data from retrospective studies of disease. *J Natl Cancer Inst* 1959;22:719-48.
15   Riley RD, Simmonds MC, Look MP. Evidence synthesis combining individual patient data and aggregate data: a systematic review identified current practice and possible methods. *J Clin Epidemiol* 2007;60:431-9.
16   McCormack K, Grant A, Scott N. Value of updating a systematic review in surgery using individual patient data. *Br J Surg* 2004;91:495-9.
17   Jeng GT, Scott JR, Burmeister LF. A comparison of meta-analytic results using literature vs individual patient data. Paternal cell immunization for recurrent miscarriage. *JAMA* 1995;274:830-4.
18   Berlin JA, Santanna J, Schmid CH, Szczech LA, Feldman HI. Individual patient- versus group-level data meta-regressions for the investigation of treatment effect modifiers: ecological bias rears its ugly head. *Stat Med* 2002;21:371-87.
19   Lambert PC, Sutton AJ, Abrams KR, Jones DR. A comparison of summary patient-level covariates in meta-regression with individual patient data meta-analysis. *J Clin Epidemiol* 2002;55:86-94.
20   Davey Smith G, Egger M, Phillips AN. Meta-analysis. Beyond the grand mean? *BMJ* 1997;315:1610-4.
21   Thompson SG, Higgins JP. Treating individuals 4: can meta-analysis help target interventions at individuals most likely to benefit? *Lancet* 2005;365:341-6.
22   Ioannidis JP, Rosenberg PS, Goedert JJ, O'Brien TR. Meta-analysis of individual participants' data in genetic epidemiology. *Am J Epidemiol* 2002;156:204-10.
23   Trusheim MR, Berndt ER, Douglas FL. Stratified medicine: strategic and economic implications of combining drugs and clinical biomarkers. *Nat Rev Drug Discov* 2007:287-93.
24   Hernandez AV, Eijkemans MJ, Steyerberg EW. Randomized controlled trials with time-to-event outcomes: how much does prespecified covariate adjustment increase power? *Ann Epidemiol* 2006;16:41-8.
25   Altman DG, Vergouwe Y, Royston P, Moons KGM. Prognosis and prognostic research: validating a prognostic model. *BMJ* 2009;338:b605.
26   Royston P, Parmar MKB, Sylvester R. Construction and validation of a prognostic model across several studies, with an application in superficial bladder cancer. *Stat Med* 2004;23:907-26.
27   Stewart LA, Clarke MJ for the Cochrane Working Group. Practical methodology of meta-analyses (overviews) using updated individual patient data. *Stat Med* 1995;14:2057-79.
28   Look MP, van Putten WL, Duffy MJ, Harbeck N, Christensen IJ, Thomssen C, et al. Pooled analysis of prognostic impact of urokinase-type plasminogen activator and its inhibitor PAI-1 in 8377 breast cancer patients. *J Natl Cancer Inst* 2002;94:116-28.
29   Early Breast Cancer Trialists' Collaborative Group. Effects of radiotherapy and of differences in the extent of surgery for early breast cancer on local recurrence and 15-year survival: an overview of the randomised trials. *Lancet* 2005;366:2087-106.
30   Moher D, Liberati A, Tetzlaff J, Altman DG for the PRISMA Group. Preferred reporting items for systematic reviews and meta-analyses: the PRISMA statement. *BMJ* 2009;339:b2535.
31   Stroup DF, Berlin JA, Morton SC, Olkin I, Williamson GD, Rennie D, et al for the Meta-analysis Of Observational Studies in Epidemiology (MOOSE) group. Meta-analysis of observational studies in epidemiology: a proposal for reporting. *JAMA* 2000;283:2008-12.
32   Wang JG, Staessen JA, Franklin SS, Fagard R, Gueyffier F. Systolic and diastolic blood pressure lowering as determinants of cardiovascular outcome. *Hypertension* 2005;45:907-13.
33   Vickers AJ, Altman DG. Statistics notes: analysing controlled trials with baseline and follow-up measurements. *BMJ* 2001;323:1123-4.
34   Abrams KR, Gillies CL, Lambert PC. Meta-analysis of heterogeneously reported trials assessing change from baseline. *Stat Med* 2005;24:3823-44.
35   Higgins JP, Thompson SG, Spiegelhalter DJ. A re-evaluation of random-effects meta-analysis. *J R Stat Soc Ser A* 2009;172:137-59.
36   Stewart LA, Tierney JF. To IPD or not to IPD? Advantages and disadvantages of systematic reviews using individual patient data. *Eval Health Prof* 2002;25:76-97.
37   Hutchon DJ. Publishing raw data and real time statistical analysis on e-journals. *BMJ* 2001;322:530.
38   Chia S, Bryce C, Gelmon K. The 2000 EBCTCG overview: a widening gap. *Lancet* 2005;365:1665-6.
39   Baigent C, Keech A, Kearney PM, Blackwell L, Buck G, Pollicino C, et al. Efficacy and safety of cholesterol-lowering treatment: prospective meta-analysis of data from 90,056 participants in 14 randomised trials of statins. *Lancet* 2005;366:1267-78.

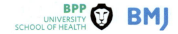

An IV for the RCT: using instrumental variables to adjust for treatment contamination in randomised controlled trials

Jeremy B Sussman, Robert Wood Johnson Foundation clinical scholar[1][2],
Rodney A Hayward, professor of medicine and public health[1][2]

[1]Robert Wood Johnson Clinical Scholars Program, Department of Internal Medicine, University of Michigan, Ann Arbor, Michigan, USA

[2]Department of Veterans Affairs, Veterans Affairs Health Services Research and Development Center of Excellence, Veterans Affairs Ann Arbor Healthcare System, Ann Arbor, Michigan, USA

Correspondence to: J B Sussman
jeremysu@med.umich.edu

Cite this as: BMJ 2010;340:c2073

DOI: 10.1136/bmj.c2073

http://www.bmj.com/content/340/bmj.c2073

ABSTRACT

Although the randomised controlled trial is the "gold standard" for studying the efficacy and safety of medical treatments, it is not necessarily free from bias. When patients do not follow the protocol for their assigned treatment, the resultant "treatment contamination" can produce misleading findings. The methods used historically to deal with this problem, the "as treated" and "per protocol" analysis techniques, are flawed and inaccurate. Intention to treat analysis is the solution most often used to analyse randomised controlled trials, but this approach ignores this issue of treatment contamination. Intention to treat analysis estimates the effect of recommending a treatment to study participants, not the effect of the treatment on those study participants who actually received it. In this article, we describe a simple yet rarely used analytical technique, the "contamination adjusted intention to treat analysis," which complements the intention to treat approach by producing a better estimate of the benefits and harms of receiving a treatment. This method uses the statistical technique of instrumental variable analysis to address contamination. We discuss the strengths and limitations of the current methods of addressing treatment contamination and the contamination adjusted intention to treat technique, provide examples of effective uses, and discuss how using estimates generated by contamination adjusted intention to treat analysis can improve clinical decision making and patient care.

Introduction

The recent European Randomized Study of Screening for Prostate Cancer[1] concluded that 1400 patients would need prostate specific antigen screening in order to prevent one death from prostate cancer. This number will be used in meta-analyses, cost effectiveness analyses, and clinical guidelines. But is it accurate? In the study, nearly 20% of people assigned to receive prostate specific antigen screening didn't undergo a single test in 10 years. In a similar American randomised controlled trial,[2] 40% of participants who weren't supposed to receive prostate specific antigen screening were actually tested. Both these trials were analysed and interpreted as though all participants followed the treatment they were randomised to. If participants had in fact adhered to their assigned intervention as randomised, would the results have been different? Are the results accurate when it comes to advising individual patients whether they should be screened?

Randomised controlled trials are the "gold standard" for examining the efficacy and safety of medical interventions because they are considered free from bias. However, what

was seen in the recent prostate specific antigen trials is common in randomised controlled trials and makes the published data less reliable. When study participants do not receive the treatment to which they were randomised, the flaw called "treatment contamination" is created. Treatment contamination can occur through treatment non-adherence (not receiving the recommended intervention because of treatment intolerance or patient preference) and treatment crossover (receiving the intervention intended for the other group in a trial). Just as non-adherence is common in clinical practice, treatment contamination in randomised controlled trials is not a small or infrequent problem—some of our largest trials have contamination of more than 30%.[3][4][5][6]

In this paper, we describe a method called the "contamination adjusted intention to treat" (CA ITT) analysis that better estimates the benefits of receiving a treatment. CA ITT analysis uses an established statistical technique called instrumental variables (IVs) analysis to adjust for the bias created by contamination. CA ITT analyses could be an excellent complement to traditional analyses but are rarely used in clinical trials, which have traditionally emphasised analytical simplicity.[7][8][9][10] We outline the problem of treatment contamination and how it is currently addressed, describe IVs and CA ITT, how they can be used in clinical trials, and summarise the benefits and limitations of the CA ITT technique.

Background: What do we do now, and what's wrong with it?

How to address treatment contamination in randomised controlled trials has been debated for years. The most commonly used approaches historically are the "as treated" and "per protocol" techniques, which have appropriately fallen out of favour (table). In as treated analyses, participants are analysed entirely on the basis of treatment

SUMMARY POINTS

- When patients in a clinical trial do not follow the protocol for their assigned treatment, the resultant "treatment contamination" can produce misleading findings
- The older methods used to deal with this problem, the "as treated" and "per protocol" analysis techniques, are flawed and inaccurate
- Intention to treat analysis estimates the effect of recommending a treatment to study participants, not the effect of receiving the treatment
- A technique that we call "contamination adjusted intention to treat analysis" can complement the intention to treat approach by producing a better estimate of the benefits and harms of receiving a treatment
- The contamination adjusted intention to treat analysis uses the statistical technique of instrumental variable analysis to address contamination

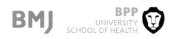

GLOSSARY

- **As treated:** Method of analysis for randomised controlled trials in which all patients are analysed on the basis of the treatment ultimately received, regardless of the treatment to which they were randomly assigned.
- **Contamination adjusted intention to treat:** Method of analysis for randomised controlled trials in which all patients are analysed as they were randomised and then the result adjusted for treatment contamination by using an instrumental variable.
- **Crossover:** When a study participant receives the intervention for the group to which he or she has not been assigned.
- **Instrumental variable:** An analytical technique, traditionally used in non-randomised research studies, that uses a variable associated with the factor under study but not directly associated with the outcome variable or any potential confounders.
- **Intention to treat:** Method of analysis for randomised controlled trials in which all patients are analysed as they were randomised, regardless of behaviour or treatment received.
- **Loss to follow-up:** When a participant in a study is not involved in the outcome assessment. This issue is not addressed in this paper.
- **Non-adherence:** When a study participant does not receive the assigned therapy, whatever the cause and no matter how legitimate the reason. Non-adherence is often used differently in clinical practice from in experimental research.
- **Per protocol:** Method of analysis for randomised controlled trials in which individuals are included in the analysis only if they followed the assigned protocol and are removed from the analysis entirely if they do not follow protocol.
- **Treatment contamination:** Any time the study participant does not follow the protocol for the assigned treatment. In a study with no treatment contamination, the results of the intention to treat and contamination adjusted intention to treat analyses will be identical.

treat analysis, sometimes called "analyse as randomised" analysis,[14] [15] participants are analysed on the basis of the treatment arm to which they were initially assigned, regardless of their ultimate treatment exposure. Intention to treat analysis avoids the flaws of the as treated and per protocol approaches and should always be the initial analysis of a randomised controlled trial. However, intention to treat analysis ignores treatment contamination altogether. What often goes unappreciated is the fact that intention to treat analysis answers the question: "how much do study participants benefit from being assigned to a treatment group?" This can be important information to policy makers and health planners, but patients and clinicians generally want to know the answer to a different question: "what are the risks and benefits of receiving a treatment?"

Using instrumental variables to help us understand results of randomised controlled trials

When physicians were investigating whether maternal smoking leads to poor birth outcomes, they determined that evidence from traditional longitudinal studies was unreliable because smokers and non-smokers are behaviourally different in so many ways aside from smoking status. A solution to this problem was found through tobacco taxes. Throughout the 1970s and 1980s, American states had many and varied increases in tobacco taxes that clearly altered smoking rates across states. Increases in cigarette taxes seem unlikely to affect birth outcomes other than through the effect on smoking. Researchers used a statistical technique known as IV analysis to estimate the impact of smoking on birth outcomes by comparing birth outcomes and changes in smoking rates with state changes in cigarette taxes.[16]

IV techniques were designed to learn from natural experiments (that is, changes in people's environments or exposures unrelated to their individual choices or behaviours), in which an unbiased "instrument" (such as change in tobacco taxation level) makes the exposure of interest (such as an individual's smoking habits) more or less likely but has no other effect, either directly or indirectly, on the outcome. IV analysis assesses how the instrument predicts the exposure and the outcome, then uses that information to understand how the exposure predicts the outcome. This type of two stage analysis is used often in the social sciences and is becoming common in observational studies in medicine.[17] [18] [19] [20] Medical examples of IVs in observational studies include comparing the outcomes among patients whose doctors prefer first generation (conventional) versus second generation (atypical) antipsychotics,[19] analysing the effects of dramatic changes in copayment on medication adherence and

received (that is, according to their behaviour, not their random assignment). In per protocol analyses, participants who fail to follow the protocol are simply dropped from the study (that is, included or excluded according to their behaviour). Although these approaches seem reasonable, people's behaviours are strongly non-random, with non-adherents generally being less healthy and less health conscious than those who adhere to treatment.[11] [12] Analysing trial data by behaviour removes the benefit of randomisation, yielding results that are generally biased.[11] [12] [13]

Guidelines now recommend that randomised controlled trials use intention to treat analysis.[14] [15] In intention to

Different methods of analysing a randomised controlled trial

	Explanation	Benefits	Negatives
As treated	Analyses by treatment received	Easy to calculateTries to address patient oriented question	Results in non-random omission bias
Per protocol	Omits all participants who do not follow protocol	Easy to calculateTries to address patient oriented question	Results in non-random omission bias
Intention to treat	Analyses by randomisation, ignores whether treatment received	Easy to assessProvides good estimate of the effect of recommending a treatment to study population	Underestimates value of receiving the treatment
Contamination adjusted intention to treat	Analyses by randomisation, adjusts for whether treatment received	Provides good estimate of an individual's risks and benefits of receiving a treatment[1]	Overestimates population level treatment benefitsSomewhat more difficult calculation

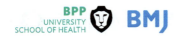

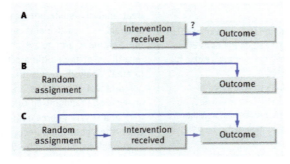

Fig 1 Analysis of randomised controlled trials. In per protocol and as treated analyses (A), random assignment is ignored, creating less reliable results. In intention to treat analyses (B), only the effect of randomisation is assessed, not the effect of receiving the intervention. The two stage contamination adjusted intention to treat approach (C) uses assignment and intervention received to calculate the effect of receiving the treatment

subsequent health outcomes among patients with chronic heart failure,[21] and using distance from a catheterisation lab to approximate the benefit of intensive therapy for heart attacks.[17] Even the random assortment of genetic information has been used as an IV called "Mendelian randomisation"—a genetic variant acts as an instrumental variable to help disentangle the confounded causal relation between phenotype and disease.[22]

Despite their theoretical appeal, valid IVs are uncommon. The most common IV in medicine is randomisation within a randomised controlled trial that has treatment contamination. IV analysis can bridge the gap between the more policy focused question posed by intention to treat analyses and the patient focused question of biological efficacy.[8 23 24]

The concept behind a CA ITT analysis is quite simple. The randomised controlled trial is treated as an IV, with treatment assignment as the "instrument." The effect of treatment assignment on outcome observed (intention to treat analysis) is adjusted by the percentage of assigned participants who ultimately receive the treatment (contamination adjustment). This way the effect of treatment receipt on the risk of the outcome can be obtained (fig). If a patient stops taking a medication early, the measured non-adherence can be adjusted for with CA ITT and the biases of as treated and per protocol analyses can be avoided. The intention to treat and the CA ITT estimates provide complementary information, and both results are important in their own right.[7 8 24 25 26 27 28] IV estimators are available in most major statistical packages.

Loss to follow-up, where a patient does not participate in planned follow-up evaluations in a trial or cannot be evaluated at all, is also a major cause of bias in randomised controlled trials, but is a separate and statistically more difficult problem (for a discussion of this topic, see Dunn et al[10]).

Real world examples
CA ITT analysis has been used for randomised controlled trials in the past, but rarely, and has gone by several different names, including "complier average causal effects,"[9 23] IVs,[29 30] efficacy estimator,[31] and preference based analysis.[26] For example, one study found that vitamin A supplementation in malnourished children reduced mortality by 41% when a traditional intention to treat analysis was used.[31] Once the high mortality rate of the treatment non-adherents was accounted for, however, receiving supplements was found to reduce mortality by two thirds (72%). A recent CA ITT analysis determined that faecal occult blood testing reduces mortality from colorectal cancer by 25% if the patient returns the sample cards, rather than by 19%, the value associated with being randomised to receive the test kit.[32]

Adjusting randomised trials for treatment contamination could allow more nuanced understanding of the medical literature. For example, the 1994 Scandinavian Simvastatin Survival Study (4S)[33] found a 20% greater effect of simvastatin on cardiac events than did the 2002 Heart Protection Study (HPS).[34] Although other explanations are possible, differences in treatment contamination clearly played a role. The Heart Protection Study, which unlike the Scandinavian Simvastatin Survival Study occurred after statins were in general use, had much higher treatment contamination. This difference alone would account for almost all of the difference between the intention to treat estimates reported in these two trials.

What are the benefits and limitations of CA ITT estimates?
The primary benefit of CA ITT analysis is improved accuracy in estimating the size of treatment benefit for a patient who receives the treatment. Why is this important? The exact effect size of a treatment is relevant whenever you weigh a treatment against negative consequences like side effects, against treatment costs in cost effectiveness analyses, or against another treatment. For example, if many patients stop taking a weight loss drug because of side effects, an intention to treat analysis would measure early treatment side effects appropriately but assess long term weight loss and side effects quite poorly. Patients and clinicians would be better informed by having information on both estimates: the proportion of people who stop the medicine because of side effects; and the degree of weight loss and side effects in patients who continue taking the medication. The comparative effectiveness of two chemotherapeutic regimens with different contamination rates could similarly be misleading to patients and clinicians.[8 32]

In addition, the estimate of benefit in many cost effectiveness analyses is based on the outcome of an intention to treat analysis, but the estimated treatment cost assumes 100% adherence. This disparity will result in underestimation of the treatment's cost effectiveness and will particularly disadvantage effective but costly treatments.

CA ITT analysis of randomised controlled trials has some limitations. Treatment contamination is not always assessed in clinical trials and can be quite difficult to measure, especially in trials of medications for chronic conditions. Partial contamination and adherence can complicate analysis substantially. Most importantly, the CA ITT technique assumes that if non-adherents had received the treatment, the treatment would have had the same medical effect as it did in adherents. If non-adherent or crossover patients exhibit a different treatment benefit from adherents, a CA ITT analysis will be biased. This issue increases the need to accurately assess heterogeneity of treatment effect among adherents.[35] However, although the assumptions of CA ITT can potentially be violated, the assumptions are more reasonable than those of standard intention to treat analysis—that patients who cross over to active treatment get no benefit and those who fail to receive an assigned intervention benefit as though they did receive it.

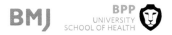

Advanced IV analysis

There are more detailed IV adjustment techniques than the CA ITT technique described here that can account for complicating factors such as partial contamination (for example, partial medication adherence or early dropout),[29] [36] time dependent contamination (such as in surgery trials where control group participants have surgery late in the study),[29] participants lost to follow-up,[37] and non-adherence in randomised equivalency studies (that is, comparing two active treatment arms).[26] These techniques, although sometimes significantly more complicated than CA ITT, have a strong theoretical basis and can substantially improve the reliability of results.

Conclusion

Randomised controlled trials in which no control participants cross over to active treatment and all those randomised to active treatment tolerate and adhere to their assigned treatment do not need to be analysed using CA ITT. However, trials do not often proceed like this and are unlikely to do so more often in the future, so an intention to treat analysis will rarely provide an accurate estimate of treatment benefits for those receiving a treatment.

In major trials, efforts should be taken to limit and quantify treatment contamination with close follow-up of study participants, surveys to assess and optimise adherence, and use of intermediate measures of adherence and effectiveness (such as following change in low density lipoprotein in cholesterol trials that are powered for survival). However, contamination is not always just a nuisance factor—it can demonstrate important factors such as how well patients tolerate treatment side effects.

Once deviations from random assignments occur, regardless of the reason, scientists running trials should examine how treatment contamination has affected their results. Although traditional intention to treat analysis (that is, the effect of recommending the treatment to study participants) should still be used for the primary analysis of a randomised controlled trial, the CA ITT approach is also important because it better estimates the efficacy of the treatment in patients who actually receive it.

The authors thank Michelle Heisler, David Kent, and Joshua Angrist for comments on earlier versions of this work.

Contributors: RAH conceived of the idea for this article and was involved in every stage of writing and editing. JBS was involved in all stages of research review, writing, and editing. Both authors act as guarantors.

Funding: This work was supported in part by the Robert Wood Johnson Clinical Scholars Program, the Department of Veteran Affairs Cooperative Studies Program (CSP #465 FS), and the Measurement Core of the Michigan Diabetes Research & Training Center (NIDDK of The National Institutes of Health [P60 DK-20572]). None of the funders had any role in the design or conduct of the study; collection, management, analysis, or interpretation of the data; or preparation, review, or approval of the manuscript.

Competing interests: Both authors have completed the Unified Competing Interest form at www.icmje.org/coi_disclosure.pdf (available on request from the corresponding author) and declare: (1) No financial support for the submitted work from anyone other than their employer; (2) No financial relationships with commercial entities that might have an interest in the submitted work; (3) No spouses, partners, or children with relationships with commercial entities that might have an interest in the submitted work; (4) No non-financial interests that may be relevant to the submitted work.

Provenance and peer review: Not commissioned; externally peer reviewed.

1   Schroder FH, Hugosson J, Roobol MJ, Tammela TL, Ciatto S, Nelen V, et al. Screening and prostate-cancer mortality in a randomized European study. *N Engl J Med* 2009;360:1320-8.

2   Andriole GL, Crawford ED, Grubb RL 3rd, Buys SS, Chia D, Church TR, et al. Mortality results from a randomized prostate-cancer screening trial. *N Engl J Med* 2009;360:1310-9.

3   Calverley PM, Anderson JA, Celli B, Ferguson GT, Jenkins C, Jones PW, et al. Salmeterol and fluticasone propionate and survival in chronic obstructive pulmonary disease. *N Engl J Med* 2007;356:775-89.

4   Weinstein JN, Lurie JD, Tosteson TD, Hanscom B, Tosteson AN, Blood EA, et al. Surgical versus nonsurgical treatment for lumbar degenerative spondylolisthesis. *N Engl J Med* 2007;356:2257-70.

5   Packer M, Fowler MB, Roecker EB, Coats AJ, Katus HA, Krum H, et al. Effect of carvedilol on the morbidity of patients with severe chronic heart failure: results of the carvedilol prospective randomized cumulative survival (COPERNICUS) study. *Circulation* 2002;106:2194-9.

6   Jackson RD, LaCroix AZ, Gass M, Wallace RB, Robbins J, Lewis CE, et al. Calcium plus vitamin D supplementation and the risk of fractures. *N Engl J Med* 2006;354:669-83.

7   Rubin DR. Inference and missing data. *Biometrika* 1976;63:581-92.

8   Cuzick J, Edwards R, Segnan N. Adjusting for non-compliance and contamination in randomized clinical trials. *Stat Med* 1997;16:1017-29.

9   Dunn G. Estimating the causal effects of treatment. *Epidemiol Psychiatr Soc* 2002;11:206-15.

10 Dunn G, Maracy M, Tomenson B. Estimating treatment effects from randomized clinical trials with noncompliance and loss to follow-up: the role of instrumental variable methods. *Stat Methods Med Res* 2005;14:369-95.

11 Simpson SH, Eurich DT, Majumdar SR, Padwal RS, Tsuyuki RT, Varney J, et al. A meta-analysis of the association between adherence to drug therapy and mortality. *BMJ* 2006;333:15.

12 Granger BB, Swedberg K, Ekman I, Granger CB, Olofsson B, McMurray JJ, et al. Adherence to candesartan and placebo and outcomes in chronic heart failure in the CHARM programme: double-blind, randomised, controlled clinical trial. *Lancet* 2005;366:2005-11.

13 Schiffner R, Schiffner-Rohe J, Gerstenhauer M, Hofstadter F, Landthaler M, Stolz W. Differences in efficacy between intention-to-treat and per-protocol analyses for patients with psoriasis vulgaris and atopic dermatitis: clinical and pharmacoeconomic implications. *Br J Dermatol* 2001;144:1154-60.

14 Altman DG. Better reporting of randomised controlled trials: the CONSORT statement. *BMJ* 1996;313:570-1.

15 Straus SE. *Evidence-based medicine: how to practise and teach EBM* . 3rd ed. Elsevier/Churchill Livingstone, 2005.

16 Evans WN, Ringel JS. Can higher cigarette taxes improve birth outcomes? *J Public Econ* 1999;72:135-54.

17 McClellan M, McNeil BJ, Newhouse JP. Does more intensive treatment of acute myocardial infarction in the elderly reduce mortality? Analysis using instrumental variables. *JAMA* 1994;272:859-66.

18 Schneeweiss S, Seeger JD, Landon J, Walker AM. Aprotinin during coronary-artery bypass grafting and risk of death. *N Engl J Med* 2008;358:771-83.

19 Schneeweiss S, Setoguchi S, Brookhart A, Dormuth C, Wang PS. Risk of death associated with the use of conventional versus atypical antipsychotic drugs among elderly patients. *CMAJ* 2007;176:627-32.

20 Hearst N, Newman TB, Hulley SB. Delayed effects of the military draft on mortality. A randomized natural experiment. *N Engl J Med* 1986;314:620-4.

21 Cole JA, Norman H, Weatherby LB, Walker AM. Drug copayment and adherence in chronic heart failure: effect on cost and outcomes. *Pharmacotherapy* 2006;26:1157-64.

22 Sheehan NA, Didelez V, Burton PR, Tobin MD. Mendelian randomisation and causal inference in observational epidemiology. *PLoS Med* 2008;5:e177.

23 Angrist JD, Imbens GW, Rubin DR. Identification of causal effects using instrumental variables. *J Am Stat Assoc* 1996;91:444-55.

24 Greenland S. An introduction to instrumental variables for epidemiologists. *Int J Epidemiol* 2000;29:722-9.

25 Glasziou PP. Meta-analysis adjusting for compliance: the example of screening for breast cancer. *J Clin Epidemiol* 1992;45:1251-6.

26 Walter SD, Guyatt G, Montori VM, Cook R, Prasad K. A new preference-based analysis for randomized trials can estimate treatment acceptability and effect in compliant patients. *J Clin Epidemiol* 2006;59:685-96.

27 Bang H, Davis CE. On estimating treatment effects under non-compliance in randomized clinical trials: are intent-to-treat or instrumental variables analyses perfect solutions? *Stat Med* 2007;26:954-64.

28 Mealli F, Imbens GW, Ferro S, Biggeri A. Analyzing a randomized trial on breast self-examination with noncompliance and missing outcomes. *Biostatistics* 2004;5:207-22.

29 Bond SJ, White IR, Sarah Walker A. Instrumental variables and interactions in the causal analysis of a complex clinical trial. *Stat Med* 2007;26:1473-96.

30 Eisenberg D, Quinn BC. Estimating the effect of smoking cessation on weight gain: an instrumental variable approach. *Health Serv Res* 2006;41:2255-66.

31 Sommer A, Zeger SL. On estimating efficacy from clinical trials. *Stat Med* 1991;10:45-52.

32 Hewitson P, Glasziou P, Watson E, Towler B, Irwig L. Cochrane systematic review of colorectal cancer screening using the fecal occult blood test (hemoccult): an update. *Am J Gastroenterol* 2008;103:1541-9.

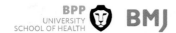

33 Randomised trial of cholesterol lowering in 4444 patients with coronary heart disease: the Scandinavian Simvastatin Survival Study (4S). *Lancet* 1994;344:1383-9.

34 Heart Protection Study Collaborative Group. MRC/BHF Heart Protection Study of cholesterol lowering with simvastatin in 20,536 high-risk individuals: a randomised placebo-controlled trial. *Lancet* 2002;360:7-22.

35 Basu A, Heckman JJ, Navarro-Lozano S, Urzua S. Use of instrumental variables in the presence of heterogeneity and self-selection: an application to treatments of breast cancer patients. *Health Econ* 2007;16:1133-57.

36 Sato T. A method for the analysis of repeated binary outcomes in randomized clinical trials with non-compliance. *Stat Med* 2001;20:2761-74.

37 Greenland S, Lanes S, Jara M. Estimating effects from randomized trials with discontinuations: the need for intent-to-treat design and G-estimation. *Clin Trials* 2008;5:5-13.

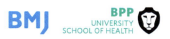

Random measurement error and regression dilution bias

Jennifer A Hutcheon, postdoctoral fellow[1], Arnaud Chiolero, doctoral candidate, fellow in public health[2][3], James A Hanley, professor of biostatistics[2]

[1]Department of Obstetrics & Gynaecology, University of British Columbia, Vancouver, Canada

[2]Department of Epidemiology, Biostatistics, and Occupational Health, McGill University, Purvis Hall, 1020 Avenue des Pins Ouest, Montreal QC, Canada H3A 1A2

[3]Institute of Social and Preventive Medicine (IUMSP), University Hospital Centre and University of Lausanne, Lausanne, Switzerland

Correspondence to: J A Hanley james.hanley@mcgill.ca

Cite this as: BMJ 2010;340:c2289

DOI: 10.1136/bmj.c2289

http://www.bmj.com/content/340/bmj.c2289

ABSTRACT

Random measurement error is a pervasive problem in medical research, which can introduce bias to an estimate of the association between a risk factor and a disease or make a true association statistically non-significant. Hutcheon and colleagues explain when, why, and how random measurement error introduces bias and provides strategies for researchers to minimise the problem

Introduction

Random measurement error is a pervasive problem in medical research and clinical practice.[1] It occurs when measurements fluctuate unpredictably around their true values and is caused by imprecise measurement tools or true biological variability, or both. For instance, when blood pressure is assessed with a sphygmomanometer, random error may arise from imprecise measurement due to rounding error or from true diurnal or day to day variation in pressure.[2][3] Hence, a blood pressure reading obtained at a single occasion may differ by an unpredictable (random) amount from an individual's usual blood pressure.[3]

Random measurement error differs from systematic measurement error.[4] Systematic error occurs when the measurement error, after multiple measurements, does not average out to zero. The measurements are consistently wrong in a particular direction—for example, they tend to be higher than the true values. In the case of blood pressure measurement, systematic error may be due to improper calibration of the sphygmomanometer or improper arm cuff size, and averaging multiple blood pressure measurements will not help estimate true blood pressure.

While the impact of systematic error is generally well appreciated by researchers and addressed in epidemiological and clinical studies, the impact of random measurement error is often less well appreciated. Since the total error in a variable with random measurement error averages out to zero, many people assume that the effects of random measurement error on the estimate of the association between an exposure (risk factor) and an outcome (disease) obtained from a regression model will also cancel out (that is, have no effect on the estimate).

Others have observed that random measurement error can bias the regression slope coefficient downwards towards the null, a phenomenon known as attenuation or regression dilution bias.[5][6][7]

In reality, the estimate of the association between an exposure and an outcome is attenuated by random measurement error in some situations but remain unchanged in others. In this article we use a simple example to show when, to what extent, and why random measurement error affects the estimates produced by regression models to assess the association between two variables. In particular, we describe how the effect of random measurement differs depending on whether the measurement error is in the exposure or outcome variable. We also make recommendations for dealing with random measurement error in the design and analysis of studies.

Example

For illustrative purposes, we consider the simplistic case of a study conducted in four hypothetical individuals. The aim of this study is to assess the association between the exposure variable systolic blood pressure and the outcome variable left ventricular mass index (LVMI).[8] It is well known that elevated blood pressure is associated with a large LVMI.[8] Imagine that both variables are measured without measurement error and are perfectly correlated, so that all four observations fall along the regression line. The regression slope, or coefficient (β), is 1.00 g/m²/mm Hg (see appendix on bmj.com for the detailed calculation). In other words, for every 1 mm Hg difference in systolic blood pressure, LVMI is an average of 1 g/m² higher. The table shows the systolic blood pressure and LVMI values measured for each individual, with no errors (section a) and with random errors in the exposure and outcome variables (sections b and c). Figure 1 shows the relation between exposure and outcome variable in diagrammatic form.

Random measurement error in the exposure (X) variable
Suppose that systolic blood pressure was measured with random errors of ±10 or ±20 mm Hg (see values in section b of table). The regression slopes estimating the association between systolic blood pressure and LVMI flatten with increasing measurement error (fig 1, panel b). As measurement error in systolic blood pressure increases, the observations become spread further apart on the X axis. While the systolic blood pressure values without measurement error range from 120 to 160 mm Hg, the horizontal range (along the X axis) increases to 100-170 mmHg with ±20 mm Hg error. The vertical range of the observations (along the Y axis), however, remains constant. Since the regression line is fitted by minimising the vertical distance between observations and their predicted values, the best fit line becomes increasingly flattened ("stretched out") in order to accommodate the increased horizontal spread of the observations. The slope β decreases from 1.00 to 0.71 g/m²/mm Hg with ±10 mm Hg random error, and to 0.38 g/m²/mm Hg with ±20 mm Hg random error.

SUMMARY POINTS

- The bias introduced by random measurement error will be different depending on whether the error is in an exposure variable (risk factor) or outcome variable (disease)
- Random measurement error in an exposure variable will bias the estimates of regression slope coefficients towards the null
- Random measurement error in an outcome variable will instead increase the standard error of the estimates and widen the corresponding confidence intervals, making results less likely to be statistically significant
- Increasing sample size will help minimise the impact of measurement error in an outcome variable but will only make estimates more precisely wrong when the error is in an exposure variable

In an extreme case, the spread of observations along the X axis could become so large that the estimate of the best-fit regression line would be virtually flat, resulting in a complete attenuation of the association between systolic blood pressure and LVMI.

The extent of the bias in the estimate of the error-prone regression slope (β^*) for a variable measured with random error (X^*) is quantified in fig 2.

The ratio of variation in error-free (true) X values to the variation in the observed error-prone (observed) values is known as the reliability coefficient, attenuation factor, or intra-class correlation. Because the variation in observed values is greater than the variation in error-free values due to random error, the ratio variation(X)/variation(X^*) will be lower than 1, and the new estimate of the coefficient β^*

will be reduced in proportion, a typical case of regression dilution bias.

In practice, the use of an exposure variable (X) measured with random error results in underestimating (or even missing altogether) an association. A well known example is the underestimation of the association between usual blood pressure and the risk of cardiovascular disease.[6] Blood pressure is most often estimated based on a limited number of readings (for example, office measurements), which leads to an imperfect approximation of usual blood pressure. The presence of random measurement error in estimates of usual blood pressure may underestimate the relative risk of cardiovascular disease due to elevated blood pressure by up to 60%.[6] It explains, at least in part, why risk of cardiovascular disease is more strongly associated with blood pressure estimates using 24 hour, ambulatory blood pressure measurements (based on numerous readings, hence with less random error) than office blood pressure (based on fewer readings).[3]

Measurement error in the outcome (Y) variable
What if the exposure variable, systolic blood pressure, was measured without error, but the outcome variable, LVMI, had random measurement error? Would a similar attenuation of the estimated regression coefficient be seen?

Suppose that LVMI (Y) was measured with a random error of ±10 g/m² or ±20 g/m² (values in section c of the table). When these error-prone LVMI values are regressed on systolic blood pressure, we see that the vertical distance (along the Y axis) between each observation and the regression line increases (panel c of fig 1). However, although the total vertical distance between each observation and the regression line is increased, the slope of the line that is able to minimise these distances is identical. As a result, no attenuation of the estimate of the regression coefficient occurs, and it remains constant at β=1.00 g/m²/mm Hg. The increased vertical distance between observed and predicted values is reflected instead in the increased standard errors around the estimate for β, which increase from 0 with no measurement error to 0.45 with ±10 g/m² error and to 0.89 with ±20 g/m² error.

Why does the slope not flatten in this situation?
The equation for a regression model with no error can be expressed as $Y = \beta_0 + \beta X + \varepsilon$ (equation 1), where the error term ε represents the variability in Y that is not explained by the model's exposure variable (X).

When Y is measured with error, Y is replaced in equation 1 with the observed (error-prone) variable Y^*, which is equal to Y + random error. It can be shown that rearranging terms yields $Y^* = \beta_0 + \beta X + \varepsilon + $ random error (equation 2). The random measurement error is simply added to the existing error term (ε) and, as a result, increases the total amount of unexplained variance in the regression model. The standard error for the estimate of β is therefore increased, with a correspondingly wider confidence interval. If a confidence interval is widened enough to include zero (for example, an estimate of the slope of 0.4, but with a 95% confidence interval from −0.1 to 0.9), the exposure would no longer be considered a statistically significant risk factor for the outcome of interest. The estimate of the regression coefficient β, however, is not affected.

In practice, although the regression coefficient itself will be unbiased when there is random measurement error in the outcome variable, the increased standard error

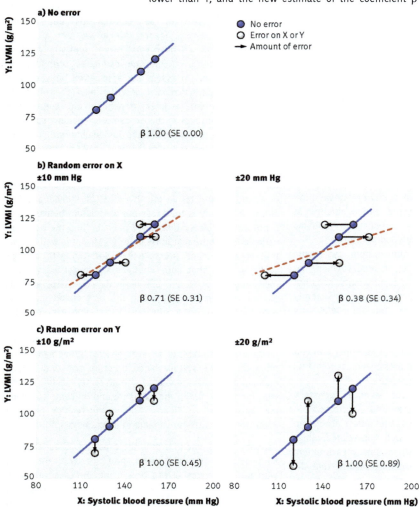

Fig 1 Effect of random measurement error on relation between systolic blood pressure (exposure) and left ventricular mass index (LVMI) (outcome). With no random measurement error (panel a), the slope (β) of the line describes the error-free association between blood pressure (X) and LVMI (Y); when blood pressure is measured with a random error of ±10 or ±20 mm Hg (panel b), there is attenuation of the slope; when LVMI is measured with a random error of ±10 or ±20 g/m² (panel c), there is increase in variability but no change in slope

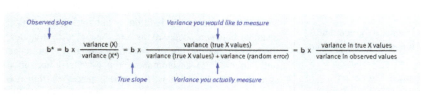

Fig 2 Degree of bias in a regression slope in the presence of random measurement error in the exposure variable (X)

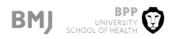

- **Random measurement error**—This occurs when the recorded values of a study variable fluctuate randomly around the true values, such that some recorded values will be higher than the true values and other recorded values will be lower
- **Linear regression model**—Statistical model used to evaluate the relation between one or more exposure variables and an outcome that is measured on a continuous scale (such as weight, blood glucose concentration, or bone mineral density). The linear relation between an exposure (X) and outcome (Y) is described by the regression equation $E(Y) = \beta_0 + \beta_1 X$, where $E(Y)$ is the expected (average) value of the variable Y, β_0 is the intercept (the average value of the outcome Y when the exposure X has a value of zero), and β_1 is the slope of the line
- **Regression slope**—The slope of the line between an exposure and outcome variable in a linear regression model. It provides an estimate of the association between an exposure and outcome variable. For instance, a slope estimate of 2 would mean that for every 1 unit difference in the exposure (X) variable, the outcome (Y) variable would be, on average, higher by 2 units. The estimate of the regression slope is also referred to as the "beta coefficient estimate" or "slope coefficient estimate"
- **Regression dilution bias**—A statistical phenomenon whereby random measurement error in the values of an exposure variable (X) causes an attenuation or "flattening" of the slope of the line describing the relation between the exposure (X) and an outcome (Y) of interest

could result in an association being overlooked because of lack of statistical significance. In essence, random measurement error in the outcome variable (Y) makes a study underpowered to detect a true effect of an exposure.

For example, ultrasound estimates of fetal weight are prone to a large degree of random measurement error (±10-15%).[9] This error reduces the value of the estimated fetal weight in making appropriate clinical decisions, such as the timing of delivery for macrosomia. It could also influence conclusions of studies aimed at understanding determinants of fetal growth. If a researcher assesses the effects of maternal stress on fetal growth by estimating the relation between maternal cortisol levels (X) and fetal weight (Y),[10] the 95% confidence intervals associated with the estimate of the slope β of the relation between the two variables will be widened due to the measurement error in estimated fetal weight. If the confidence interval is widened enough to include zero, the researcher would conclude that the association between maternal cortisol and fetal weight is not statistically significant, irrespective of the value of the slope itself.

Spirometry readings are another type of measurement prone to substantial random error, which is introduced by imprecise equipment, variability in technician skill, and participant behaviour.[11] Consequently, confidence intervals around the estimated slope would also be widened in studies assessing determinants of respiratory status if the outcome is measured using spirometry.

In summary, the impact of random measurement error will be different depending on whether the error is in the exposure (X) or the outcome (Y) variable:

- Random measurement error in the exposure variable (X) will bias the regression coefficient (slope) towards the null (regression dilution bias, attenuation)
- Random measurement error in the outcome variable (Y) will have minimal effect on the regression coefficient, but will decrease the precision of the estimate (that is, increase the standard error).

The impact of random measurement error on measures of association is not restricted to cases where the outcome of interest is a continuous variable; it also occurs when the outcome of interest is a binary variable (such as disease versus no disease) or a survival time. For example, using home blood pressure measurements as the exposure (X), the hazard ratio for cardiovascular diseases (the outcome Y) was 1.020/unit of mm Hg based one measurement versus 1.035/unit of mm Hg based on the average of eight measurements.[12] Of note, if correlation is used to assess an association between two variables, the correlation coefficient will be reduced if random error occurs either in X or in Y.

Additional bias beyond the effects of random measurement error can be introduced if the degree of random error differs according to case or control status (or exposed v unexposed status). The impact of this "differential" measurement error, and strategies to minimise it, are described elsewhere.[13] For a comprehensive treatment of measurement error, including what to do if there is measurement error in confounder variables, we recommend the textbook of Carroll et al.[14]

Recommendations for researchers

The best strategy for dealing with random measurement error is to minimise it in the first place at the study design stage, either by investing in instruments capable of more precise measurements or obtaining repeated measurements from an individual to better estimate the true values.

With random measurement error in the exposure (X) variable, increasing the sample size will not minimise the bias from random error. Increasing the sample size will only make the estimates more precisely wrong.

If estimates of the extent of measurement error can be obtained from internal validation studies or the literature[15] (using the reliability coefficient R), the regression coefficients can be corrected for the expected downward bias. Several authors have reviewed different statistical approaches to correct biased regression coefficients.[16][17][18] However, these approaches rely on assumptions that may often not be met and are difficult to verify.[19] The heated debate over the validity of "de-attenuated" estimates of the association between 24 hour sodium excretion in urine and blood pressure in the Intersalt study in the *BMJ*,[20][21][22][23][24] for example, serves to underline the limitations of addressing measurement error in the analysis stage of a study. Correction for regression dilution bias requires a clear understanding of not only the extent of the random error but also the degree to which the error may be correlated with error in other variables. Any correlation in the errors, as was argued might occur between 24 hour sodium excretion and blood pressure, would produce highly inflated estimates of the association between sodium and blood pressure. These corrections for regression dilution bias may be better used for exploratory or sensitivity analyses.

If the outcome (Y) variable is prone to random measurement error, researchers should increase either the sample size or the number of measurements taken per subject to account for the increased standard error of the coefficient estimate. This increase will compensate for the precision lost as a result of random error.

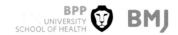

Values of exposure variable systolic blood pressure and outcome variable left ventricular mass index (LVMI) with different degrees of random measurement error

Random measurement error	Systolic blood pressure (mm Hg)	LVMI (g/m²)
a) No error in exposure or outcome variable		
	120	80
	130	90
	150	110
	160	120
b) Random error in exposure variable (X)		
Error of ±10 mm Hg	110	80
	140	90
	160	110
	150	120
Error of ±20 mm Hg	100	80
	150	90
	170	110
	140	120
c) Random error in outcome variable (Y)		
Error of ±10 g/m²	120	70
	130	100
	150	120
	160	110
Error of ±20 g/m²	120	60
	130	110
	150	130
	160	100

The increase in number of subjects required can be estimated by the formula n/R, where n is the sample size required if no measurement error exists and R is the reliability coefficient. For example, if a sample size of 100 patients is required with error-free measurements, the use of error-prone measurements with a reliability coefficient of $R = 0.6$ would increase the number of patients required to detect the same effect to $n/R = 100/0.6 = 167$ patients.[25] For cases where increasing the number of measurements per patient is preferable to increasing the number of patients, the Spearman-Brown formula for stepped up reliability can be used to estimate the number of repeated measurements per subject required to achieve a desired level of precision.[26] [27] [28]

Contributors: All authors contributed to the conception and drafting of the manuscript and approved the final version of the manuscript for publication. Table and figures were produced by AC. JAHutcheon is guarantor for the article.

Details of funding: JAHutcheon was supported by a doctoral research award from the Canadian Institutes of Health Research. AC was supported by a grant from the Swiss National Science Foundation (PASMA-115691/1) and by a grant from the Canadian Institutes of Health Research. JAHanley was supported by the Natural Sciences and Engineering Research Council of Canada and the Fonds québécois de la recherche sur la nature et les technologies. The work in this study was independent of funders.

Competing interests: All authors have completed the Unified Competing Interest form at www.icmeje.org/coi_disclosure.pdf (available on request from the corresponding author) and declare that (1) none of the authors has support from any companies for the submitted work; (2) none of the authors has relationships with any company that might have an interest in the submitted work in the previous 3 years; (3) their spouses, partners, or children have no financial relationships that may be relevant to the submitted work; and (4) none of the authors has any non-financial interests that may be relevant to the submitted work.

1 Bland JM, Altman DG. Measurement error. *BMJ* 1996;313:744.
2 Rose G. Standardisation of observers in blood pressure measurement. *Lancet* 1965;285:673-4.
3 Pickering TG, Shimbo D, Haas D. Ambulatory blood-pressure monitoring. *N Engl J Med* 2006;354:2368-74.
4 Last JM, ed. *A dictionary of epidemiology* . 4th ed. Oxford University Press, 2001.
5 Spearman C. The proof and measurement of association between two things. *Am J Psychol* 1904;15:72-101.
6 MacMahon S, Peto R, Cutler J, Collins R, Sorlie P, Neaton J, et al. Blood pressure, stroke, and coronary heart disease. Part 1, prolonged differences in blood pressure: prospective observational studies corrected for the regression dilution bias. *Lancet* 1990;335:765-74.
7 Liu K. Measurement error and its impact on partial correlation and multiple linear regression analyses. *Am J Epidemiol* 1988;127:864-74.
8 Den Hond E, Staessen JA, on behalf of the APTH THOP investigators. Relation between left ventricular mass and systolic blood pressure at baseline in the APTH and THOP trials. *Blood Press Monit* 2003;8:173-5.
9 Dudley NJ. A systematic review of the ultrasound estimation of fetal weight. *Ultrasound Obstet Gynecol* 2005;25:80-9.
10 Diego MA, Jones NA, Field T, Hernandez-Reif M, Schanberg S, Kuhn C, et al. Maternal psychological distress, prenatal cortisol, and fetal weight. *Psychosom Med* 2006;68:747-53.
11 Miller MR, Hankinson J, Brusasco V, Burgos F, Casaburi R, Coates A, et al. Standardisation of spirometry. *Eur Respir J* 2005;26:319-38.
12 Stergiou GS, Parati G. How to best monitor blood pressure at home? Assessing numbers and individual patients. *J Hypertens* 2010;28:226-8.
13 Greenland S, Lash TL. Bias analysis. In: Rothman KJ, Greenland S, Lash TL, eds. *Modern epidemiology* . 3rd ed. Lippincott, Williams & Wilkins, 2008:345-80.
14 Carroll RJ, Ruppert D, Stefanski LA. *Measurement error in nonlinear models* . Chapman and Hall/CRC Press, 1995.
15 Whitlock G, Clarke T, Vander Hoorn S, Rodgers A, Jackson R, Norton R, et al. Random errors in the measurement of 10 cardiovascular risk factors. *Eur J Epidemiol* 2001;17:907-9.
16 Knuiman MW, Divitini ML, Buzas JS, Fitzgerald PEB. Adjustment for regression dilution in epidemiological regression analyses. *Ann Epidemiol* 1998;8:56-63.
17 Rosner B, Speigelman D, Willett WC. Correction of logistic regression relative risk estimates and confidence intervals for random within-person measurement error. *Am J Epidemiol* 1992;136:1400-13.
18 Andersen PK, Liestol K. Attenuation caused by infrequently updated covariates in survival analysis. *Biostatistics* 2003;4:633-49.
19 Frost C, White IR. The effect of measurement error in risk factors that change over time in cohort studies: do simple methods overcorrect for "regression dilution"? *Int J Epidemiol* 2005;34:1359-68.
20 Elliott P, Stamler J, Nichols R, Dyer AR, Stamler R, Kesteloot H, et al, for the Intersalt Cooperative Research Group. Intersalt revisited: further analyses of 24 hour sodium excretion and blood pressure within and across populations. *BMJ* 1996;312:1249-53.
21 Dyer AR, Elliott P, Marmot M, Kesteloot H, Stamler R, Stamler J, for the Intersalt Steering and Editorial Committee. Strength and importance of the relation of dietary salt to blood pressure. *BMJ* 1996;312:1661-4.
22 Davey Smith G, Phillips AN. Inflation in epidemiology: "The proof and measurement of association between two things" revisited. *BMJ* 1996;312:1659-64.
23 Day NE. Epidemiological studies should be designed to reduce correction needed for measurement error to a minimum. *BMJ* 1997;315:484.
24 Davey Smith G, Phillips AN. Correction for regression dilution bias in Intersalt study was misleading. *BMJ* 1997;315:484.
25 Fitzmaurice G. Measurement error and reliability. *Nutrition* 2002;18:112-4.
26 Perkins DO, Wyatt RJ, Bartko JJ. Penny-wise and pound-foolish: the impact of measurement error on sample size requirements in clinical trials. *Biol Psychiatry* 2000;47:762-6.
27 Spearman C. Correlation calculated from faulty data. *Br J Psychol* 1910;3:271-95.
28 Brown W. Some experimental results in the correlation of mental abilities. *Br J Psychol* 1910;3:296-322.

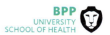

The double jeopardy of clustered measurement and cluster randomisation

Michael S Kramer, professor[1][2], Richard M Martin, professor[3][4], Jonathan A C Sterne, professor[3], Stanley Shapiro, professor[2], Mourad Dahhou, statistician[1], Robert W Platt, associate professor[1][2]

epartment of Pediatrics, McGill
niversity Faculty of Medicine,
ontreal, Canada

epartment of Epidemiology and
ostatistics, McGill University
aculty of Medicine

epartment of Social Medicine,
niversity of Bristol, Bristol

MRC Centre for Causal Analysis,
niversity of Bristol

orrespondence to: M S Kramer,
ontreal Children's Hospital, 2300
pper Street (Les Tourelles),
ontreal, Quebec H3H 1P3 michael.
amer@mcgill.ca

te this as: BMJ 2009;339:b2900

OI: 10.1136/bmj.b2900

ttp://www.bmj.com/content/339/
mj.b2900

ABSTRACT

Michael S Kramer and colleagues suggest that double clustering might explain the negative results of some cluster randomised trials and describe some strategies for avoiding the problem

Cluster randomised trials have become popular for evaluating health service and public health interventions. The clusters are groups of individuals, such as families, schools, clinics, hospitals, or entire communities. Cluster randomised trials provide the rigours of randomisation, while reducing treatment "contamination"; contact between subjects randomised to two (or more) interventions may expose them to both interventions and thus reduce differences in outcome between the groups.[1][2] In addition, cluster randomisation is often more feasible than individual randomisation because group dynamics can make it easier to change practices or behaviours within an overall group than to change practices or behaviours among individuals within the same group.

But cluster randomisation also has some disadvantages. Primary among these is reduced statistical power due to within cluster correlation of outcomes. In other words, individuals within the same cluster are more likely to experience the same study outcome than those in other clusters, irrespective of treatment allocation. This within cluster correlation is usually assessed with the intraclass correlation coefficient (ICC). This coefficient is a measure of how much more similar the values of an outcome are within the same cluster than among different clusters randomised to the same treatment. It is formally defined as the ratio of the between cluster variance to the total variance. If all variation within each treatment group is "explained" by differences within clusters, and no variation is observed between clusters (that is, in the absence of clustering), the ICC=0.[3] Statistical power depends on the degree of clustering; the larger the ICC, the greater the reduction in statistical power. If ICC=0, a cluster randomised trial has the same statistical power as an individually randomised trial with the same number of participants; if ICC=1, the power is reduced to that of an individually randomised trial in which the sample size is equal to the number of clusters.

A second disadvantage of cluster randomisation can occur if the number of clusters is small. Despite proper randomisation, imbalance can occur in potentially confounding baseline factors that differ by chance across clusters. Such imbalance may require multivariable statistical adjustment, but adjustment cannot remove imbalance in factors that are unmeasured or imprecisely measured.

Although the advantages and limitations of cluster randomised trials are now well known, the consequences of clustered measurement have received far less attention. Observer level clustering of outcomes in individually randomised trials has been discussed,[4] but we recently encountered the "double jeopardy" that arises when clustered measurement occurs in cluster randomised trials. This problem, which we discuss below, deserves wider recognition by trialists and clinicians participating in the design, conduct, and interpretation of cluster randomised trials.

Clustered measurement

In many studies, including both experimental (randomised) and observational studies, measurement of the outcome is naturally clustered. Measurement can be clustered because of either the observer (the person who measures the outcome) or the measuring instrument. The number of observers is often far lower than the number of participants in the study. For measurements susceptible to systematic (non-random) error, clustering among study participants measured by the same observer will occur if some observers tend to measure systematically higher or lower values than other observers, irrespective of the true value of the measurement. Such clustered measurement will lead to intracluster correlation, but the cluster is now defined as the group of individuals whose outcome is measured by the same observer.[4] This type of clustered measurement can also occur when several unstandardised measuring instruments are used for different participants, even with the same observer—for example, use of several inadequately calibrated sphygmomanometers for measuring blood pressure.

Combined clustering: "double jeopardy"

Clustered measurement can occur in any type of study. When measurements are clustered within the same groupings that serve as the units for cluster randomisation, however, a pernicious problem arises: the variation due to clustered measurement becomes inseparable from that due to clustered randomisation. Examples include a single teacher who obtains outcome measurements in a school where the school is the unit of randomisation or a clinician who is responsible for measuring outcome in a practice, clinic, or hospital where those sites are the units of randomisation. The conflation of clustered measurement with cluster randomisation can greatly increase the

SUMMARY POINTS

- Clustered measurement occurring in cluster randomised trials will reduce the precision of the results
- Random allocation of observers or a single observer will avoid clustered measurement but may be impossible for large, geographically dispersed clusters
- All studies should use standardised measurement techniques and ensure adequate training of observers
- Pilot studies and monitoring of initial data can identify difficulties in outcome measurement
- Despite these steps some systematic measurement differences may remain

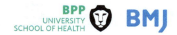

intraclass correlation and hence reduce statistical power. If the number of clusters is small, double clustering can also inflate or deflate true treatment differences if systematically higher measurements occur more frequently by chance in one treatment group than in the other.

Recent example

To show how measurement error and clustering can affect the precision of treatment effects in cluster randomised trials, we review our recent experience with the Promotion of Breastfeeding Intervention Trial, a cluster randomised trial of a breastfeeding promotion intervention carried out in the Republic of Belarus.[5] The units of randomisation were maternity hospitals and one affiliated polyclinic (outpatient clinic) per maternity hospital. These hospitals and clinics were spread across the country. The initial period of follow-up was for 12 months, with a subsequent follow-up at age 6.5 years for 13 889 (81.5%) of the 17 046 children originally randomised. The effects of the intervention on the 6.5 year outcomes have been reported.[6 7 8 9 10]

Here, we contrast the results we obtained for three of these outcomes: body mass index (weight (kg)/(height (m)^2), triceps skinfold thickness, and verbal IQ score. The paediatricians were trained to measure all outcomes at a week long training session on a sample of school aged children living in a residential facility near Minsk. Each participating paediatrician was also given a training video (for the anthropometric measures) and detailed written instructions in Russian.[8] All anthropometric measurements were obtained in duplicate and averaged. Standard administration and scoring of the Wechsler Abbreviated Scale of Intelligence test was demonstrated by, and practised under the supervision of local child psychologists and psychiatrists with experience in IQ testing in children; during the training session, high interpaediatrician agreement was achieved on repeat testing of the same children.[10]

The figure shows the (crude) means of the three outcomes for each of the 31 clusters (polyclinics), in ascending order. The 31 means range from 14.7 to 16.2 for body mass index, 4.3 to 14.4 mm for triceps skinfold thickness, and 82 to 130 points for verbal IQ. The digital read out weight scale is the least susceptible to between clinic differences, and adequate attention to positioning the child and placing the horizontal stadiometer bar on the child's head can minimise systematic errors in measuring height. These features of measurement explain why mean body mass index does not vary greatly by polyclinic.

In contrast, the ranges in means for triceps skinfold thickness and verbal IQ were too wide to be explained by true geographic differences. It is not credible that average triceps skinfold thicknesses in 6.5 year old children would vary 3.5-fold among the 31 polyclinics (especially given the narrow observed range of body mass index) or that true average verbal IQ scores would vary by nearly 50 points. Instead, these differences are likely to reflect systematic measurement differences among the 31 polyclinics. Despite our efforts to standardise measurements across paediatricians and polyclinics, variability in technique for separating subcutaneous fat from muscle (for triceps skinfold thickness) and in acceptance of definitions of words and explanations of similarities between words (for verbal IQ) seems to have led to systematic differences between polyclinics.

The table shows the means in the experimental and control groups and the ICC for the same three outcome

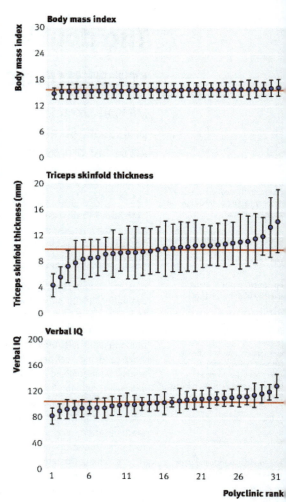

Fig Mean (±1 SD) body mass index (top), triceps skinfold thickness (middle), and verbal IQ (bottom) in 31 participating polyclinics, in ascending order. Red horizontal lines depict the means of the 31 polyclinic means for each outcome.

measurements. The ICC for body mass index was quite low, reflecting the consistency in measurement. The ICCs for triceps skinfold thickness and verbal IQ were both high, reflecting the large differences in means among the 31 polyclinics, although the ICC for triceps skinfold was lower than for verbal IQ because of higher variation within polyclinics; the SD was about 40% of the mean for the triceps skinfold compared with 15% of the mean for verbal IQ. The mean values for body mass index and for triceps skinfold thickness were similar in the experimental and control groups, but because the ICC was much lower for body mass index the 95% confidence interval around the cluster adjusted difference in means was also much narrower. The cluster adjusted difference in mean verbal IQ scores was large (7.5 points higher in the experimental than in the control group), but because the ICC was high, the 95% CI was wide.

The effect of within polyclinic clustering on the precision (width of the confidence interval) of the estimated treatment differences can be shown by carrying out an intention to treat analysis without the cluster adjustment—that is, based on the individual as the unit of analysis. Such an analysis erroneously assumes that ICC=0. The estimated treatment differences are 0.1 (95% confidence interval 0.02 to 0.1) for body mass index (owing to rounding errors, this is larger than the crude difference), −0.1 (−0.2 to 0.1) mm for triceps skinfold thickness, and 10.0 (9.4 to 10.5) for verbal IQ. The

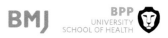

Results of intention to treat analysis for body mass index, triceps skinfold thickness, and verbal IQ at 6.5 year follow-up				
Outcome	Mean (SD) value in experimental group	Mean (SD) value in control group	ICC	Mean (95% CI) cluster adjusted difference
Body mass index	15.6 (1.7)	15.6 (1.7)	0.03	0.1 (−0.2 to 0.3)
Triceps skinfold (mm)	9.9 (4.1)	10.0 (3.6)	0.18	−0.4 (−1.8 to 1.0)
Verbal IQ	108.7 (16.4)	98.7 (16.0)	0.31	7.5 (0.8 to 14.3)

ICC=Intraclass correlation coefficient.

confidence intervals are too narrow, providing overly precise estimates of the treatment effect, because they do not account for the clustered randomisation or measurement.

What can be done to minimise double clustering?

Some of the strategies we suggest for minimising double clustering can and should be incorporated into the design and conduct of all cluster randomised trials. Others, however, may be difficult or impossible to implement because of logistical obstacles.

One strategy is to randomly allocate observers across clusters. Such an approach may not be feasible, however, if observers and trial participants are geographically dispersed, as in our trial. Another potential solution is to use a single observer with proved measurement validity and precision to assess the outcome in all clusters. That approach is analogous to using a single, highly accurate laboratory to analyse blood or other biological samples obtained from multiple study sites. But in trials with large numbers of participants or wide geographical dispersion this may be difficult or impossible to achieve.

A third strategy is to standardise measurement techniques and ensure adequate training of observers. The trial's manual of procedures is an important training tool and reference guide, but for some types of measurement (such as triceps skinfold and verbal IQ in our study), systematic differences across clusters are likely to persist despite these efforts. A pilot study can identify difficulties in outcome measurement before starting the main trial. The pilot study can detect "outlier" observers and attempt to modify their behaviour, but this is unlikely to eliminate systematic differences for some types of measurement. Finally, initial data collection should always be monitored closely to identify observers who may require additional training and instruments that require repair or replacement. We incorporated this approach in our trial, and it should be feasible in all cluster randomised trials. It will, however, add to the costs and logistical difficulties of the trial when the clusters are numerous and geographically dispersed.

Conclusion

Cluster randomisation is a powerful tool for rigorously testing the efficacy of health services and public health interventions. A major problem can occur, however, when outcome measurements are subject to systematic errors that are clustered within the same units that serve as the clusters for randomisation.

We suspect that double clustering may have occurred more often than recognised in the past and could partly explain the negative results of some previous cluster randomised trials. Future CONSORT statements for cluster randomised trials[11] should recommend that reports contain text (or a table) summarising the distributions of the cluster means for each study outcome and describe design features (if any) used to reduce clustered measurement. Investigators should be aware of the potential for double clustering and implement study procedures that minimise its risk.

Contributors: MSK, SS, and RWP contributed to obtaining funding for this project and to the design, analysis, interpretation, and writing or revision of the manuscript. RMM and JACS had major roles in the interpretation of the analysis and in the writing and revision of the manuscript. MD performed the statistical analysis and contributed to its interpretation. MSK is guarantor.

Funding: Supported by a grant from the Canadian Institutes of Health Research. RWP is a career investigator (chercheur-boursier) of the Fonds de la recherche en santé du Québec. RMM was supported by grant number FOOD-DT-2005-007036 from the European Union's project on early nutrition programming: long-term efficacy and safety of trials.

Competing interests: None declared.

Provenance and peer review: Not commissioned; externally peer reviewed.

1   Donner A, Klar N. *Design and analysis of cluster randomisation trials in health research* . London: Arnold, 2000.
2   Ukoumunne OC, Gulliford MC, Chinn S, Sterne JAC, Burney PGJ. Methods for evaluating area-wide and organisation based interventions in health and health care: a systematic review. *Health Technol Assess* 1999;3:iii-92.
3   Kirkwood BR, Sterne JAC. *Essential medical statistics* . 2nd ed. Oxford: Blackwell Science, 2003.
4   Lee KJ, Thompson SG. Clustering by health professional in individually randomised trials. *BMJ* 2005;330:142-4.
5   Kramer MS, Chalmers B, Hodnett ED, Sevkovskaya Z, Dzikovich I, Shapiro S, et al. Promotion of breastfeeding intervention trial (PROBIT): a randomized trial in the Republic of Belarus. *JAMA* 2001;285:413-20.
6   Kramer MS, Matush L, Vanilovich I, Platt RW, Bogdanovich N, Sevkovskaya Z, et al. Does prolonged and exclusive breastfeeding reduce the risk of allergy and asthma? New evidence from a large randomised trial. *BMJ* 2007;335:815-20.
7   Kramer MS, Vanilovich I, Matush L, Bogdanovich N, Zhang X, Shishko G, et al. The effect of prolonged and exclusive breastfeeding on dental caries in early school-age children: new evidence from a large randomised trial. *Caries Res* 2007;41:484-8.
8   Kramer MS, Matush L, Vanilovich I, Platt RW, Bogdanovich N, Sevkovskaya Z, et al. Effects of prolonged and exclusive breastfeeding on child height, weight, adiposity, and blood pressure at age 6.5 years: new evidence from a large randomized trial. *Am J Clin Nutr* 2007;86:1717-21.
9   Kramer MS, Fombonne E, Igumnov S, Vanilovich I, Matush L, Mironova E, et al. Effects of prolonged and exclusive breastfeeding on child behavior and maternal adjustment: evidence from a large randomized trial. *Pediatrics* 2008;121:e435-440.
10 Kramer MS, Aboud F, Mironova E, Vanilovich I, Platt RW, Matush L, et al. Breastfeeding and child cognitive development: new evidence from a large randomized trial. *Arch Gen Psychiatry* 2008;65:578-84.
11 Campbell MK, Elbourne DR, Altman DG, for the CONSORT Group. CONSORT statement: extension to cluster randomised trials. *BMJ* 2004;328:702-8.

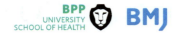

Implementation research: what it is and how to do it

David H Peters, professor[1], Taghreed Adam, scientist[2], Olakunle Alonge, assistant scientist[1], Irene Akua Agyepong, specialist public health[3], Nhan Tran, manager[4]

[1]Johns Hopkins University Bloomberg School of Public Health, Department of International Health, 615 N Wolfe St, Baltimore, MD 21205, USA

[2]Alliance for Health Policy and Systems Research, World Health Organization, CH-1211 Geneva 27, Switzerland

[3]University of Ghana School of Public Health/Ghana Health Service, Accra, Ghana

[4]Alliance for Health Policy and Systems Research, Implementation Research Platform, World Health Organization, CH-1211 Geneva 27, Switzerland

Correspondence to: D H Peters dpeters@jhsph.edu

Cite this as: BMJ 2013;347:f6753

DOI: 10.1136/bmj.f6753

http://www.bmj.com/content/347/bmj.f6753

ABSTRACT

Implementation research is a growing but not well understood field of health research that can contribute to more effective public health and clinical policies and programmes. This article provides a broad definition of implementation research and outlines key principles for how to do it

The field of implementation research is growing, but it is not well understood despite the need for better research to inform decisions about health policies, programmes, and practices. This article focuses on the context and factors affecting implementation, the key audiences for the research, implementation outcome variables that describe various aspects of how implementation occurs, and the study of implementation strategies that support the delivery of health services, programmes, and policies. We provide a framework for using the research question as the basis for selecting among the wide range of qualitative, quantitative, and mixed methods that can be applied in implementation research, along with brief descriptions of methods specifically suitable for implementation research. Expanding the use of well designed implementation research should contribute to more effective public health and clinical policies and programmes.

Defining implementation research

Implementation research attempts to solve a wide range of implementation problems; it has its origins in several disciplines and research traditions (supplementary table A). Although progress has been made in conceptualising implementation research over the past decade,[1] considerable confusion persists about its terminology and scope.[2] [3] [4]

SUMMARY POINTS

- Implementation research has its origins in many disciplines and is usefully defined as scientific inquiry into questions concerning implementation—the act of fulfilling or carrying out an intention
- In health research, these intentions can be policies, programmes, or individual practices (collectively called interventions)
- Implementation research seeks to understand and work in "real world" or usual practice settings, paying particular attention to the audience that will use the research, the context in which implementation occurs, and the factors that influence implementation
- A wide variety of qualitative, quantitative, and mixed methods techniques can be used in implementation research, which are best selected on the basis of the research objective and specific questions related to what, why, and how interventions work
- Implementation research may examine strategies that are specifically designed to improve the carrying out of health interventions or assess variables that are defined as implementation outcomes
- Implementation outcomes include acceptability, adoption, appropriateness, feasibility, fidelity, implementation cost, coverage, and sustainability

The word "implement" comes from the Latin "implere," meaning to fulfil or to carry into effect.[5] This provides a basis for a broad definition of implementation research that can be used across research traditions and has meaning for practitioners, policy makers, and the interested public: "Implementation research is the scientific inquiry into questions concerning implementation—the act of carrying an intention into effect, which in health research can be policies, programmes, or individual practices (collectively called interventions)."

Implementation research can consider any aspect of implementation, including the factors affecting implementation, the processes of implementation, and the results of implementation, including how to introduce potential solutions into a health system or how to promote their large scale use and sustainability. The intent is to understand what, why, and how interventions work in "real world" settings and to test approaches to improve them.

Principles of implementation research

Implementation research seeks to understand and work within real world conditions, rather than trying to control for these conditions or to remove their influence as causal effects. This implies working with populations that will be affected by an intervention, rather than selecting beneficiaries who may not represent the target population of an intervention (such as studying healthy volunteers or excluding patients who have comorbidities).

Context plays a central role in implementation research. Context can include the social, cultural, economic, political, legal, and physical environment, as well as the institutional setting, comprising various stakeholders and their interactions, and the demographic and epidemiological conditions. The structure of the health systems (for example, the roles played by governments, non-governmental organisations, other private providers, and citizens) is particularly important for implementation research on health.

Implementation research is especially concerned with the users of the research and not purely the production of knowledge. These users may include managers and teams using quality improvement strategies, executive decision makers seeking advice for specific decisions, policy makers who need to be informed about particular programmes, practitioners who need to be convinced to use interventions that are based on evidence, people who are influenced to change their behaviour to have a healthier life, or communities who are conducting the research and taking action through the research to improve their conditions (supplementary table A). One important implication is that often these actors should be intimately involved in the identification, design, and conduct phases of research and not just be targets for dissemination of study results.

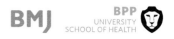

Table 1 Implementation outcome variables

Implementation outcome	Working definition*	Related terms†
Acceptability	The perception among stakeholders (for example, consumers, providers, managers, policy makers) that an intervention is agreeable	Factors related to acceptability (for example, comfort, relative advantage, credibility)
Adoption	The intention, initial decision, or action to try to employ a new intervention	Uptake, utilisation, intention to try
Appropriateness	The perceived fit or relevance of the intervention in a particular setting or for a particular target audience (for example, provider or consumer) or problem	Relevance, perceived fit, compatibility, perceived usefulness or suitability
Feasibility	The extent to which an intervention can be carried out in a particular setting or organisation	Practicality, actual fit, utility, trialability
Fidelity	The degree to which an intervention was implemented as it was designed in an original protocol, plan, or policy	Adherence, delivery as intended, integrity, quality of programme delivery, intensity or dosage of delivery
Implementation cost	The incremental cost of the implementation strategy (for example, how the services are delivered in a particular setting). The total cost of implementation would also include the cost of the intervention itself	Marginal cost, total cost‡
Coverage	The degree to which the population that is eligible to benefit from an intervention actually receives it.	Reach, access, service spread or effective coverage (focusing on those who need an intervention and its delivery at sufficient quality, thus combining coverage and fidelity), penetration (focusing on the degree to which an intervention is integrated in a service setting)
Sustainability	The extent to which an intervention is maintained or institutionalised in a given setting	Maintenance, continuation, durability, institutionalisation, routinisation, integration, incorporation

Adapted from references 6 and 33.

*Original definitions referred to individual "innovations or evidence-based practices." This table uses the term "intervention" so that the definitions are more broadly applicable to programmes and policies. The original authors used the term "penetration" rather than "coverage."

†Other terms are more commonly found in implementation literature on large scale programmes and policies.[8,34-36]

‡Cost data also provide numerators for measures of efficiency and specifically measures of cost-utility, cost-benefit, or cost effectiveness.

Implementation outcome variables

Implementation outcome variables describe the intentional actions to deliver services.[6] These implementation outcome variables—acceptability, adoption, appropriateness, feasibility, fidelity, implementation cost, coverage, and sustainability—can all serve as indicators of the success of implementation (table 1). Implementation research uses these variables to assess how well implementation has occurred or to provide insights about how this contributes to one's health status or other important health outcomes.

Implementation strategies

Curran and colleagues defined an "implementation intervention" as a method to "enhance the adoption of a 'clinical' intervention," such as the use of job aids, provider education, or audit procedures.[7] The concept can be broadened to any type of strategy that is designed to support a clinical or population and public health intervention (for example, outreach clinics and supervision checklists are implementation strategies used to improve the coverage and quality of immunisation).

A review of ways to improve health service delivery in low and middle income countries identified a wide range of successful implementation strategies (supplementary table B).[8] Even in the most resource constrained environments, measuring change, informing stakeholders, and using information to guide decision making were found to be critical to successful implementation.

Implementation influencing variables

Other factors that influence implementation may need to be considered in implementation research. Sabatier summarised a set of such factors that influence policy implementation (clarity of objectives, causal theory, implementing personnel, support of interest groups, and managerial authority and resources).[9]

The large array of contextual factors that influence implementation, interact with each other, and change over time highlights the fact that implementation often occurs as part of complex adaptive systems.[10] Some implementation strategies are particularly suitable for working in complex systems. These include strategies to provide feedback to key stakeholders and to encourage learning and adaptation by implementing agencies and beneficiary groups. Such strategies have implications for research, as the study methods need to be sufficiently flexible to account for changes or adaptations in what is actually being implemented.[8 11] Research designs that depend on having a single and fixed intervention, such as a typical randomised controlled trial, would not be an appropriate design to study phenomena that change, especially when they change in unpredictable and variable ways.

Another implication of studying complex systems is that the research may need to use multiple methods and different sources of information to understand an implementation problem. Because implementation activities and effects are not usually static or linear processes, research designs often need to be able to observe and analyse these sometimes iterative and changing elements at several points in time and to consider unintended consequences.

Implementation research questions

As in other types of health systems research, the research question is the king in implementation research. Implementation research takes a pragmatic approach, placing the research question (or implementation problem)

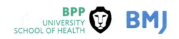

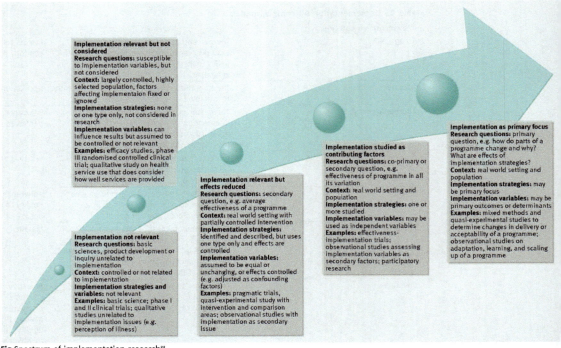

Fig Spectrum of implementation research[33]

as the starting point to inquiry; this then dictates the research methods and assumptions to be used. Implementation research questions can cover a wide variety of topics and are frequently organised around theories of change or the type of research objective (examples are in supplementary table C).[12] [13]

Implementation research can overlap with other types of research used in medicine and public health, and the distinctions are not always clear cut. A range of implementation research exists, based on the centrality of implementation in the research question, the degree to which the research takes place in a real world setting with routine populations, and the role of implementation strategies and implementation variables in the research (figure).

A more detailed description of the research question can help researchers and practitioners to determine the type of research methods that should be used. In table 2, we break down the research question first by its objective: to explore, describe, influence, explain, or predict. This is followed by a typical implementation research question based on each objective. Finally, we describe a set of research methods for each type of research question.

Much of evidence based medicine is concerned with the objective of influence, or whether an intervention produces an expected outcome, which can be broken down further by the level of certainty in the conclusions drawn from the study. The nature of the inquiry (for example, the amount of risk and considerations of ethics, costs, and timeliness), and the interests of different audiences, should determine the level of uncertainty.[8] [14] Research questions concerning programmatic decisions about the process of an implementation strategy may justify a lower level of certainty for the manager and policy maker, using research methods that would support an adequacy or plausibility inference.[14] Where a high risk of harm exists and sufficient time and resources are available, a probability study design might be more appropriate, in which the result in an area where the intervention is implemented is compared with

areas without implementation with a low probability of error (for example, $P < 0.05$). These differences in the level of confidence affect the study design in terms of sample size and the need for concurrent or randomised comparison groups.[8] [14]

Implementation specific research methods

A wide range of qualitative and quantitative research methods can be used in implementation research (table 2). The box gives a set of basic questions to guide the design or reporting of implementation research that can be used across methods. More in-depth criteria have also been proposed to assess the external validity or generalisability of findings.[15] Some research methods have been developed specifically to deal with implementation research questions or are particularly suitable to implementation research, as identified below.

KEY QUESTIONS TO ASSESS RESEARCH DESIGNS OR REPORTS ON IMPLEMENTATION RESEARCH[33]

- Does the research clearly aim to answer a question concerning implementation?
- Does the research clearly identify the primary audiences for the research and how they would use the research?
- Is there a clear description of what is being implemented (for example, details of the practice, programme, or policy)?
- Does the research involve an implementation strategy? If so, is it described and examined in its fullness?
- Is the research conducted in a "real world" setting? If so, is the context and sample population described in sufficient detail?
- Does the research appropriately consider implementation outcome variables?
- Does the research appropriately consider context and other factors that influence implementation?
- Does the research appropriately consider changes over time and the level of complexity of the system, including unintended consequences?

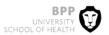

Table 2   Type of implementation research objective, implementation question, and research methods

Objective	Description	Implementation question	Research methods and data collection approaches
Explore	Explore an idea or phenomenon to make hypotheses or generalisations from specific examples	What are the possible factors and agents responsible for good implementation of a health intervention? For enhancing or expanding a health intervention?	Qualitative methods: grounded theory, ethnography, phenomenology, case studies and narrative approaches; key informant interviews, focus groups, historical reviews
			Quantitative: network analysis, cross sectional surveys
			Mixed methods: combining qualitative and quantitative methods
Describe	Identify and describe the phenomenon and its correlates or possible causes	What describes the context in which implementation occurs? What describes the main factors influencing implementation in a given context?	Quantitative: cross sectional (descriptive) surveys, network analysis
			Qualitative methods: ethnography, phenomenology, case studies and narrative approaches; key informant interviews, focus groups, historical reviews
			Mixed methods: both qualitative and quantitative inquiry with convergence of data and analyses
Influence	Test whether an intervention produces an expected outcome		
With adequacy	With sufficient confidence that the intervention and outcomes are occurring	Is coverage of a health intervention changing among beneficiaries of the intervention?	Before-after or time series in intervention recipients only; participatory action research
With plausibility	With greater confidence that the outcome is due to the intervention	Is a health outcome plausibly due to the implemented intervention rather than other causes?	Concurrent, non-randomised cluster trials: health intervention implemented in some areas and not in others; before-after or cross sectional study in programme recipients and non-recipients; typical quality improvement studies
With probability	With a high (calculated) probability that the outcome is due to the intervention	Is a health outcome due to implementation of the intervention?	Partially controlled trials: pragmatic and cluster randomised trials; health intervention implemented in some areas and not in others; effectiveness-implementation hybrids
Explain	Develop or expand a theory to explain the relation between concepts, the reasons for the occurrence of events, and how they occurred	How and why does implementation of the intervention lead to effects on health behaviour, services, or status in all its variations?	Mixed methods: both qualitative and quantitative inquiry with convergence of data and analyses
			Quantitative: repeated measures of context, actors, depth and breadth of implementation across subunits; network identification; can use designs for confirmatory inferences; effectiveness-implementation hybrids
			Qualitative methods: case studies, phenomenological and ethnographic approaches with key informant interviews, focus groups, historical reviews
			Participatory action research
Predict	Use prior knowledge or theories to forecast future events	What is the likely course of future implementation?	Quantitative: agent based modelling; simulation and forecasting modelling; data extrapolation and sensitivity analysis (trend analysis, econometric modelling)
			Qualitative: scenario building exercises; Delphi techniques from opinion leaders

Adapted from references 8, 14, and 33.

Pragmatic trials

Pragmatic trials, or practical trials, are randomised controlled trials in which the main research question focuses on effectiveness of an intervention in a normal practice setting with the full range of study participants.[16] This may include pragmatic trials on new healthcare delivery strategies, such as integrated chronic care clinics or nurse run community clinics. This contrasts with typical randomised controlled trials that look at the efficacy of an intervention in an "ideal" or controlled setting and with highly selected patients and standardised clinical outcomes, usually of a short term nature.

Effectiveness-implementation hybrid trials

Effectiveness-implementation hybrid designs are intended to assess the effectiveness of both an intervention and an implementation strategy.[7] These studies include components of an effectiveness design (for example, randomised allocation to intervention and comparison arms) but add the testing of an implementation strategy, which may also be randomised. This might include testing the effectiveness of a package of delivery and postnatal care in under-served areas, as well testing several strategies for providing the care. Whereas pragmatic trials try to fix the intervention under study, effectiveness-implementation hybrids also intervene and/or observe the implementation process as it actually occurs. This can be done by assessing implementation outcome variables.

Quality improvement studies

Quality improvement studies typically involve a set of structured and cyclical processes, often called the plan-do-study-act cycle, and apply scientific methods on a continuous basis to formulate a plan, implement the plan, and analyse and interpret the results, followed by an iteration of what to do next.[17 18] The focus might be on a clinical process, such as how to reduce hospital acquired infections in the intensive care unit, or management processes such as how to reduce

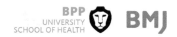

waiting times in the emergency room. Guidelines exist on how to design and report such research—the Standards for Quality Improvement Reporting Excellence (SQUIRE).[17]

Speroff and O'Connor describe a range of plan-do-study-act research designs, noting that they have in common the assessment of responses measured repeatedly and regularly over time, either in a single case or with comparison groups.[18] Balanced scorecards integrate performance measures across a range of domains and feed into regular decision making.[19] [20] Standardised guidance for using good quality health information systems and health facility surveys has been developed and often provides the sources of information for these quasi-experimental designs.[21] [22] [23]

Participatory action research

Participatory action research refers to a range of research methods that emphasise participation and action (that is, implementation), using methods that involve iterative processes of reflection and action, "carried out with and by local people rather than on them."[24] In participatory action research, a distinguishing feature is that the power and control over the process rests with the participants themselves. Although most participatory action methods involve qualitative methods, quantitative and mixed methods techniques are increasingly being used, such as for participatory rural appraisal or participatory statistics.[25] [26]

Mixed methods

Mixed methods research uses both qualitative and quantitative methods of data collection and analysis in the same study. Although not designed specifically for implementation research, mixed methods are particularly suitable because they provide a practical way to understand multiple perspectives, different types of causal pathways, and multiple types of outcomes—all common features of implementation research problems.

Many different schemes exist for describing different types of mixed methods research, on the basis of the emphasis of the study, the sampling schemes for the different components, the timing and sequencing of the qualitative and quantitative methods, and the level of mixing between the qualitative and quantitative methods.[27] [28] Broad guidance on the design and conduct of mixed methods designs is available.[29] [30] [31] A scheme for good reporting of mixed methods studies involves describing the justification for using a mixed methods approach to the research question; describing the design in terms of the purpose, priority, and sequence of methods; describing each method in terms of sampling, data collection, and analysis; describing where the integration has occurred, how it has occurred, and who has participated in it; describing any limitation of one method associated with the presence of the other method; and describing any insights gained from mixing or integrating methods.[32]

Conclusion

Implementation research aims to cover a wide set of research questions, implementation outcome variables, factors affecting implementation, and implementation strategies. This paper has identified a range of qualitative, quantitative, and mixed methods that can be used according to the specific research question, as well as several research designs that are particularly suited to implementation research. Further details of these concepts can be found in

a new guide developed by the Alliance for Health Policy and Systems Research.[33]

Contributors: All authors contributed to the conception and design, analysis and interpretation, drafting the article, or revising it critically for important intellectual content, and all gave final approval of the version to be published. NT had the original idea for the article, which was discussed by the authors (except OA) as well as George Pariyo, Jim Sherry, and Dena Javadi at a meeting at the World Health Organization (WHO). DHP and OA did the literature reviews, and DHP wrote the original outline and the draft manuscript, tables, and boxes. OA prepared the original figure. All authors reviewed the draft article and made substantial revisions to the manuscript. DHP is the guarantor.

Funding: Funding was provided by the governments of Norway and Sweden and the UK Department for International Development (DFID) in support of the WHO Implementation Research Platform, which financed a meeting of authors and salary support for NT. DHP is supported by the Future Health Systems research programme consortium, funded by DFID for the benefit of developing countries (grant number H050474). The funders played no role in the design, conduct, or reporting of the research.

Competing interests: All authors have completed the ICMJE uniform disclosure form at www.icmje.org/coi_disclosure.pdf and declare: support for the submitted work as described above; NT and TA are employees of the Alliance for Health Policy and Systems Research at WHO, which is supporting their salaries to work on implementation research; no financial relationships with any organisations that might have an interest in the submitted work in the previous three years; no other relationships or activities that could appear to have influenced the submitted work.

Provenance and peer review: Invited by journal; commissioned by WHO; externally peer reviewed.

1   Brownson RC, Colditz GA, Proctor EK, eds. Dissemination and implementation research in health: translating science to practice. Oxford University Press, 2012.
2   Ciliska D, Robinson P, Armour T, Ellis P, Brouwers M, Gauld M, et al. Diffusion and dissemination of evidence-based dietary strategies for the prevention of cancer. Nutr J 2005;4(1):13.
3   Remme JHF, Adam T, Becerra-Posada F, D'Arcangues C, Devlin M, Gardner C, et al. Defining research to improve health systems. PLoS Med 2010;7:e1001000.
4   McKibbon KA, Lokker C, Mathew D. Implementation research. 2012. http://whatiskt.wikispaces.com/Implementation+Research.
5   The compact edition of the Oxford English dictionary. Oxford University Press, 1971.
6   Proctor E, Silmere H, Raghavan R, Hovmand P, Aarons G, Bunger A, et al. Outcomes for implementation research: conceptual distinctions, measurement challenges, and research agenda. Adm Policy Ment Health 2010;38:65-76.
7   Curran GM, Bauer M, Mittman B, Pyne JM, Stetler C. Effectiveness-implementation hybrid designs: combining elements of clinical effectiveness and implementation research to enhance public health impact. Med Care 2012;50:217-26.
8   Peters DH, El-Saharty S, Siadat B, Janovsky K, Vujicic M, eds. Improving health services in developing countries: from evidence to action. World Bank, 2009.
9   Sabatier PA. Top-down and bottom-up approaches to implementation research. J Public Policy 1986;6(1):21-48.
10   Paina L, Peters DH. Understanding pathways for scaling up health services through the lens of complex adaptive systems. Health Policy Plan 2012;27:365-73.
11   Gilson L, ed. Health policy and systems research: a methodology reader. World Health Organization, 2012.
12   Tabak RG, Khoong EC, Chambers DA, Brownson RC. Bridging research and practice: models for dissemination and implementation research. Am J Prev Med 2012;43:337-50.
13   Improved Clinical Effectiveness through Behavioural Research Group (ICEBeRG). Designing theoretically-informed implementation interventions. Implement Sci 2006;1:4.
14   Habicht JP, Victora CG, Vaughn JP. Evaluation designs for adequacy, plausibility, and probability of public health programme performance and impact. Int J Epidemiol 1999;28:10-8.
15   Green LW, Glasgow RE. Evaluating the relevance, generalization, and applicability of research. Eval Health Prof 2006;29:126-53.
16   Swarenstein M, Treweek S, Gagnier JJ, Altman DG, Tunis S, Haynes B, et al, for the CONSORT and Pragmatic Trials in Healthcare (Practihc) Groups. Improving the reporting of pragmatic trials: an extension of the CONSORT statement. BMJ 2008;337:a2390.
17   Davidoff F, Batalden P, Stevens D, Ogrince G, Mooney SE, for the SQUIRE Development Group. Publication guidelines for quality improvement in health care: evolution of the SQUIRE project. Qual Saf Health Care 2008;17(suppl I):i3-9.
18   Speroff T, O'Connor GT. Study designs for PDSA quality improvement research. Q Manage Health Care 2004;13(1):17-32.
19   Peters DH, Noor AA, Singh LP, Kakar FK, Hansen PM, Burnham G. A balanced scorecard for health services in Afghanistan. Bull World Health Organ 2007;85:146-51.

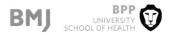

20   Edward A, Kumar B, Kakar F, Salehi AS, Burnham G. Peters DH. Configuring balanced scorecards for measuring health systems performance: evidence from five years' evaluation in Afghanistan. *PLOS Med* 2011;7:e1001066.

21   Health Facility Assessment Technical Working Group. Profiles of health facility assessment method, MEASURE Evaluation, USAID, 2008.

22   Hotchkiss D, Diana M, Foreit K. How can routine health information systems improve health systems functioning in low-resource settings? Assessing the evidence base. MEASURE Evaluation, USAID, 2012.

23   Lindelow M, Wagstaff A. Assessment of health facility performance: an introduction to data and measurement issues. In: Amin S, Das J, Goldstein M, eds. Are you being served? New tools for measuring service delivery. World Bank, 2008:19-66.

24   Cornwall A, Jewkes R. "What is participatory research?" *Soc Sci Med* 1995;41:1667-76.

25   Mergler D. Worker participation in occupational health research: theory and practice. *Int J Health Serv* 1987;17:151.

26   Chambers R. Revolutions in development inquiry. Earthscan, 2008.

27   Creswell JW, Plano Clark VL. Designing and conducting mixed methods research. Sage Publications, 2011.

28   Tashakkori A, Teddlie C. Mixed methodology: combining qualitative and quantitative approaches. Sage Publications, 2003.

29   Leech NL, Onwuegbuzie AJ. Guidelines for conducting and reporting mixed research in the field of counseling and beyond. *Journal of Counseling and Development* 2010;88:61-9.

30   Creswell JW. Mixed methods procedures. In: Research design: qualitative, quantitative and mixed methods approaches. 3rd ed. Sage Publications, 2009.

31   Creswell JW, Klassen AC, Plano Clark VL, Clegg Smith K. Best practices for mixed methods research in the health sciences. National Institutes of Health, Office of Behavioral and Social Sciences Research, 2011.

32   O'Cathain A, Murphy E, Nicholl J. The quality of mixed methods studies in health services research. *J Health Serv Res Policy* 2008;13:92-8.

33   Peters DH, Tran N, Adam T, Ghaffar A. Implementation research in health: a practical guide. Alliance for Health Policy and Systems Research, World Health Organization, 2013.

34   Rogers EM. Diffusion of innovations. 5th ed. Free Press, 2003.

35   Carroll C, Patterson M, Wood S, Booth A, Rick J, Balain S. A conceptual framework for implementation fidelity. *Implement Sci* 2007;2:40.

36   Victora CG, Schellenberg JA, Huicho L, Amaral J, El Arifeen S, Pariyo G, et al. Context matters: interpreting impact findings in child survival evaluations. *Health Policy Plan* 2005;20(suppl 1):i18-31.

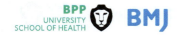

A multicomponent decision tool for prioritising the updating of systematic reviews

Yemisi Takwoingi, research fellow[1], Sally Hopewell, senior research fellow[2][3], David Tovey, editor in chief of the Cochrane Library[4], Alex J Sutton, professor of medical statistics[5]

[1]Public Health, Epidemiology and Biostatistics, University of Birmingham, Edgbaston, Birmingham B15 2TT, UK

[2]Centre for Statistics in Medicine, University of Oxford, Oxford, UK

[3]INSERM, U738, Paris, France

[4]Cochrane Editorial Unit, London, UK

[5]Department of Health Sciences, University of Leicester, Leicester, UK

Correspondence to: Y Takwoingi
y.takwoingi@bham.ac.uk

Cite this as: BMJ 2013;347:f7191

DOI: 10.1136/bmj.f7191

http://www.bmj.com/content/347/bmj.f7191

ABSTRACT

There is no formal consensus on when to update a systematic review, and updating too frequently can be an inefficient use of resources and introduce bias. A multicomponent tool could help researchers decide when is best to update such reviews

Evidence evolves as new research becomes available, and thus systematic reviews should be kept up to date to maintain their relevance and validity. However, the decision to update a systematic review should be made carefully because updating is potentially resource intensive, and updating too soon could introduce bias.[1] In contrast, if reviews are not updated frequently enough, doctors and policy makers could act on evidence that is out of date. There is currently no consensus on when to initiate updating.[2]

Traditionally, the Cochrane Collaboration used a biennial updating policy,[3] yet many Cochrane reviews are out of date (fig 1); only about 20% of reviews are updated every two years. As of February 2013, the *Cochrane Database of Systematic Reviews*, published in the *Cochrane Library*, contained 5418 reviews.[4] This number implies that 2700 Cochrane reviews will need to be updated per year to comply with the updating policy, in addition to producing new reviews. Despite the emphasis on Cochrane reviews in this paper, updating is a common challenge, and methods are needed to prioritise reviews that are most in need of updating.

A methodological review of different methods for identifying when to update a systematic review found that existing methods were not comprehensive because they only considered either qualitative or quantitative techniques.[5] We describe a multicomponent (that is, including both qualitative and quantitative components) updating decision tool that can be used to determine when to prioritise one or more systematic reviews for updating. We provide a brief overview of the initial development and evaluation of the two complementary components, describe how they have been improved and integrated to produce the decision tool, and give illustrative examples of its implementation.

Development and evaluation of the qualitative decision tree

In 2007, the Cochrane Opportunities Fund supported a project to develop a strategic and evidence based approach to guide decisions of whether and when to update Cochrane reviews.[6] An international steering committee was established to provide guidance and support to the project. A decision tree comprising a series of qualitative signals of the need to update and an updating checklist were developed. A pilot study evaluated their validity and reliability, and the results of the pilot and input from users and methodological experts were used to refine the decision tree. The full report of the project is available online.[7]

Development and evaluation of the quantitative tool

The initial quantitative approach[8] adapted work on sample size methods for designing new studies to update existing meta-analyses.[9][10] The scope of the approach was broadened by compiling a candidate list of quantitative signals (web fig 1), based on existing[11] and new signals.[12] The signals were categorised into those that can be evaluated "immediately" and those that require simulation methods to compute. Many signals on this list are self explanatory, or are based on quantities described elsewhere (that is, Barrowman's new participant ratio[13] and the I^2 statistic[14]). The web appendix provides further details, and additional information is available elsewhere.[15] Although in a small evaluation two signals performed well,[8] we were aware that a comprehensive approach including qualitative signals relevant to the entire review was essential.

Development and evaluation of the multicomponent updating decision tool

The two approaches outlined above were developed independently. Subsequently, a collaboration began between both development groups and the Cochrane Editorial Unit. The quantitative tool prioritised a portfolio of systematic reviews, on the basis of the signals or the total number of signals triggered, and further work was required to establish an optimal combination of signals. Thus, a principal task in developing the multicomponent tool involved developing a statistical prediction tool based on a prediction equation (box 1), derived from using signals from the candidate list. We developed the prediction tool using a sample of Cochrane reviews (web fig 2). The web appendix describes the development of the prediction tool with further details available elsewhere.[15] We modified the qualitative decision tree and integrated the prediction tool to produce the first version of the multicomponent updating decision tool.[15]

The Cochrane Airways Group piloted this decision tool on 21 of their most cited systematic reviews or reviews

SUMMARY POINTS

- There is no consensus on appropriate methods for deciding when to update systematic reviews
- A decision tool was developed to replace an approach based on an arbitrary and rigid time period with a priority based approach
- The tool broadly consists of three criteria: clinical question answered or no longer relevant, new relevant factors to consider, and availability of new studies
- The decision tool can help identify reviews most sensitive to change and thus minimise unnecessary updating and waste of resources

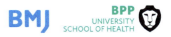

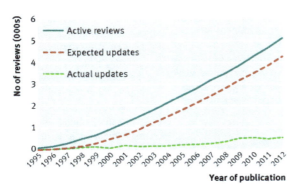

Fig 1 Number of active and updated reviews published in the *Cochrane Library* from 1995 to 2012. Active reviews are the total number of published reviews excluding reviews that have been withdrawn. Therefore, it is expected that these reviews will be considered for updating within two years of the last date of publication

with the most website hits (Welsh E, Karner C, Stovold E, Cates C, 20th Cochrane Colloquium, Auckland, New Zealand, 2012). It took five days to evaluate the 21 reviews, and eight reviews were identified that required updating (that is, with conclusions most likely to change). Consequently, resources that would have been wasted updating reviews less likely to benefit from updating were saved. The tool was considered easy to use, and it provided a structured and transparent way to assess and prioritise Cochrane reviews for updating. Challenges were encountered: for example, screening records for complex interventions, screening topics outside the screener's comfort zone, and evaluating the possibility that updating the risk of bias would change the conclusions of the review. Nonetheless, the tool gave an opportunity to have these discussions and focused the debate. Specialists can be consulted on discreet questions if needed. The evaluation highlighted the need for clear and detailed guidance to enhance consistency in the assessment of subjective elements and appropriate application of the statistical prediction element of the tool. Therefore, we revised the guidance developed for Cochrane Review Groups, and the document is available on request from the editor in chief's office, known as the Cochrane Editorial Unit (ceu@cochrane.org). Following feedback, we further refined the tool to create the updating decision tool summarised in fig 2.

Overview of the multicomponent updating decision tool

Our decision tool has three steps (fig 2), and an assessment is required at each step.

Step 1: Is the clinical question already answered by the available evidence or is the clinical question deemed no longer relevant?

If it is expected that there will never be any further information that could change the findings of the review, the current evidence is deemed conclusive, or that the clinical question is deemed no longer relevant, this should be noted. A decision can be made to flag the review as "Current question; no longer being updated" or "Historical question; no longer being updated" as appropriate.

Step 2: Are there any new factors relevant to the existing review?

These might include:

- Information from existing included studies—for example, information about new treatment regimens, population subgroups, harms, economic data, or outcome measures,

including data from ongoing studies or previously missing data
- New methodology—for example, new statistical techniques, or changes in methodological guidance
- Response to feedback from users of the review
- Inclusion in policy decision making or clinical practice guidelines—for example, it might be important to update a review to include it in a new clinical guideline. If any such factors (termed updating signals) are identified, then a judgment is made on whether a signal for updating is likely or unlikely to change the results or conclusions of the review.

This step will involve a degree of subjectivity and should involve all members of the review team or editorial team (or both).

Step 3: Are there new studies?

If new studies are identified that are relevant to the primary outcome on which the conclusions of the review are based—and thus could be included in the main meta-analysis of this outcome in the review—then the statistical prediction tool can be applied. The probability (given as a percentage) of this new evidence changing the conclusions of the systematic review is based on the size and number of new studies added. Our results (web fig 3 and web appendix) indicated that a threshold probability of around 50% is suggestive of the need to update a systematic review, but any threshold can be chosen. If the new studies identified are not eligible to be included in a meta-analysis but still provide new information, then a judgment will need to be made about their likely effect on the conclusions of the review.

Documentation and presentation of decisions

To provide clarity and transparency for readers, the decision made at each step of the tool should be carefully documented together with reasons for the decisions. If an updating signal is deemed unlikely to change the conclusions of a systematic review, then the decision can be made not to update the review. For Cochrane reviews, such decisions (citing any new studies) can be documented in the "What's new" table that shows readers the current status of the review, and the review can be flagged as "Current question; considered to be up to date." For other systematic reviews, authors will need to explore avenues of dissemination with journals or publishers.

Alternatively, if a signal is deemed likely to change the conclusions of a systematic review, and there is a review team available, the review should be updated as soon as possible. If a review team is not currently available then the review should be flagged as a "Priority for updating." We retrospectively applied the tool to two Cochrane reviews to illustrate its use (boxes 2 and 3; tables 1 and 2 compare the out of date and updated reviews considered)

Discussion

The unification of two approaches has produced a comprehensive and practical tool that can aid updating systematic reviews at the appropriate time by identifying priority updates. We believe that the decision tool has a role in improving the efficiency of the systematic review process; the task of updating can be managed methodically and limited resources used more efficiently. The tool can also be used to objectively compare systematic reviews that have new studies to determine which review(s) should have the highest updating priority. The statistical prediction

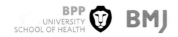

BOX 1 PREDICTION EQUATION FOR ESTIMATING THE PROBABILITY OF CONCLUSIONS CHANGING AFTER THE ADDITION OF NEW STUDIES TO AN EXISTING META-ANALYSIS

The prediction equation uses two signals: the ratio of the total weight of the new studies to the total weight of the old studies (weight ratio) in an updated meta-analysis; and the number of new studies (web table and web appendix provide more details).

The equation is:

Estimated p=invlogit(0.1207+0.4101×weight ratio+0.1836×number of new trials)

Where p is the estimated probability that conclusions will change when the review is updated; and invlogit is the inverse logit function, which is calculated as:

invlogit(x)=exp(x)÷(1+exp(x))

The prediction equation was implemented in user friendly software to calculate this probability for a single meta-analysis or each meta-analysis in a portfolio of reviews. We plan to describe elsewhere full details of this flexible software—"metarank"— implemented as a macro in Stata software, version 11.0. The code and user guide can be obtained from the corresponding author.

element of the decision tool can rank reviews in order of the probability that conclusions will change instead of using a threshold probability to assign priority. Ideally, reviews within similar clinical or topic areas should be compared.

This work contributed to the strategic session on Cochrane content at the Cochrane Collaboration's 2012 mid-year meeting. After the meeting, it was recommended that the current "one size fits all" guidance for updating every two years should be replaced in favour of prioritising updates using methods such as the updating decision tool, although no single prioritisation method should be prescribed.[16] This recommendation is comparable with the approach adopted by *BMJ Clinical Evidence*, which has replaced an annual updating policy with a tailored updating schedule based on the content of the review, availability of new studies, and popularity of the review with their readers.[17]

The updating decision tool has limitations. The prediction component should not be used if studies included in the main meta-analysis in the earlier version of a review are excluded in the updated version. Prediction models are also typically overoptimistic when developed and the tool will benefit from evaluation in a wider cohort of reviews to assess the accuracy of predictions of the need to update. Updating is an iterative process, and we have not yet

BOX 2 APPLYING THE DECISION TOOL TO A COCHRANE REVIEW WITH A HIGH PRIORITY FOR UPDATING

Table 1 compares the main characteristics of the out of date and updated reviews.

Application of the decision tool to the out of date version of the review

- Step 1: Is the clinical question already answered by the available evidence or is the clinical question deemed no longer relevant? No
- Step 2: Are there any new factors relevant to the existing review to consider? No
- Step 3: Are there new studies? Yes

There were 37 new studies of ibuprofen versus placebo, as well as existing meta-analyses of the primary outcome. When 12 of the new studies were included in the meta-analysis of the primary outcome for the 200 mg dose, the prediction tool gave a probability that conclusions would change of 96%.

The new studies also provided data for additional analyses. These included the secondary outcome, which was the use of rescue treatment (proportion of participants using rescue treatment; time to use of rescue treatment), and sensitivity analyses (pain model, dental v other types of surgery; dose response in dental studies, 200 mg v 400 mg; salt preparation, standard ibuprofen v ibuprofen lysine, arginine, and "soluble").
Decision: Flag the review as "High priority for updating."

Current status and abridged history of the review in the *Cochrane Library*

Review content assessed as up to date: 11 May 2009.
Publication status and date: Stable (no update expected for reasons given in "What's new"), published in issue 6, 2012.

"What's new" table entry

Date: 25 April 2012.
Event: Review declared as stable.
Description: Although new studies on ibuprofen may be published, they are unlikely to affect the results of this review; therefore, the authors suggest that there should be no need to update this review for at least five years.

History

Date: 11 May 2009.
Event: New citation required and conclusions changed.
Description: Information from 37 new studies with 5595 participants was added, giving a total of 72 studies and 9186 participants. Numbers needed to treat for at least 50% pain relief over 4-6 h were not significantly changed. Additional information are provided on the proportion of participants requiring rescue treatment and median or mean time to use of rescue treatment, with higher doses giving slightly better results. Pain model and ibuprofen formulation could both affect the result, with dental impaction models and soluble ibuprofen salts producing better efficacy estimates. A dose response was shown in dental pain.

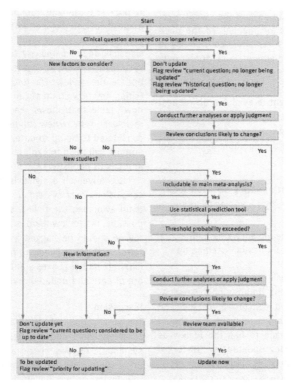

Fig 2 Multicomponent updating decision tool for prioritising systematic review updates. The decision made at each step of the tool should be carefully documented together with reasons for the decisions, thus ensuring transparency and reproducibility. The decision nodes have been numbered to aid the documentation process

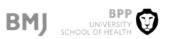

Table 1 Applying the decision tool to a Cochrane review with a high priority for updating: summary of out of date and updated reviews

Characteristic	Out of date version	Updated version
Citation	Collins S, Moore RA, McQuay HJ, Wiffen PJ, Rees J, Derry S. Single dose oral ibuprofen for acute postoperative pain in adults. *Cochrane Database Syst Rev* 1999;1: CD001548	Derry CJ, Derry S, Moore RA, McQuay HJ. Single dose oral ibuprofen for acute postoperative pain in adults. *Cochrane Database Syst Rev* 2009;3: CD001548
Included studies	35	72
Primary outcome	Proportion with .50% pain relief over 4-6 h	Proportion with .50% pain relief over 4-6 h
Comparisons (no of studies)	Ibuprofen v placebo (n=35); diclofenac v placebo (n=6); diclofenac v ibuprofen (n=2)	Ibuprofen v placebo (n=72); comparisons involving diclofenac are no longer in the review
Ibuprofen dose (no of studies)	Mainly 200 mg (n=8) and 400 mg (n=31)	Mainly 200 mg (n=20) and 400 mg (n=61)
Participants	Adults (n=2214 on ibuprofen; n=1377 on placebo)	Adults (n=5804 on ibuprofen; n=3382 on placebo)
Findings (risk ratio (95% CI))	200 mg (707 participants): 4.7 (3.2 to 6.9); 400 mg (2817 participants): 3.4 (3.0 to 3.9)	200 mg (2690 participants): 4.6 (3.9 to 5.6); 400 mg (6475 participants): 3.9 (3.6 to 4.4)
Authors' conclusions	Both drugs work well. Choosing between them is an issue of dose, safety, and cost.	The substantial amount of high quality evidence shows that ibuprofen is an effective analgesic in treating postoperative pain. Numbers needed to treat for 200 mg and 400 mg ibuprofen did not change significantly from the previous review even when a substantial amount of new information was added. New information is provided on retreatment.

BOX 3 APPLYING THE DECISION TOOL TO A COCHRANE REVIEW WITH A LOW PRIORITY FOR UPDATING

Table 2 compares the main characteristics of the out of date and updated reviews.

Application of the decision tool to the out of date version of the review

- Step 1: Is the clinical question already answered by the available evidence or is the clinical question deemed no longer relevant? No
- Step 2: Are there any new factors relevant to the existing review to consider? No
- Step 3: Are there new studies? Yes

There were six new studies, as well as existing meta-analyses of the primary outcome. When three of the new studies were included in the meta-analysis of the primary outcome shown above, the prediction tool gave a probability that conclusions would change of 45%. Only one of the other three new studies contributed data (329 participants) to any of the other meta-analyses in the review.

Decision: Do not update yet. Flag review as "Current question; considered to be up to date."

Current status and abridged history of the review in the *Cochrane Library*

Review content assessed as up to date: 12 July 2009.

Publication status and date: New search for studies and content updated (no change to conclusions), published in issue 4, 2009.

"What's new" table entry

Date: 9 July 2009.

Event: New search has been performed.

Description: The review has been updated to include six new trials involving 4209 participants, bringing the total number of included trials to 10 involving 26865 participants. The background and discussion sections have been updated to include new material of relevance. The main conclusions are essentially unchanged from the previous version of the review.

History

Date: 18 August 2008.

Event: Amended.

Description: Converted to new review format.

developed criteria to establish when enough evidence has accrued on a given topic and systematic review that it is deemed decisive and not worth conducting further primary research. This factor should be investigated in a future study.

The use of the tool depends on monitoring the literature for new evidence. Tsafnat and colleagues have suggested the possibility of automation of systematic reviews leading to best currently available evidence at the push of a button.[18] Therefore, we can foresee a seamless and "on demand" approach to updating if the tool is linked with innovative methods, such as machine learning techniques for identifying relevant new studies. We also anticipate a role for the quantitative component of the decision tool beyond updating. The quantitative component can be extended to calculate the likelihood of future studies overturning the conclusions of a new systematic review. This assessment will take into account ongoing studies and provide explicit information on further research needed, such as the number and size of new studies.[10] This information can be added to the review to show the robustness of its conclusions and potential "shelf life." It can also provide justification for new clinical trials.

Systematic reviews are not equal—the rate at which evidence accumulates and the effect of new evidence on conclusions may differ. The decision tool can promote channelling limited resources into updating systematic reviews that are most sensitive to change, thus improving the quality and reliability of healthcare decisions made on the basis of current evidence. We believe that this priority based approach that minimises unnecessary updating is more sustainable than an approach based on an arbitrary time period.

We thank Rachel Marshall from the Cochrane Editorial Unit for the helpful advice given during this project; Kirsty Loudon, Mike Clarke, David Moher, Simon French, Anne Eisinga, and Rob Scholten for their valuable input into the earlier development of the qualitative component of the decision tool; and Emma Welsh, managing editor of the Cochrane Airways Group and who led the pilot study of the decision tool, and her team for sharing their experience of using the tool. The views expressed in this article are those of the authors and do not necessarily represent the views of the Cochrane Collaboration.

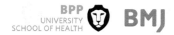

Table 2 Applying the decision tool to a Cochrane review with a low priority for updating: summary of out of date and updated reviews

Characteristic	Out of date version	Updated version
Citation	Hankey G, Sudlow CLM, Dunbabin DW. Thienopyridine derivatives (ticlopidine, clopidogrel) versus aspirin for preventing stroke and other serious vascular events in high vascular risk patients. *Cochrane Database Syst Rev* 2000;1:CD001246	Sudlow CLM, Mason G, Maurice JB, Wedderburn CJ, Hankey GJ. Thienopyridine derivatives versus aspirin for preventing stroke and other serious vascular events in high vascular risk patients. *Cochrane Database Syst Rev* 2009;4:CD001246
Included studies	4	10
Primary outcome	Measure of effectiveness: composite outcome of stroke, myocardial infarction, or death from a vascular cause	Measure of effectiveness: composite outcome of stroke, myocardial infarction, or death from a vascular cause
Comparison (no of studies)	Thienopyridines (ticlopidine, clopidogrel) v aspirin (n=4)	Thienopyridines (ticlopidine, clopidogrel) v aspirin (n=7)
Participants	Patients at high risk of vascular disease (n=11 329 on thienopyridines; n=11 327 on aspirin)	Patients at high risk of vascular disease (n=13 119 on thienopyridines; n=13 136 on aspirin)
Findings (odds ratio (95% CI))	0.91 (0.84 to 0.98); 22 656 participants	0.92 (0.85 to 0.99); 26 255 participants
Authors' conclusions	The available randomised evidence shows that the thienopyridine derivatives are modestly but significantly more effective than aspirin in preventing serious vascular events in patients at high risk (and specifically in patients with a transient ischaemic attack or ischaemic stroke), but there is uncertainty about the size of the additional benefit.	The thienopyridine derivatives are at least as effective as aspirin in preventing serious vascular events in patients at high risk, and possiblysomewhat more so. However, the size of any additional benefit is uncertain and could be negligible.
Citation	Hankey G, Sudlow CLM, Dunbabin DW. Thienopyridine derivatives (ticlopidine, clopidogrel) versus aspirin for preventing stroke and other serious vascular events in high vascular risk patients. *Cochrane Database Syst Rev* 2000;1:CD001246	Sudlow CLM, Mason G, Maurice JB, Wedderburn CJ, Hankey GJ. Thienopyridine derivatives versus aspirin for preventing stroke and other serious vascular events in high vascular risk patients. *Cochrane Database Syst Rev* 2009;4:CD001246

Contributors: All authors contributed to the idea and design of the study, drafted, and edited the manuscript. DT and SH obtained funding for the study. SH was part of the team that developed the original qualitative component. YT and AJS developed the original quantitative component. SH extracted the data, and YT conducted analyses under supervision by AJS. All authors are guarantors.

Funding: This project was funded by the National Institute for Health Research (NIHR) Cochrane-NHS Engagement Award Scheme (project no 10/4000/01). The views and opinions expressed therein are those of the authors and do not necessarily reflect those of the Department of Health.

Competing interests: All authors read and understood the BMJ policy on declaration of interests and declare financial support from the NIHR Cochrane-NHS Engagement Award Scheme.

Data sharing: No additional data available.

1 Hopewell S, Clarke M, Stewart L, Tierney J. Time to publication for results of clinical trials. *Cochrane Database Syst Rev* 2007;2:MR000011.
2 Tsertsvadze A, Maglione M, Chou R, Garritty C, Coleman C, Lux L, et al. Updating comparative effectiveness reviews: current efforts in AHRQ's effective health care program. *J Clin Epidemiol* 2011;64:1208-15.
3 Higgins JPT, Green S, Scholten RJPM. Chapter 3: Maintaining reviews: updates, amendments and feedback. In: Higgins JPT, Green S, eds. Cochrane handbook for systematic reviews of interventions. Version 5.1.0 [updated March 2011]. Cochrane Collaboration, 2011.
4 Cochrane Database of Systematic Reviews. In: The Cochrane Library, Issue 2, 2013. Wiley, 2013.
5 Moher D, Tsertsvadze A, Tricco AC, Eccles M, Grimshaw J, Sampson M, et al. When and how to update systematic reviews. *Cochrane Database Syst Rev* 2008;1:MR000023.
6 Loudon K, Hopewell S, Clarke M, Moher D, French S, Scholten R, et al. Development of a decision tool for updating Cochrane reviews. Presentation at the 16th Cochrane Colloquium: Evidence in the era of globalisation; 2008 Oct 3-7; Freiburg, Germany [abstract]. *Z Evid Qual Gesundhwes* 2008;102:24-5.
7 Hopewell S, Loudon K, Clarke MJ, Moher D, Scholten R, Eisinga A, et al. A decision tool for updating Cochrane reviews. 2013. www.

editorial-unit.cochrane.org/sites/editorial-unit.cochrane.org/files/uploads/Final%20report_Tool%20for%20updating%20Cochrane%20reviews.pdf.
8 Sutton AJ, Donegan S, Takwoingi Y, Garner P, Gamble C, Donald A. An encouraging assessment of methods to inform priorities for updating systematic reviews. *J Clin Epidemiol* 2009;62:241-51.
9 Sutton AJ, Cooper NJ, Jones DR, Lambert PC, Thompson JR, Abrams KR. Evidence-based sample size calculations based upon updated meta-analysis. *Stat Med* 2007;26:2479-500.
10 Ferreira ML, Herbert RD, Crowther MJ, Verhagen A, Sutton AJ. When is a further clinical trial justified? *BMJ* 2012;345:e5913.
11 Shojania KG, Sampson M, Ansari MT, Ji J, Garritty C, Rader T, et al. Updating systematic reviews. Technical review no 16. Publication no 07-0087. Agency for Healthcare Research and Quality, 2007.
12 Takwoingi Y, Sutton AJ, Donegan S, Garner P, Gamble C, Donald A. Prioritising the updating of systematic reviews. Presentation at the 16th Cochrane Colloquium: Evidence in the era of globalisation; 2008 Oct 3-7; Freiburg, Germany [abstract]. *Z Evid Fortbild Qual Gesundhwes* 2008;102:93.
13 Barrowman NJ, Fang M, Sampson M, Moher D. Identifying null meta-analyses that are ripe for updating. *BMC Med Res Methodol* 2003;3:13
14 Higgins JP, Thompson SG, Deeks JJ, Altman DG. Measuring inconsistency in meta-analyses. *BMJ* 2003;327:557-60.
15 Tovey D, Marshall R, Bazian Ltd, Hopewell S, Rader T. Fit for purpose: centralised updating support for high-priority Cochrane reviews. 2011. www.editorial-unit.cochrane.org/fit-purpose-centralised-updating-support-high-priority-cochrane-reviews.
16 MacLehose H, Hilton J, Tovey D, Becker L, Binder L, Chandler J, et al. The Cochrane Library: revolution or evolution? Shaping the future of Cochrane content: report of the Cochrane Collaboration's strategic session, Paris, France, 18 April 2012. www.editorial-unit.cochrane.org/sites/editorial-unit.cochrane.org/files/uploads/2012-CC-strategic-session_meeting-report.pdf.
17 Nuts, bolts, and tiny little screws: how Clinical Evidence works. 2013. www.clinicalevidence.com/x/set/static/cms/nuts-and-bolts.html.
18 Tsafnat G, Dunn A, Glasziou P, Coiera E. The automation of systematic reviews. *BMJ* 2013;346:f139.

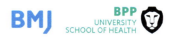

The impact of outcome reporting bias in randomised controlled trials on a cohort of systematic reviews

Jamie J Kirkham, research associate[1], Kerry M Dwan, research assistant[1],
Douglas G Altman, director, professor[2], Carrol Gamble, senior lecturer[1], Susanna Dodd,
lecturer[1], Rebecca Smyth, research associate[3], Paula R Williamson, director, professor[1]

Centre for Medical Statistics and
Health Evaluation, University of
Liverpool, Liverpool L69 3GS

Centre for Statistics in Medicine,
University of Oxford, Oxford OX2
6UD

Population, Community and
Behavioural Sciences, University of
Liverpool, Liverpool, L69 3GB

Correspondence to: P R Williamson
prw@liv.ac.uk

Cite this as: BMJ 2010;340:c365

DOI: 10.1136/bmj.c365

http://www.bmj.com/content/340/
bmj.c365

ABSTRACT

Objective To examine the prevalence of outcome reporting bias—the selection for publication of a subset of the original recorded outcome variables on the basis of the results—and its impact on Cochrane reviews.

Design A nine point classification system for missing outcome data in randomised trials was developed and applied to the trials assessed in a large, unselected cohort of Cochrane systematic reviews. Researchers who conducted the trials were contacted and the reason sought for the non-reporting of data. A sensitivity analysis was undertaken to assess the impact of outcome reporting bias on reviews that included a single meta-analysis of the review primary outcome.

Results More than half (157/283 (55%)) the reviews did not include full data for the review primary outcome of interest from all eligible trials. The median amount of review outcome data missing for any reason was 10%, whereas 50% or more of the potential data were missing in 70 (25%) reviews. It was clear from the publications for 155 (6%) of the 2486 assessable trials that the researchers had measured and analysed the review primary outcome but did not report or only partially reported the results. For reports that did not mention the review primary outcome, our classification regarding the presence of outcome reporting bias was shown to have a sensitivity of 88% (95% CI 65% to 100%) and specificity of 80% (95% CI 69% to 90%) on the basis of responses from 62 trialists. A third of Cochrane reviews (96/283 (34%)) contained at least one trial with high suspicion of outcome reporting bias for the review primary outcome. In a sensitivity analysis undertaken for 81 reviews with a single meta-analysis of the primary outcome of interest, the treatment effect estimate was reduced by 20% or more in 19 (23%). Of the 42 meta-analyses with a statistically significant result only, eight (19%) became non-significant after adjustment for outcome reporting bias and 11 (26%) would have overestimated the treatment effect by 20% or more.

Conclusions Outcome reporting bias is an under-recognised problem that affects the conclusions in a substantial proportion of Cochrane reviews. Individuals conducting systematic reviews need to address explicitly the issue of missing outcome data for their review to be considered a reliable source of evidence. Extra care is required during data extraction, reviewers should identify when a trial reports that an outcome was measured but no results were reported or events observed, and contact with trialists should be encouraged.

Selective reporting bias in a study is defined as the selection, on the basis of the results, of a subset of analyses to be reported. Selective reporting may occur in relation to outcome analyses,[1] subgroup analyses,[2] and per protocol analyses, rather than in intention to treat analyses,[3] as well as with other analyses.[4] Three types of selective reporting of outcomes exist: the selective reporting of some of the set of study outcomes, when not all analysed outcomes are reported; the selective reporting of a specific outcome—for example, when an outcome is measured and analysed at several time points but not all results are reported; and incomplete reporting of a specific outcome—for example, when the difference in means between treatments is reported for an outcome but no standard error is given.

A specific form of bias arising from the selective reporting of the set of study outcomes is outcome reporting bias, which is defined as the selection for publication of a subset of the original recorded outcome variables on the basis of the results.[5] Empirical research on randomised controlled trials shows strong evidence of an association between significant results and publication: studies that report positive or significant results (P<0.05) are more likely to be published, and outcomes that are statistically significant have higher odds of being fully reported than those that are not significant (range of odds ratios: 2.2 to 4.7).[6] An analysis of studies that compared trial publications with protocols found that 40-62% of trials changed, introduced, or omitted at least one primary outcome.[6]

The systematic review process has been developed to minimise biases and random errors in the evaluation of healthcare interventions.[7] Cochrane systematic reviews are internationally recognised as among the best sources, if not the best source, of reliable up to date information on health care.[8] [9] Meta-analysis, a statistical technique for combining results from several related but independent studies, can make important contributions to medical research—for example, by showing that there is evidence to support treatments not widely used[10] or that evidence is lacking to support treatments that are in wide use.[11]

Missing outcome data can affect a systematic review in two ways. Publication bias, where a study is not published

SUMMARY POINTS

- Empirical research indicates that statistically significant outcomes are more likely to be fully reported than non-significant results in published reports of randomised controlled trials

- Little is known about the impact of outcome reporting bias in source trial reports on the conclusions of systematic reviews

- Few review authors mentioned the potential problem of outcome reporting bias

- Outcome reporting bias was suspected in at least one trial in more than a third of reviews

- In a sensitivity analysis, nearly a fifth of statistically significant meta-analyses of the review primary outcome were affected by outcome reporting bias and a quarter would have overestimated the treatment effect by 20% or more

on the basis of its results, can lead to bias in the analysis of a particular outcome in a review, especially if the decision not to submit or publish the study is related to the results for that outcome. In a published study that has been identified by the reviewer, outcome reporting bias can arise if the outcome of interest in the review had been measured and analysed but not reported on the basis of the results.

Little is known about the impact of outcome reporting bias on systematic reviews. One previous study examined a small cohort of nine Cochrane reviews of randomised trials.[1] Although outcome reporting bias in the review primary outcome was suspected in several individual randomised trials, the impact of such bias on the conclusions drawn in the meta-analyses was minimal. This study used a very select set of reviews, however, and highlighted the need for a larger study.

In this paper we report the findings of the Outcome Reporting Bias in Trials (ORBIT) study, in which we applied a new classification system for the assessment of selective outcome reporting and evaluated the validity of the tool. We used the classification system to estimate the prevalence of outcome reporting bias and its impact on an unselected cohort of Cochrane reviews. To our knowledge, this is the first systematic empirical study of the impact of outcome reporting bias in randomised controlled trials on the results of systematic reviews.

Methods

We examined an unselected cohort of new reviews from 50 of the 51 Cochrane collaboration review groups published in three issues of the *Cochrane Library* (Issue 4, 2006, Issue 1, 2007, and Issue 2, 2007). For each review, two investigators (JJK and SD) independently examined the "types of outcome measures" section to determine whether the review specified a single primary outcome. For those reviews where either no primary outcome was detailed or multiple primary outcomes were specified, the lead reviewer was contacted and asked to select a single primary outcome from those listed. When no contact could be established or the reviewer(s) could not define a single primary outcome, two investigators (PRW and SD) independently selected and agreed upon a single primary outcome from those listed.

Assessment of systematic reviews

Two investigators (JJK and SD) scrutinised all 33 reviews from Issue 4, 2006 that specified a single primary outcome and agreed on the need for further assessment of all but two reviews. Both disagreements were related to whether the reasons for exclusion were suggestive of outcome reporting bias. Each remaining review was read by one investigator (JJK) to check whether all included trials fully reported the review primary outcome. The reason for exclusion of any trial (in the "characteristics of excluded studies" section) was also checked for any suggestion of potential outcome reporting bias. For example, a trial excluded because there was "no relevant outcome data" required further scrutiny because the relevant outcome might have been measured but not reported. Any uncertainties regarding the excluded studies were referred to PRW.

Reviews that did not identify any randomised controlled trials were not assessed further. Similarly, reviews were not assessed further if no standard definition of the primary outcome exists, because outcome reporting bias assessment in this situation would be impossible. One example is relapse in schizophrenia trials, for which definitions include a change in symptom score and hospital readmission.

Classification of randomised controlled trials in systematic reviews

For each review, an outcome matrix was constructed showing the reporting of the primary outcome and other outcomes in each trial included, distinguishing full, partial, or no reporting. An example of an outcome matrix is given in table 1. For this example, "live birth" was the review primary outcome. The matrix was completed using the information in the review and revised accordingly in light of any extra information obtained from the trial reports or through contact with the trialists. Outcomes for which the data could be included in a meta-analysis were considered to be fully reported. Such data may have been in the trial report or may have been calculated indirectly from the results. For example, the number of events may have been calculated from the proportion of events and the number of patients in the treatment group, or the standard error of the treatment effect may have been calculated from the estimate of effect and the associated P value.

A classification system was developed to assess the risk of bias when a trial was excluded from a meta-analysis, either because the data for the outcome were not reported or because the data were reported incompletely (for example, just as "not significant"). The system was refined over the initial few months of the study, but if an amendment was made all previous classifications were reviewed and adjusted as appropriate to ensure consistency of application. The categories reflect the stages of assessing whether an outcome was measured, whether an outcome was analysed, and, finally, the nature of the results presented (table 2). The system identifies whether there is evidence that the outcome was measured and analysed but only partially reported (A to D classifications), whether the outcome was measured but not necessarily analysed (E and F), if it is unclear whether the outcome was measured (G and H), or if it is clear the outcome was not measured (I).

For each classification category, an assessment was made of the risk of outcome reporting bias arising from the lack of inclusion of non-significant results. A "high risk"

Table 1 Example of a review outcome matrix displaying the information available in trial reports

Trial ID (author, year of publication)	Review primary outcome	Other review outcomes		Additional outcomes (reported in any of the eligible trials)		
		Chemical pregnancy rate	Clinical pregnancy rate	Ectopic pregnancy rate	Birth weight of baby	Reason for exclusion
	Live birth rate					
12345678.1 (Smith, 1999)	o	×		×	×	–
12345678.2 (Lowe, 2001)		o	×		×	–
12345678.3 (Biggs, 2004)	×			×		–
...						
Excluded trials						
1234578.9 (Johns, 2006)	×	×	×	×	×	No relevant outcome data
...						

Full reporting of results for treatment comparison of interest.
× *No reporting of results for treatment comparison of interest.*
o *Partial reporting of results for treatment comparison of interest.*

classification was awarded when it was either known or suspected that the results were partially or not reported because the treatment comparison was statistically non-significant (P>0.05). A "low risk" classification was awarded when it was suspected, but not actually known, that the outcome was either not measured, measured but not analysed, or measured and analysed but either partially reported or not reported for a reason unrelated to the results obtained. A "no risk" classification was reserved for cases where it was known that the outcome was not measured, known that it was measured but not analysed, or known that it was measured and analysed but the reason for partial or no reporting was not because the results were statistically non-significant. For cases where the outcome was measured but not necessarily analysed, judgment was needed as to whether it was likely (E) or unlikely (F) that the measured outcome was analysed and not reported because of non-significant results. When it was unclear whether the outcome was measured, judgment was needed as to whether it was likely that the outcome was measured and analysed but not reported on the basis of non-significant results (G) or unlikely that the outcome was measured at all (H). Trials classified as A/D/E/G, C/F/H, and B/I were assumed to be at high, low, and no risk of outcome reporting bias, respectively, in relation to the review primary outcome. Examples of each of the classifications in the ORBIT study are shown in web table A.

On the basis of all identified publications for a trial, one investigator (JJK, SD, or KD) and the corresponding review author independently classified any trial that did not report or partially reported results for the review primary outcome (table 2). All trials excluded from the review but selected for assessment were also classified. For each classification, justification for the classification was recorded in prose to supplement the category code, including verbatim quotes from the trial publication whenever possible. The agreed classification, with the justification, was then reviewed by the senior investigator (PRW). Any discrepancies were discussed until a final overall classification was agreed for each trial and the justification for the classification

documented in full. When the corresponding review author and coauthors were unable to assist with our assessments and the clinical area proved to be challenging, help was sought from medical colleagues at the University of Liverpool.

To assess how many reviewers had considered the possibility of outcome reporting bias, we searched the text of included reviews for the words "selective" and "reporting."

Accuracy of classification

For trials for which it was uncertain whether the review primary outcome had actually been measured and/or analysed (E, F, G, or H classification; table 2), the trialists were contacted via email (address obtained from either the trial report or a search of PubMed or Google) and asked to confirm whether the review primary outcome was measured and analysed. If so, the reason for not reporting the results was requested. Non-responders were contacted a second time if a reply was not received within three weeks. Trialists were not contacted if a reviewer had previously approached them for the relevant information.

Two separate sensitivity and specificity analyses were performed. The first analysis considered only G and H classifications and aimed to determine how good our classification system was at judging whether the primary outcome of interest in the review had been measured when it was not mentioned in the trial report. For this analysis only, we incorporated an extra category of G classification for trials with binary outcomes where we predicted that the outcome was measured but it was not reported because there were no events.

The second analysis compared our classifications with information from the trialists to establish whether we could predict if biased reporting had occurred. Implicitly, E and G classifications suggested that bias was likely because it was either clear or assumed that the outcome had been measured and possible that non-reporting could have been influenced by the non-significance of the result. These classifications were taken to imply bias on the basis of the lack of inclusion of non-significant results. The specificity was calculated taking F and H classifications to indicate no bias. This analysis excluded any studies classified as F that were ongoing because it is difficult to assess bias until a study is completed. Confidence intervals for sensitivity and specificity estimates were calculated using standard formulae.[12]

Amount and impact of missing trial data

The amount of missing data per review was calculated, firstly on the basis of trials that omitted data for any reason and secondly only using those trials where data omission was suspected on the basis of the results (that is, outcome reporting bias was suspected). The maximum bias bound approach was used in a sensitivity analysis[13][14] to estimate the impact of outcome reporting bias on the review meta-analysis. This approach calculates an upper bound for the bias resulting from the number of eligible studies suspected of outcome reporting bias, and assumes that on average smaller studies (lower precision) will have a higher probability of not reporting the outcome of interest than larger studies (higher precision). This method was applied only to reviews that had a single meta-analysis of the review primary outcome, because if there were multiple meta-analyses it would be difficult to ascertain to which analyses

Table 2 The Outcome Reporting Bias In Trials (ORBIT) study classification system for missing or incomplete outcome reporting in reports of randomised trials

	Description	Level of reporting	Risk of bias*
	Clear that the outcome was measured and analysed		
A	Trial report states that outcome was analysed but only reports that result was not significant (typically stating P>0.05)	Partial	High risk
B	Trial report states that outcome was analysed but only reports that result was significant (typically stating P<0.05)	Partial	No risk
C	Trial report states that outcome was analysed but insufficient data were presented for the trial to be included in meta-analysis or to be considered to be fully tabulated	Partial	Low risk
D	Trial report states that outcome was analysed but no results reported	None	High risk
	Clear that the outcome was measured		
E	Clear that outcome was measured but not necessarily analysed. Judgment says likely to have been analysed but not reported because of non-significant results	None	High risk
F	Clear that outcome was measured but not necessarily analysed. Judgment says unlikely to have been analysed but not reported because of non-significant results	None	Low risk
	Unclear whether the outcome was measured		
G	Not mentioned but clinical judgment says likely to have been measured and analysed but not reported on the basis of non-significant results	None	High risk
H	Not mentioned but clinical judgment says unlikely to have been measured at all	None	Low risk
	Clear that the outcome was not measured		
I	Clear that outcome was not measured	NA	No risk

*Risk of bias arising from the lack of inclusion of non-significant results when a trial was excluded from a meta-analysis or not fully reported in a review because the data were unavailable.

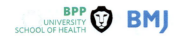

the trial with suspected outcome reporting bias would relate without discussion with a clinical expert. The impact was not assessed for trials with H or I classifications, where it was suggested that the review primary outcome had not been measured, or G classifications where the explanation was that there were no events. The impact was assessed both in terms of the percentage change in the treatment effect estimate and the change in the statistical significance of the treatment effect estimate after adjustment.

Results

Assessments of systematic reviews

The *Cochrane Library* published 309 new reviews in Issue 4, 2006, Issue 1, 2007, and Issue 2, 2007 (fig 1). We excluded 12 reviews by the Cochrane Methodology Review Group. Single primary outcomes were specified in 103 reviews, whereas lead reviewers or co-reviewers were asked to select a single primary outcome for the remaining 194 reviews. In 173 cases reviewers were willing to do so, with 127 (73%) choosing the first outcome listed. For the remaining 21 reviews a single primary outcome was selected by the research team (PRW and SD). On further scrutiny, however, 14 reviews were excluded because the review primary outcome was not well defined.

Among the remaining 283 reviews, the median number of reviews from an individual Cochrane review group was five (range 1 to 21, interquartile range (IQR) 2 to 7). The five groups with most reviews were the hepato-biliary group (21 reviews), the pregnancy and childbirth group (18), the neonatal group (14), the oral health group (13), and the menstrual disorders and subfertility group (12). The median number of randomised controlled trials per review was five (range 0 to 134, IQR 2 to 10).

A total of 126 reviews did not require further assessment: 38 did not identify any randomised controlled trials and 88 fully reported the primary outcome for all eligible trials. This left 157 reviews requiring further assessment—that is, 55% (157/283) of reviews did not include full data on the primary outcome of interest from all eligible trials.

By text searching for the words "selective" and "reporting," 20 (7%) of the 283 reviews assessed were found to have mentioned outcome reporting bias, the proportion being similar in reviews requiring and those not requiring further assessment.

Full reporting of review primary outcomes in trials

Figure 2 shows a flow diagram for the assessment of the 2562 trials included in the study cohort of 283 systematic reviews. Seventy-six trial reports could not be assessed because the articles were not in English. Seventy-one per cent (1774/2486) of the remaining trials fully reported the review primary outcome in the trial report.

Table 3 provides information on 177 trial reports that gave full data on the primary outcome of interest that was not included in the review. For 59 trials, the data were not included in the review for a reason unrelated to outcome reporting bias. For 118 trials (7% of the 1774 trials that fully reported the review primary outcome), the review primary outcome data were fully reported in the publication but were not included in the review. Information on missed outcome data was fed back to the reviewers for inclusion in a review update.

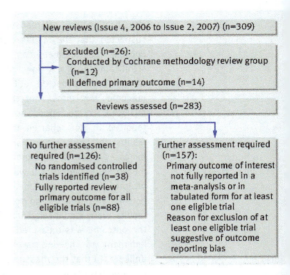

Fig 1 Flow diagram for Outcome Reporting Bias In Trials (ORBIT) study

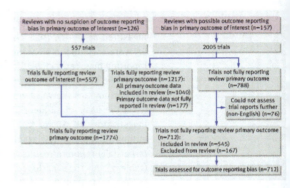

Fig 2 Assessment of randomised controlled trials within reviews

Classification of trials

For 788 (31%) of the 2562 trials included in our study, the review primary outcome was either partially reported or not reported (fig 2). Seventy-six trial reports could not be assessed because the articles were not in English, leaving 2486 assessable trials and 712 trial reports requiring a classification (545 included in reviews and 167 excluded from reviews). Table 4 shows the classification of these 712 trials.

For 155 (6%) of the 2486 assessable trials, it was clear that the review primary outcome was measured and analysed (A, B, C, or D classification), but partial reporting meant the data could not be included in a meta-analysis. Trials classified as C were grouped according to the nature of the missing data (web table B).

A total of 359 (50%) of the 712 trials with missing data were under high suspicion for outcome reporting bias (A, D, E, or G classification; table 4). The prevalence of reviews containing at least one trial with high outcome reporting bias suspicion was 34% (96/283).

Accuracy of classification

Information on whether the outcome of interest was measured and analysed was lacking in 538 trial reports (E, F, G, or H classification). We found the email addresses of 167

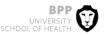

Table 3 Reasons for omission of data from trials fully reporting review primary outcome (n=177)

	Reason	Number of trials
Data not included in review for a reason unrelated to outcome reporting bias (n=59)		
Invalid measurement scales	In some reviews only certain validated measurement scales were allowed. Cases in which the primary outcome was deemed to be fully reported using a non-validated scale and there was no apparent evidence of outcome reporting bias were accepted as full reporting.	4
Poor reporting of time to event data	For inclusion in a time to event meta-analysis, the log hazard ratio and a measure of its variance is required. Although this information was not reported in these trials, enough information was reported to rule out outcome reporting bias. a. Review tabulates median time to event (no meta-analysis considered), whereas trials fully report the number of events as a binary outcome in each treatment arm (n=19) b. Review reports the number of events in a binary outcome meta-analysis, whereas the trials report the median time to event, Kaplan-Meier plot, and significance of the difference in survival curves for each treatment arm using log rank test (n=12)	31
Quality issues	The review primary outcome was fully reported in the trial report but the results were not included in the review owing to methodological shortcomings (for example, the trial was a crossover trial with no washout period). This was acceptable as full reporting if the primary outcome data were fully reported and the reasons for these shortcomings were discussed by the reviewer. These methodological shortcomings were considered to be quality issues not related to outcome reporting bias.	24
Data not included in review despite being fully reported in trial (n=118)		
Not fully reported in the review text*	The results were fully reported in the trial report but only partially reported in the review text (no meta-analysis undertaken). a. Review reported the P values only (n=19) b. Review reported the magnitude of treatment effect (group means or medians, or difference in means) but with no measure of precision or variability (confidence interval, standard deviation, or standard error for means; interquartile or other range for medians; n=7) c. Review reported the number of participants with the event for each group (or percentages) but did not give sample sizes for the denominators (n=2) d. Review reported the results from the main intervention arm only (n=1)	29
No event*	The primary outcome was not observed in any patient throughout the trial, which was mentioned in the trial report but not in the review.	31
No results reported in review*	The results were fully reported in the trial report but nothing was reported in the review. a. The outcome data were missed during data extraction (perhaps reported in a supplementary article rather than the main publication; n=42) b. The outcome data were available but extraction was not straightforward—that is, perhaps some calculation was involved before the data were in a suitable format for inclusion in a review meta-analysis (n=8) c. Trial reported results from a non-parametric analysis and review included only parametric results for use in a meta-analysis (n=8)	58

*This information was forwarded to the reviewer.

Table 4 Trials assessed for outcome reporting bias (n=712)

Classification	Number of fully published trials	Number of abstracts	Total number of trials (%)
A	23	7	30 (4)
B	2	6	8 (1)
C	113	4	117 (16)
D	0	0	0 (0)
E	113	9	122 (17)
F	24	9	33 (5)
G	192	15	207 (29)
H	148	28	176 (25)
I	15	4	19 (3)
Total	630	82	712

(31%) authors and contacted these individuals. Responses were received from 65 authors (39%): 26% (9/34) of authors whose trial had an E classification; 33% (1/3) who got an F classification; 42% (30/71) who got a G classification; and 42% (25/59) of individuals from trials with an H classification.

To determine whether the outcome of interest was measured or not, we compared our assessments against the trialists' information for 55 trials for which the outcome had not been mentioned in the trial report (G or H classification). The sensitivity for predicting that the outcome had been measured was 92% (23/25, 95% CI 81% to 100%), whereas the specificity for predicting that the outcome had not been measured was 77% (23/30, 95% CI 62% to 92%; table 5). Details of the nine incorrect classifications are provided in table 6.

To measure our judgment on whether outcome reporting bias occurred or not, we compared our assessments against the trialists' information for 62 trials for which the outcome was either clearly measured but not necessarily analysed (E and F classification) or had not been mentioned in the trial report (G or H classification). Three ongoing studies were excluded from this analysis. The sensitivity of our classification system for detecting bias was calculated to be 88% (7/8, 95% CI 65% to 100%), whereas the specificity was 80% (43/54, 95% CI 69% to 90%; table 7)

Amount and impact of missing trial data

The median amount of review primary outcome data missing from trials for any reason was 10%. For the 96 reviews that included at least one trial with a high suspicion of outcome reporting bias, the median amount of missing data was 43%.

Of the 283 reviews in our study cohort, 81 included a single meta-analysis of the review primary outcome and were included in the assessment of the impact of outcome reporting bias on the review meta-analysis. Table 8 lists the reasons for excluding reviews from the assessment of impact.

A total of 52 of the 81 reviews included in the assessment of impact included at least one trial that had a high suspicion of outcome reporting bias. In 27 of these 52 reviews, no sensitivity analysis was undertaken because classifications for all trials with missing data suggested that the review primary outcome seemed not to have been measured or it was suspected that there were no events (H and some G classifications, respectively; 17 reviews), or the reviewer or review text suggested that the missing studies

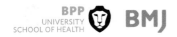

Table 5 Accuracy of judgment as to whether the review primary outcome was measured (G or H classification)

			Information from trialist		
			Primary outcome measured	Primary outcome not measured	Total
ORBIT assessment	Primary outcome measured	G classification	4	7*	11
		G classification (no event)	19	0	19
		Total	23	7	30
	Primary outcome not measured	H classification	2*	23	25
Total			25	30	55

*Reasons for these disagreements are given in table 6.

Table 6 Reasons for incorrect judgment as to whether the outcome of interest was measured in a trial (G or H classification)

ORBIT study classification	Primary outcome of interest	Information from trialist	Reason for incorrect classification
Likely to have been measured			
G	Cause specific survival	Data were not reported on this outcome, only on overall survival	We thought it possible that the cause of death would have been recorded if it was breast cancer, which patients in the trial had been diagnosed with
G	Cognitive development	No data on cognitive development, only evaluated motor development	A number of trials in this review reported on both cognitive development and motor development
G	Bone fractures*	Bone fractures not measured, only bone mineral density	Although "bone fractures" is a long term outcome, one short term trial included in the review reported no bone fractures. It was thought that all similar trials would have the ability to detect a bone fracture even though it is unlikely that an event occurred. There is also lack of consensus between experts in this field on whether it is plausible to accurately detect bone fractures using the technology used in these trials
G	Pain response to bisphosphonates	Pain was only looked at through analgesic consumption but was not measured using the visual analogue scale required for review	It was clear that pain was an outcome domain of interest in this trial, and most other included trials reported pain using a visual analogue scale scale
G	Improvement in nerve function	This outcome was not measured. The trial assessed function using only a clinician's judgment, as would happen in clinical practice. Changes in skin, motor, sensory, and autonomic function are complex to measure, and reliability of measurement varies. It is difficult to determine what changes would be considered clinically significant to individual patients, so the study was not based on such measurements	It was clear that nerve function was an outcome domain of interest in this trial. We thought that since the other two trials included in this review reported on this outcome by using validated sensory and muscle testing scores, then this outcome would have also been measured in this trial in addition to the clinical assessments. There is lack of consensus between clinical experts on the validity and reliability of using validated test scores in this clinical field
Not likely to have been measured			
H	Mean weekly alcohol consumption	Mean weekly alcohol consumption was measured in the original study, but the primary results paper had not been written at the time of the early publication cited in the review. Results still not published	This study was excluded because no prespecified outcomes were mentioned. The trial report included in the review looked only at healthcare utilisation and did not report any outcome data that suggested that the review primary outcome would have been measured
H	Live birth rate	Data were collected on live birth rate but were not complete at time of publication. All pregnancies resulted in live birth. Result still not published but data now analysed (P>0.05)	The primary end point for this trial was the number of clinical pregnancies diagnosed at 12 weeks' gestation. On the basis of the studies included in this review, it seems that trials in this area often do not follow-up to birth

*This reason applied to three separate trials within the same review.

would not have been combined with the other trials in the meta-analysis for reasons not related to outcome reporting bias (10 reviews). For the other 25 reviews that could be assessed, the maximum bias bound sensitivity analysis indicated that the statistically significant conclusions of eight of these reviews were not robust to outcome reporting bias—that is, the treatment effect estimate changed from a significant result favouring treatment (95% confidence interval excludes the null value) to a non-significant result (reviews one to eight; table 9). In a further eight analyses, the result was robust to outcome reporting bias—that is, the result for the adjusted pooled estimate was also statistically significant (P<0.05). The remaining nine analyses had non-significant treatment effect estimates for which the application of the sensitivity analysis produced no substantial change in three analyses and a change from favouring one group to moving the effect estimate closer to the null value of no difference in treatment effect in six analyses. For all the 25 reviews assessed, the median percentage change in the treatment effect estimates after the adjustment based on the maximum bias bound was 39% (IQR 18% to 67%).

Our sensitivity analysis indicates that of the 81 reviews where there was a single meta-analysis of the review primary outcome, the significance of the results was not robust to outcome reporting bias in eight (10%) cases and the treatment effect estimate was reduced by more than 20% in 19 (23%) reviews. If only the 42 meta-analyses with a statistically significant result are considered, however, then eight (19%) become non-significant after adjustment for outcome reporting bias and 11 (26%) overestimated the treatment effect estimate by 20% or more.

Discussion

Outcome reporting bias was suspected in at least one randomised controlled trial in more than a third of the systematic reviews we examined (35%), which is substantially higher than the number of reviews in which a reference to the potential for outcome reporting bias was found (7%), thus demonstrating under-recognition of the problem. We have also shown through sensitivity analysis that outcome reporting bias affects the treatment effect estimate in a substantial proportion of Cochrane reviews.

Strengths and limitations of the study

The strengths of this study are that we evaluated a large, unselected cohort of reviews, review authors were involved in the assessment of outcome reporting bias, and the authors of the trials included in the reviews were contacted for information. In addition, the textual justification for each trial classification was checked by a senior investigator.

We undertook an internal pilot study of 33 reviews to determine the level of agreement between two researchers on the need for further assessment of a review for suspicion of outcome reporting bias. Given that agreement was high, we concluded that it would be sufficient for a single reviewer to assess the remainder of the reviews, provided a second reviewer checked the reasons for excluded studies where there was uncertainty.

For the majority of trials that were missing outcome data, judgment was needed regarding the potential for outcome reporting bias. We believe we have shown that sufficiently accurate assessments are possible. This conclusion, however, rests on the assumption that the trialists we contacted provided accurate information to us. A previous study suggested that trialists may be reluctant to admit selective reporting.[15] In our study, the response

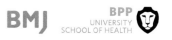

Table 7 Accuracy of judgment as to whether outcome reporting bias occurred (E, F, G, or H classification)

ORBIT assessment		Information from trialist		Total
		Bias	No bias	
	High risk	7(4* + 3†)	11(7‡ + 4§)	18
	Low risk	1¶	43(24** + 19††)	44
Total		8	54	62

*Review primary outcome measured but not analysed owing to small number of events.
†Review primary outcome measured and analysed but result not significant (P>0.05; one case), or result analysed but trialist would not share significance of result until article published (two cases).
‡Review primary outcome not measured (all incorrectly predicted—see all G classifications, table 6).
§Review primary outcome measured but not analysed because it was not a specific end point in the trial (one case), was measured in a small subset of patients in one treatment arm but not analysed (one case), or was analysed but favoured intervention (P<0.05; two cases).
¶See "Live birth rate" example, table 6.
**Review primary outcome not measured.
††Review primary outcome measured but no events recorded.

Table 8 Reasons for excluding reviews from the assessment of impact

Reason	Number of reviews
Total number of reviews identified	309
Preliminary exclusions	
Study by Cochrane methods group	12
Primary outcome not well defined	14
Total number reviews included in the study	283
Exclusions from assessment of impact	
Review identified no randomised controlled trials	38
Language restrictions	2
No meta-analysis	45
Primary outcome measured in different ways (for example, weight might have been reported as BMI or change in weight)	20
Longitudinal study	15
Studies not combined owing to clinical heterogeneity	4
Review included several meta-analyses (owing to different intervention comparisons)	78
Total number of reviews included in assessment of impact	81

rate for those trialists for whom an email address was obtained was similar in trials with a high risk classification and those with a low risk classification. If response bias was operating, we would expect the sensitivity of our classifications to be underestimated (as a result of trialists with high risk classifications being less likely to respond if they have selectively reported outcomes) and the specificity overestimated (as a result of trialists with low risk classifications being more likely to respond if they have not selectively reported outcomes). With such response bias, the number of selectively reported trials in a review would be underestimated; thus the impact of outcome reporting bias on the conclusions of the reviews studied here may have been underestimated.

Our classifications of trials for outcome reporting bias facilitated an assessment of the robustness of review conclusions to such bias.[13] [14] The maximum bias bound approach was the method chosen to examine this source of bias because it can be applied to any outcome type. Although only 81 (29%) of the 283 reviews studied comprised a single meta-analysis of the primary outcome of interest and were thus included in the assessment, there is no reason to believe the results of this assessment would not be generalisable to those reviews containing multiple meta-analyses of the primary outcome relating to different treatment comparisons. However, a limitation of our study is that it has not examined how the impact of outcome reporting bias should be assessed in reviews that do not include a meta-analysis.

Comparison with other studies
We are only aware of one previous study that used similar methods to examine the prevalence of outcome reporting bias and its impact on systematic reviews.[1] This study used a highly selected set of nine reviews, however, in which 10 or more trials had been included in the meta-analysis of a binary outcome. Although outcome reporting bias of the primary outcome of interest was suspected in several individual randomised trials, the impact of such bias on the conclusions drawn in the meta-analyses was minimal. The findings from that study, in terms of the potential for outcome reporting bias to impact on the conclusions of a review and the degree of impact being related to the amount of missing outcome data, were similar to the current study.

A second study of meta-analyses in Cochrane reviews demonstrated a weak positive association between the amount of outcome data missing from the source trial reports and the treatment effect estimate.[16] Our study goes further by reviewing excluded studies and classifying the likelihood of outcome reporting bias in a review on the basis of the individual trial reports.

Implications for systematic reviews
The reliability of systematic reviews can be improved if more attention is paid to outcome data missing from the source trial reports. Trials should not be excluded because there is "no relevant outcome data" as the outcome data may be missing as a direct result of selective outcome reporting. Increasing the accuracy of data extraction, possibly by involving a second reviewer, could reduce the amount of missing data. If a high proportion of data is missing, reviewers should be encouraged to contact the trialists to confirm whether the outcome was measured and analysed and, if so, obtain the results. More than a third of the trialists contacted in this study responded to requests for information, 60% within a day and the remainder within three weeks. Similar response rates were observed with trials published in the past five years compared with those published earlier. In addition, some review authors did not declare when a trial report stated that no events were observed in any group. We believe that reviewers should report all such data in their review.

Review authors will need to use their judgment regarding the potential for outcome reporting bias. Unfortunately, we believe there are few practical alternatives to this approach, since to do nothing is unacceptable and to contact trialists for the information or data is recommended but is not always feasible or successful. To support their judgment, reviewers should justify fully in the text of their report the classification assigned and should include verbatim quotes from the trial publication whenever possible.

The classification system that we used in this study has been presented and applied by participants during workshops that we have developed and delivered at international Cochrane colloquia and the UK Cochrane meetings. The feedback from these workshops has so far not indicated any major shortcomings of this classification system or that any additional categories are required. Adoption of the new Cochrane risk of bias tool,[11] which includes a judgment of the risk of selective outcome reporting, should also help to raise awareness of outcome reporting bias.

If a sensitivity analysis used to assess the impact of outcome reporting bias on an individual review shows

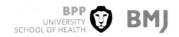

Table 9 Sensitivity analysis to assess the robustness of the conclusions of the review to outcome reporting bias (n=25 reviews)

Review	Intervention*	Number of trials with results fully reported in meta-analysis (n)	Number of eligible trials missing from meta-analysis and suspected of outcome reporting bias (m)	Proportion of missing data (%)†	Original pooled estimate (95% confidence interval)	Conclusion	Adjusted pooled estimate (95% confidence interval)‡	Change in estimate (%)
1	Active treatment v placebo/nothing	6	3	45	HR 0.57 (0.39 to 0.82)	Favours active treatment	HR 0.73 (0.51 to 1.06)§	37¶
2	Active treatment v placebo/nothing	4	4	11	RR 0.49 (0.26 to 0.90)	Favours active treatment	RR 0.79 (0.42 1.46)§	59
3	Active treatment v placebo/nothing	3	3	81	WMD 0.39 (0.11 to 0.67)	Favours active treatment	WMD 0.21 (−0.07 to 0.49)§	46
4	Active treatment v placebo/nothing	4	2	20	SMD 0.66 (0.20 to 1.12)	Favours active treatment	SMD 0.41 (−0.05 to 0.88)§	38
5	Active treatment v placebo/nothing	9	4	10	RR 0.49 (0.32 to 0.74)	Favours active treatment	RR 0.67 (0.45 to 1.02)§	35
6	Active treatment 1 v active treatment 2	29	9	18	RD -0.04 (−0.07 to −0.01)	Favours active treatment 1	RD −0.02 (−0.05 to 0.01)§	50
7	Active treatment 1 v active treatment 2	5	1	7	RR 0.27 (0.09 to 0.81)	Favours active treatment 2	RR 0.38 (0.13 to 1.12)§	15
8	Active treatment v placebo/nothing	14	1	3	RR 0.31 (0.11 to 0.91)**	Favours active treatment	RR 0.39 (0.13 to 1.12)§	12
9	Active treatment v placebo/nothing	1	4	78	WMD 1.09 (0.48 to 1.70)	Favours active treatment	WMD 0.66 (0.05 to 1.27)	39
10	Active treatment v placebo/nothing	2	1	30	WMD 0.42 (0.14 to 0.69)	Favours active treatment	WMD 0.31 (0.03 to 0.58)	26
11	Active treatment 1 v active treatment 2	1	9	81	RR 0.55 (0.40 to 0.76)	Favours active treatment 1	RR 0.63 (0.46 to 0.87)	18
12	Active treatment 1 v active treatment 2	21	1	2	OR 0.24 (0.18 to 0.30)	Favours active treatment 1	OR 0.25 (0.19 to 0.32)	1
13	Active treatment 1 v active treatment 2	4	1	18	RD −0.17 (−0.24 to −0.10)	Favours active treatment 1	RD −0.09 (−0.21 to −0.07)	47
14	Active treatment v placebo/nothing	34	16	50	WMD −1.27 (−1.58 to −0.97)	Favours active treatment	WMD −0.79 (−1.10 to −0.49)	38
15	Active treatment v placebo/nothing	13	3	11	RR 0.62 (0.52 to 0.75)	Favours active treatment	RR 0.69 (0.58 to 0.83)	18
16	Active treatment v placebo/nothing	9	3	44	WMD 3.70 (−1.19 to 8.60)	Favours active treatment	WMD 0.69 (−4.20 to 5.59)	81
17	Active treatment v placebo/nothing	13	3	19	SMD −0.87 (−1.37 to −0.36)	Favours active treatment	SMD −0.57 (−1.08 to −0.06)	34
18	Active treatment 1 v active treatment 2	13	2	8	RR 0.85 (0.68 to 1.07)	Favours active treatment 1	RR 0.93 (0.73 to 1.17)	53
19	Active treatment v placebo/nothing	2	1	66	Peto's OR 1.51 (0.79 to 2.87)	Favours active treatment	Peto's OR 1.17 (0.61 to 2.23)	67
20	Active treatment 1 v active treatment 2	9	2	17	RR 0.77 (0.48 to 1.22)	Favours active treatment 1	RR 0.99 (0.62 to 1.57)	96
21	Active treatment v placebo/nothing	2	1	67	WMD 0.38 (−0.39 to 1.15)§	Favours placebo/nothing	WMD 0.08 (−0.69 to 0.85)	79
22	Active treatment 1 v active treatment 2	1	1	18	RR 1.13 (0.85 to 1.49)	Favours active treatment 2	RR 1.01 (0.76 to 1.33)	92
23	Active treatment v placebo/nothing	3	1	50	RR 1.15 (0.80 to 1.65)	Favours placebo/nothing	RR 1.00 (0.70 to 1.44)	100
24	Active treatment 1 v active treatment 2	13	1	1	RD −0.03 (−0.1 to 0.03)	Favours active treatment 1	RD −0.01 (−0.08 to 0.05)	67
25	Active treatment v placebo/nothing	4	1	20	OR 1.12 (0.72 to 1.73)	Favours placebo/nothing	OR 0.98 (0.64 to 1.52)	13

*"Placebo/nothing" implies that the intervention was given as an add on therapy—that is, patients in both arms received standard care.

†Calculated as participants in trials missing from meta-analysis and suspected of outcome reporting bias divided by participants in trials missing from meta-analysis and suspected of outcome reporting bias plus participants in trials with results fully reported.

‡The maximum bias bound was calculated and then added to or subtracted from the original pooled estimate to move it closer towards the null.

§Indicates loss of significance.

¶Calculated as (0.73−0.57)/(1−0.57).

**Subtotals not combined in review; subtotals combined here for this analysis.

Abbreviations: HR, hazard ratio; OR, odds ratio; RD, risk difference; RR, relative risk; SMD, standardised mean difference; WMD, weighted mean difference.

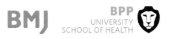

that the results are not robust to outcome reporting, the review conclusions may need to be amended. Even if the results appear robust, the reviewer should still consider the potential for bias caused by unpublished studies. An example of this approach is described in a recent tutorial paper (Dwan KM et al, submitted manuscript, 2009).

Implications for trials

Recent long term initiatives could reduce the problem of outcome reporting bias in trials. For example, registration of randomised controlled trials before initiation[17] and advance publication of detailed protocols document that the trials exist and ensure their planned outcomes are specified. Reviewers can search registries to locate unpublished trials eligible to be included in a systematic review. Trialists should be encouraged to describe all changes to the outcomes stated in the protocol.

The standardisation of outcome measures in specific clinical areas, if implemented, will reduce the potential for bias.[18 19] In our sample, 18% (51/283) of reviews contained at least one trial where it was either clear or suspected that the review primary outcome was not measured (H or I classification). This represents 31 790 (4%) of the 836 689 trial patients studied. There was a missed opportunity to measure a core outcome in these individuals because this study focused on review primary outcomes.

A recent review of trial funders' guidelines[20] has identified gaps in relation to outcome reporting bias. Current recommendations, however, state that all prespecified primary and secondary outcomes should be fully reported; any changes to the prespecified outcomes from the protocol should be explained in the final report; and the choice of outcomes included in the final report should not be based on the results.[20]

The members of the World Health Organization International Clinical Trials Registry Platform working group on the reporting of findings of clinical trials have proposed that "the findings of all clinical trials must be made publicly available."[21] From 2008, the US Food and Drug Administration Act has required that results from clinical trials are made publicly available on the internet in a "registry and results databank" within a year of completion of the trial, whether the results have been published or not.[22] US public law requires "a table of demographic and baseline characteristics of the study participants as well as a table of primary and secondary outcome measures for each arm of the clinical trial, including the results of scientifically appropriate tests of the statistical significance."

We hope that such strategies, coupled with activities to raise awareness of the issues, will reduce the prevalence of outcome reporting bias in clinical research.

Future research

Our study undoubtedly underestimates the influence of outcome reporting bias on this cohort of Cochrane reviews. Review primary outcomes are less likely to be prone to outcome reporting bias than secondary outcomes as primary outcomes are usually chosen on the basis of clinical importance—thus increasing the measurement and reporting of the outcome—or because they are the most frequently reported variables. In an associated study, a sample of trialists identified in this study was interviewed about differences between the trial protocol and the trial report in order to understand outcome reporting bias across all primary and secondary outcomes (Smyth R et al, submitted manuscript, 2009). Future work is planned to assess the prevalence and impact of outcome reporting bias across all outcomes in a cohort of reviews.

In reviews that do not include a meta-analysis, outcome reporting bias may still be operating and may affect the conclusions. Guidance is needed on how to address this problem.

The authors are grateful to the many Cochrane reviewers who collaborated in some way to make this research possible. Their input includes defining the review primary outcome of interest, forwarding trial reports from their reviews, and establishing the outcome reporting bias classification for particular trials within their reviews. We thank the Cochrane Steering Group, and Cochrane statisticians and clinicians from the University of Liverpool who have provided expert knowledge when further assistance was required. We also acknowledge the trialists who answered specific queries about the reporting of outcomes in their trials. Finally, we thank Steve Taylor for undertaking some of the assessments and Chris Braithwaite for designing the study database.

Contributors: PRW, DGA, and CG designed the study protocol and developed the classification system for assessing outcome reporting bias in trials. The study case report form was designed by JJK, SD, and PRW. JJK contacted all review authors to confirm the chosen review primary outcome for use in the study. PRW and SD identified and agreed on the review primary outcome when no contact with the review authors was achieved. Assessments of outcome reporting bias (including obtaining trial reports and completing the outcome reporting bias classifications and justifications with the guidance from the systematic reviewers) were completed by JJK, SD, and KMD. All assessment justifications were checked by PRW. All the data were entered into the database by JJK. JJK and RS contacted trialists to verify if the review primary outcome was measured and/or analysed when outcome reporting bias was suspected. JJK and KMD undertook the data analysis under the supervision of PRW. JJK prepared the initial manuscript. JJK, PRW, DGA, and KMD were all involved in the substantial revision of this manuscript. All authors commented on the final manuscript before submission. PRW is the guarantor for the project.

Funding: The Outcome Reporting Bias In Trials (ORBIT) project was funded by the Medical Research Council (grant number G0500952). The funders had no role in the study design, data collection and analysis, decision to publish, or preparation of this manuscript.

Competing interests: PRW, CG, DGA, KMD, and RS are members of the Cochrane Collaboration. JJK and SD declare no competing interests.

Ethical approval: No ethics committee opinion was required for this study.

Provenance and peer review: Not commissioned; externally peer reviewed.

1   Williamson PR and Gamble C. Identification and impact of outcome selection bias in meta-analysis. *Stat Med* 2005;24:1547-61.
2   Hahn S, Williamson PR, Hutton JL, Garner P, Flynn EV. Assessing the potential for bias in meta-analysis due to selective reporting of subgroup analyses within studies. *Stat Med* 2000;19:3325-36.
3   Moreno SG, Sutton AJ, Turner EH, Abrams KR, Cooper NJ, Palmer TM, et al. Novel methods to deal with publication biases: secondary analysis of antidepressant trials in the FDA trial registry database and related trial publications. *BMJ* 2009;339:b2981.
4   Higgins JPT, Green S, eds. *Cochrane handbook for systematic reviews of interventions: version 5.0.1* . The Cochrane Collaboration, 2008.
5   Hutton JL, Williamson PR. Bias in meta-analysis due to outcome variable selection within studies. *Appl Stat* 2000;49:359-70.
6   Dwan K, Altman DG, Arnaiz JA, Bloom J, Chan A, et al. Systematic review of the empirical evidence of study publication bias and outcome reporting bias. *PloS ONE* 2008;3:e3081.
7   Egger M, Davey Smith G, Altman DG. *Systematic reviews in healthcare: meta-analysis in context.* 2nd ed. BMJ Books, 2001.
8   Shea B, Moher D, Graham I, Pham B, Tugwell P. A comparison of the quality of Cochrane reviews and systematic reviews published in paper-based journals. *Eval Health Prof* 2002;25:116-29.
9   Moher D, Tetzlaff J, Tricco AC, Sampson M, Altman DG. Epidemiology and reporting characteristics of systematic reviews. *PLoS Med* 2007;4:e78.
10   Clarke MJ, Hopewell S, Juszczak E, Eisinga A, Kjeldstrom M. Compression stockings for preventing deep vein thrombosis in airline passengers. *Cochrane Database Syst Rev* 2006;(2):CD004002.
11   Alderson P, Bunn F, Lefebvre C, Li Wan Po A, Li L, Roberts I, et al. Human albumin solution for resuscitation and volume expansion in critically ill patients. *Cochrane Database Syst Rev* 2004;(4):CD001208.
12   Altman DG. Diagnostic tests. In: Altman DG, Machin D, Bryant TN, Gardner MJ, eds. *Statistics with confidence* . 2nd ed. BMJ Books, 2000.
13   Williamson PR, Gamble C. Application and investigation of a bound for outcome reporting bias. *Trials* 2007;8:9.
14   Copas J, Jackson D. A bound for publication bias based on the fraction of unpublished studies. *Biometrics* 2004;60:146-53.
15   Chan A, Altman D. Identifying outcome reporting bias in randomised trials on PubMed: review of publications and survey of authors. *BMJ* 2005;330:753.

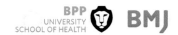

16   Furukawa TA, Watanabe N, Omori IM, Montori VM, Guyatt GH. Association between unreported outcomes and effect size estimates in Cochrane meta-analyses. *JAMA* 2007;297:468-70.

17   World Health Organization. *World Health Organization international clinical trials registry platform: unique ID assignment* . WHO, 2005.

18   Sinha I, Jones L, Smyth RL, Williamson PR. A systematic review of studies that aim to determine which outcomes to measure in clinical trials in children. *PLoS Med* 2008;5:96.

19   Clarke M. Standardising outcomes in paediatric clinical trials. *PLoS Med* 2008;5:e120.

20   Dwan K, Gamble C, Williamson PR, Altman DG. Reporting of clinical trials: a review of research funders' guidelines. *Trials* 2008;9:66.

21   Ghersi D, Clarke M, Berlin J, Gulmezoglu M, Kush R, Lumbiganon P, et al. Reporting the findings of clinical trials: a discussion. *Bull World Health Organ* 2008;86:492-3.

22   United States Code (2008) US Public Law 110-85: Food and Drug Administration Amendments Act 2007. http://frwebgate. access.gpo.gov/cgi-bin/getdoc.cgi?dbname=110_cong_public_ laws&docid=f:publ085.110.pdf.

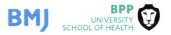

Assessing equity in systematic reviews: realising the recommendations of the Commission on Social Determinants of Health

Peter Tugwell, professor[1], Mark Petticrew, chair in public health evaluation[2], Elizabeth Kristjansson, associate professor[3], Vivian Welch, research coordinator[4], Erin Ueffing, coordinator[5], Elizabeth Waters, Jack Brockhoff chair of child public health[6], Josiane Bonnefoy, assistant professor[7], Antony Morgan, associate director[8], Emma Doohan, project manager[8], Michael P Kelly, director[8]

Department of Medicine and Institute of Population Health, University of Ottawa, Ottawa Hospital Research Institute, Ottawa, Ontario, Canada

Department of Social and Environmental Health Research, Faculty of Public Health and Policy, London School of Hygiene and Tropical Medicine, London, UK

School of Psychology, Institute of Population Health, University of Ottawa

Ottawa Hospital Research Institute, Institute of Population Health, University of Ottawa

Campbell and Cochrane Equity Methods Group, Institute of Population Health, University of Ottawa

The McCaughey Centre, Melbourne School of Population Health, University of Melbourne, Melbourne, Australia

School of Public Health, Faculty of Medicine, University of Chile, Santiago, Chile

Centre for Public Health Excellence, National Institute for Health and Clinical Excellence, London, UK

Correspondence to: P Tugwell
tugwellb@uottawa.ca

Cite this as: BMJ 2010;341:c4739

DOI: 10.1136/bmj.c4739

http://www.bmj.com/content/341/bmj.c4739

ABSTRACT

A group from the Cochrane Collaboration, Campbell Collaboration, and the World Health Organization Measurement and Evidence Knowledge Network has developed guidance on assessing health equity effects in systematic reviews of healthcare interventions. This guidance is also relevant to primary research

Background to health inequalities and inequities

The terms health inequalities and health inequities are used in different ways in different societies and by different authors.[1] We use the term inequity in preference to inequality, following the definitions articulated by Whitehead.[2] She describes health inequality as: "measurable differences in health experience and health outcomes between different population groups—according to socioeconomic status, geographical area, age, disability, gender or ethnic group." She defines health inequity as differences in opportunity for different population groups which result in, for example, unequal life chances, access to health services, nutritious food, adequate housing, etc. These differences may be measurable; they are also judged to be unfair and unjust.[2] The World Health Organization's Commission on the Social Determinants of Health (CSDH) has further defined health equity as "the absence of unfair and avoidable or remediable differences in health among social groups."[3]

The need for adequate reporting of health equity effects

The CSDH final report recognised that tackling health inequities requires a firm evidence base.[4] The Measurement and Evidence Knowledge Network of the CSDH recommended systematic reviews (which use explicit methods to summarise evidence from multiple primary studies) as one source of evidence for public policy decisions about equity.[5] In response to this recommendation, the Cochrane Collaboration and Campbell Collaboration formed a working group to investigate the necessary tailoring of methods of systematic reviews. The Cochrane Collaboration aims to help policy makers, practitioners, and the public make informed decisions about health interventions by preparing, updating, and promoting the accessibility of systematic reviews. The Campbell Collaboration has a focus on evidence related to the wider determinants of health, covering systematic reviews of the effectiveness of social and behavioural interventions in education, crime and justice, and social welfare.[6]

Process of developing recommendations

This article is the product of four years of methodology research and meetings of the Campbell and Cochrane Equity Methods Group and the Measurement and Evidence Knowledge Network, which included international leaders in systematic reviews and health equity. We held four working sessions (see box 1) with mixed methods experts, social scientists, economists, experts in systematic reviews, experts in public health and health equity, experts from low and middle income countries, and policy advisers who use systematic reviews. For the evidence base, we drew heavily on the extensive work done by the members of the Measurement and Evidence Knowledge Network, who participated in our working sessions. We developed draft guidance, with panel members reviewing the evidence and then working through each component at the meetings to allow input from all participants. Written comments were solicited from those unable to attend. After these meetings and publication of the Measurement and Evidence Knowledge Network's final report,[5] the coordinating group (the authors of the present paper) held five conference calls to revise the challenges and recommendations and prepare the present paper.

SUMMARY POINTS

- The Commission on Social Determinants for Health has recommended assessment of health equity effects of public policy decisions
- This article provides guidance on assessing equity for users and authors of systematic reviews of interventions
- Particular challenges occur in seven components of such reviews: (1) developing a logic model, (2) defining disadvantage and for whom interventions are intended, (3) deciding on appropriate study design(s), (4) identifying outcomes of interest, (5) process evaluation and understanding context, (6) analysing and presenting data, and (7) judging applicability of results
- Greater focus on health equity in systematic reviews may improve their relevance for both clinical practice and public policy making

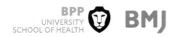

BOX 1 TIMELINE OF DEVELOPMENT OF RECOMMENDATIONS FOR REPORTING OF HEALTH EQUITY EFFECTS

- *2005*—Launch of Commission on Social Determinants of Health (CSDH)
- *2005*—Measurement and Evidence Knowledge Network (MEKN) established
- *April 2006*—First MEKN meeting (Santiago)
- *December 2006*—First Campbell and Cochrane Equity Methods Group meeting (Oslo)
- *February 2007*—Second Campbell and Cochrane Equity Methods Group meeting (Ottawa)
- *March 2007*—Second MEKN meeting (London)
- *May 2007*—Third Campbell and Cochrane Equity Methods Group meeting (London)
- *October 2007*—MEKN makes "evidence-based recommendations" to CSDH on reviews of equity
- *August 2008*—Final CSDH report
- *October 2008*—Fourth Campbell and Cochrane Equity Methods Group meeting (Freiburg)
- *2009*—MEKN and Cochrane and Campbell Equity Working Group discussions

Challenges and recommendations

We identified challenges in seven components of systematic reviews of intervention studies that address equity: (1) developing a logic model, (2) defining disadvantage and for whom interventions are intended, (3) deciding on appropriate study design(s), (4) identifying outcomes of interest, (5) process evaluation and understanding context, (6) analysing and presenting data, and (7) judging applicability of results (box 2).

1. Developing a logic model

All too often, associations of dubious relevance are found, and intermediate or surrogate outcomes are reported that have unclear relationships to the critical equity health and wellbeing endpoints. We recommend that a logic model be developed; this is a schematic that shows the hypothesised relation between interventions and their intended outcomes.[15] For example, it can describe how policy interventions may work in different populations. Logic models should address societal and contextual factors that may influence the successful implementation of an intervention.[16]

2. Defining disadvantage and for whom interventions are intended

To tackle the social determinants of health, the social structure in which the interventions occur must be understood. The Measurement and Evidence Knowledge Network report stresses key axes of social stratification (class, status, education, occupation, income and assets, gender, race, ethnicity, caste, tribes, religion, national origins, age, and residence), while the Campbell and Cochrane Equity Methods Group and the Cochrane Public Health Review Group use the acronym PROGRESS (place of residence, race/ethnicity, occupation, gender, religion, education, socioeconomic status, and social capital).[17] [18] [19] Additional PROGRESS axes such as age, sexual orientation, and disability have been proposed.[20]

These stratifiers interact, overlap, and cluster together in their implications. Their implications on inequities are dependent on context, so authors of equity oriented systematic reviews must strive to understand and explore the mediating effect of context. When details on relevant axes of social differentiation are not reported, proxy measures can be considered.

Reviewers must also assess whether the studied intervention is universal or targeted. Universal approaches aim at the whole population, but may have differential effects at different levels of the socioeconomic gradient. Targeted interventions are aimed at specific groups, usually the most disadvantaged. Both are relevant, but the reviewer must carefully assess each study's definition of disadvantage and whether the "disadvantaged" individuals are truly disadvantaged in that context. For universal interventions, the reviewer needs to analyse outcomes, where possible with data from the primary studies, by categories of disadvantage (such as high or low income) to determine whether differential effects exist. This is not relevant for targeted interventions, but these interventions also require a thoughtful approach. One concern is that stigmatisation may result from being targeted. To reduce stigmatisation (and for other ethical and practical reasons), some interventions may target groups instead of individuals (such as whole classes of pupils for school feeding programmes).

3. Deciding on the appropriate study design(s)

The *Cochrane Handbook* reflects the founding philosophy of the Cochrane Collaboration that the evidence be searched systematically: it "focuses particularly on systematic reviews of randomised trials because they are more likely to provide unbiased information than other study designs."[21] However, the recent chapters on non-randomised studies and public health and health promotion retain the emphasis on the pivotal systematic searching but extend this focus to ensure the evidence optimally reflects the context in which programmes are implemented.[22] Likewise, the Measurement and Evidence Knowledge Network report states: "Taking an evidence-based approach does not mean relying on or privileging only one kind of method, such as the randomised controlled trial. It does not mean that there is only one hierarchy of evidence, and it does not mean an epistemological rejection of subjective positions or methods."[5]

When moving beyond establishing the efficacy of drugs and vaccines, narrow inclusion criteria that focus only on randomised controlled trials risk overlooking relevant studies. This will exclude, for example, most upstream interventions that address health inequities. Most population-level interventions have not yet been subject to controlled studies, but other designs do provide an evidence base to inform practice and policy, as the tobacco pricing example in box 2 shows.[10] Systematic reviewers must therefore consider the "fitness for purpose" of criteria for evidence inclusion, considering which study designs will provide meaningful evidence to answer the review question.

4. Identifying the appropriate outcomes

The *Cochrane Handbook* recommends that systematic reviews include all outcomes likely to be meaningful to the public, practitioners, and policy makers.[21] In the case of equity-focused reviews, outcomes important to disadvantaged people should be included when available. In specifying important outcomes, attention should be given to measures of wellbeing and not simply to measures of morbidity and mortality. Although much work has been done recently to produce better measures of wellbeing,[23] [24] their application in intervention studies in the main remains

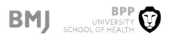

BOX 2 RECOMMENDATIONS FOR APPLYING THE EQUITY LENS TO SYSTEMATIC REVIEWS

1. Develop a logic model

- Equity oriented systematic reviews should include a logic model to elucidate hypotheses for how the intervention (whether a policy or a programme) was expected to work, and how factors associated with disadvantage (social stratification) might interact with the hypothesised mechanisms of action. Reviews should incorporate input from relevant stakeholders in defining the research question(s) and developing the logic model.
- *Example*—Logic models were developed by the Canadian Collaboration for Immigrant and Refugee Health to guide systematic reviews on interventions for immigrants and refugees.[7]

2. Define disadvantage and for whom interventions are intended

- Equity oriented systematic reviews should define population selection criteria based on the question being asked. The reviewer must consider whether a group is truly disadvantaged in the study setting. In the case of targeted interventions, the population sample should be restricted to disadvantaged populations or settings in which most people are disadvantaged. In the case of universal interventions, the reviewer must be able to present data that are stratified by one or more axes of differentiation. When data on disadvantage are not available, proxy measures may be considered.
- *Example*—Baseline nutritional status was identified as a proxy for socioeconomic disadvantage in a Campbell-Cochrane systematic review of a school feeding programme.[8]

3. Decide on the appropriate study design(s)

- Equity oriented systematic reviews should define selection criteria for study designs according to their "fitness for purpose" rather than following an evidence hierarchy.[9] The rationale for the fitness for purpose should be clearly stated and explained.
- *Example*—A systematic review of the effects of tobacco pricing on smoking behaviour did not find controlled trials but did find informative observational studies. Nine of 42 studies examined aspects of equity (such as lower versus higher income smokers, ethnicity): these suggested that pricing might have a greater effect in people with lower incomes.[10] This observational evidence base is informative about the differential effects of a major tobacco control intervention, whereas reviewing the evidence from randomised controlled trials alone would produce an "empty review"—a review with little to say about the policies' effects.

4. Identify the appropriate outcomes

- Equity oriented systematic review outcomes should be chosen based on importance and relevance of outcomes across "PROGRESS+" categories (place of residence, race/ethnicity, occupation, gender, religion, education, socioeconomic status, and social capital—plus age, sexual orientation, and disability).
- *Example*—Including "Return to work" as an outcome after tuberculosis treatment might not be meaningful to a person who has little chance of employment because of social disadvantage.

5. Evaluate processes and understand context

- In equity oriented systematic reviews, a process evaluation should be undertaken, using qualitative methods to assess why, how, when, and under what circumstances an intervention is most likely to be effective. This requires extracting sufficient information from primary studies, and possibly obtaining additional grey literature on the intervention. Furthermore, systematic reviews could include additional historical and contemporary material to enrich an analysis of contextual factors that may enhance or limit the effectiveness of the intervention.
- *Example*—In school feeding programmes, was the energy value of the food supplements sufficient to change outcomes?[8]

6. Analyse and present the data

- Equity oriented systematic reviews should analyse data on gaps, gradients, and targeted interventions based on the fitness for purpose of the summary measure and availability of data (see Evans et al[11] for a thorough discussion of gap and gradient analysis). Where possible, both relative and absolute measures should be presented.[12]
- *Example*—The harvest plot can be used to analyse the presence of gradients in effect size from complex and diverse studies.[13]

7. Discuss applicability of findings

- Equity oriented systematic reviews should discuss the applicability, transferability, and external validity of findings according to accepted criteria as well as consider context (such as using theory and judgment). Thorough attention to understanding context and process evaluation will aid judgments about applicability.
- *Example*—A Cochrane review assessing the equity implications of training lay health workers concluded that, even though 32 of 48 studies were conducted in high income countries, their findings might well be applicable to lower income countries more generally because the findings were consistent across all settings.[14]

---

atheoretical. Given the complex nature of wellbeing, the Measurement and Evidence Knowledge Network report calls for reviewers to take a more robust approach to the conceptualisation of it and its associated constructs (such as quality of life, social cohesion, and community integration) so that important links between wellbeing and physical outcomes can be made explicit and more easily understood.[25]

Intermediate outcomes also may be appropriate, but only insofar as they predict important health outcomes,[26] and this link should be shown in the logic model (No 1 above); data on adverse effects should always be included where available.

5. Process evaluation and understanding context

Another challenge is ensuring appropriate assessments of process and implementation and of wider contextual issues that could explain the study findings.

Process evaluation assesses the intervention's quality and any interaction with disadvantage. It elucidates how the intervention or programme was delivered, the mechanisms of effect, for whom it worked, in which respects, and under what circumstances.[21] Diverse methods are available to conduct a process evaluation, including structured checklists and qualitative analysis of the context and quality of the intervention as delivered. The fidelity of an intervention describes the extent to which the programme was delivered as planned, and whether the plans were sufficient to achieve the desired outcomes. The population to whom the intervention is actually delivered is also important, since the failure of programmes to reach the poorest in society is well documented.[27]

Understanding context—The context within which a study is undertaken is vital to effectiveness; changes in the wider economic context (such as recession) can override the impact of smaller scale interventions (such as community kitchens). Furthermore, intervention effectiveness may differ beyond the contexts in which the intervention was originally developed. Thus, reviewers should always carefully extract, synthesise, and discuss evidence on the context's impact on effectiveness and implications for transferring the intervention to other settings. However, in bringing different sources of evidence together, they must ensure that the different study designs are clearly linked with the appropriate research question articulated in the study's protocol. In this instance, process evaluations will not be competing with randomised controlled trials (from a hierarchical point of view) but can be assessed against the same broad principles of evidence based public health, including transparency of approach and relevance or applicability to the context of the population being studied.

6. Data analysis and presentation

Equity oriented reviews need to present evidence on outcomes in disadvantaged populations. The Measurement and Evidence Knowledge Network report reviews three ways in which health inequities are conventionally described— health disadvantage, health gaps, and health gradients.[5] Health disadvantage focuses on differences between distinct segments of the population or between societies. The health gaps approach focuses on the differences between the most disadvantaged and other groups (often the least disadvantaged). The health gradient approach addresses

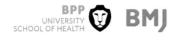

health differences that exist across the whole population spectrum—that is, it focuses on systematically patterned gradients in health inequalities. The Measurement and Evidence Knowledge Network focused on the gradient approach because it considered a society-wide approach to health inequities.

The choice of summary measure for gradient and gap analysis and presentation in systematic reviews needs to fit the research question and be comprehensible and useable for the target audience. Subgroup comparisons should be specified a priori.[21] Analysis needs to consider that disadvantaged people may be under-represented in the primary studies.[27]

7. Applicability of findings

The key component of applicability is the transferability of findings: will effectiveness in controlled conditions transfer to real world settings,[28] how much has cultural or political context shaped the original studies' designs and their subsequent interpretation,[5] and will interventions that are effective in one setting work in different contexts? Thus, applicability relates to the context within which the primary data were collected and the setting to which they will be extrapolated.[29] Conditional cash transfers are one example: they worked well in Latin America, where there is adequate infrastructure, but have failed in sub-Saharan Africa.[30]

Conclusions

In this article we provide guidance to assist authors conducting and writing equity oriented systematic reviews, editors and reviewers considering such articles for publication, and readers critically appraising published articles.

The strengths of our approach are inclusiveness (by enabling geographical, methodological, and disciplinary diversity) and assessment of the feasibility of the guidance using published systematic reviews as case studies. It also places the focus strongly on the quality of primary studies, and on extending the range of information to be extracted from them. This requires a paradigm shift in the generation and synthesis of evidence.

The limitations of our approach include the focus on Cochrane and Campbell reviews, which comprise only 20% of published systematic reviews.[31] The selection of participants in the meetings was based on purposive and opportunistic invitations to individuals with expertise or specific interest in equity related methods. This was not designed to be representative, but rather to identify key issues in developing guidance. Moreover, the list of issues is not exhaustive, nor is it the final word: we intend it to stimulate methodological development, discussion, and practice in this field.

Equity focused reviews require deeper investigation of primary studies. This needs great care in extracting data on outcomes and study quality, and a deeper consideration of the implementation theory, process, and context. Although these data are not always available to the systematic reviewer, it is essential to seek them, and to ask that authors of primary studies report them.

We acknowledge the contributions of participants in the equity meetings in Oslo, Ottawa, Dublin, Vancouver, and London (listed at www.equity.cochrane.org). We also thank Marion Doull, Ronald Labonte, Johan Mackenbach, Jessie McGowan, Andy Oxman, and Helen Roberts for their valuable comments on drafts of our manuscript.

Contributors: PT initiated the paper. All authors contributed to the development of the manuscript. All authors made significant contributions to a series of drafts of the manuscript, and all saw and approved the final version. PT had final responsibility for the decision to submit for publication; he is the guarantor for the article. There were no professional medical writers involved in this paper.

Funding: PT and VW have support from the Canadian Agency for Drugs and Technology for Health (CADTH) for the submitted work; the Campbell and Cochrane Equity Methods Group is funded by the Canadian Institutes of Health Research (CIHR); PT is funded by a Canadian Research Chair Tier 1 Award. VW was supported by a CIHR doctoral award. None of the funders had input or influence on the content or conclusions of this paper; the final decision to publish rested with the authors and the guarantor, PT.

Competing interests: PT and MP are joint convenors of the Campbell and Cochrane Equity Methods Group; EU is the salaried coordinator. VW is a research coordinator with the Methods Group. JB, AM, and MPK were members of the Measurement and Evidence Knowledge Network of the Commission for Social Determinants of Health, and ED was a project manager on the same knowledge network. EW is the coordinating editor of the Cochrane Public Health Review Group. All authors have completed the Unified Competing Interest form at http://www.icmje.org/coi_disclosure.pdf (available on request from the corresponding author) and declare that (1) PT and VW have support from the Canadian Agency for Drugs and Technology for Health (CADTH) for the submitted work; the Campbell and Cochrane Equity Methods Group is funded by the Canadian Institutes of Health Research (CIHR); PT is funded by a Canadian research chair tier 1 award; VW was supported by a CIHR doctoral award; (2) the authors have no relationships with companies that might have an interest in the submitted work in the previous 3 years; (3) their spouses, partners, or children have no financial relationships that may be relevant to the submitted work; and (4) the authors have no non-financial interests beyond those stated above that may be relevant to the submitted work.

Provenance and peer review: Not commissioned; externally peer reviewed.

1   Leon DA, Walt G, Gilson L. Recent advances: international perspectives on health inequalities and policy. BMJ 2001;322:591-4.
2   Whitehead M. The concepts and principles of equity and health. Int J Health Serv 1992;22:429-45.
3   Solar O, Irwin A. Towards a conceptual framework for analysis and action on the social determinants of health. WHO, Commission on Social Determinants of Health, 2007.
4   Commission on Social Determinants of Health. Final report. Closing the gap in a generation: health equity through action on the social determinants of health. CSDH, 2008. http://whqlibdoc.who.int/publications/2008/9789241563703_eng.pdf
5   Kelly MP, Morgan A, Bonnefoy J, Butt J, Bergman V. The social determinants of health: developing an evidence base for political action. Final report to World Health Organization Commission on the Social Determinants of Health from Measurement and Evidence Knowledge Network. 2007. www.who.int/social_determinants/resources/mekn_report_100ct07.pdf.
6   Davies P, Boruch R. The Campbell Collaboration. Does for public policy what Cochrane does for health. BMJ 2001;323:294-5.
7   Tugwell P, Pottie K, Welch V, Ueffing E, Chambers A, Feightner J. Evaluation of evidence-based literature and formation of recommendations for the Clinical Preventive Guidelines for Immigrants and Refugees in Canada. CMAJ 2010, doi:10.1503/cmaj.090289.
8   Kristjansson EA, Robinson V, Petticrew M, MacDonald B, Krasevec J, Janzen L, et al. School feeding for improving the physical and psychosocial health of disadvantaged elementary school children. Cochrane Database Syst Rev 2007;1:CD004676.
9   Petticrew M, Roberts H. Evidence, hierarchies, and typologies: horses for courses. J Epidemiol Community Health 2003;57:527-9.
10 Thomas S, Fayter D, Misso K, Ogilvie D, Petticrew M, Sowden A, et al. Population tobacco control interventions and their effects on social inequalities in smoking: systematic review. Tob Control 2008;17:230-7.
11 Evans T, Whitehead M, Diderichsen F, Bhuiya A, Wirth M, eds. Challenging inequities in health: from ethics to action. Oxford University Press, 2001.
12 Carling CL, Kristoffersen DT, Montori VM, Herrin J, Schunemann HJ, Treweek S, et al. The effect of alternative summary statistics for communicating risk reduction on decisions about taking statins: a randomized trial. PLoS Med 2009;6:e1000134.
13 Lewin SA, Dick J, Pond P, Zwarenstein M, Aja G, van Wyk BE, et al. Lay health workers in primary and community health care. Cochrane Database Syst Rev 2005;1:CD004015.
14 Ogilvie D, Fayter D, Petticrew M, Sowden A, Thomas S, Whitehead W, et al. The harvest plot: A method for synthesising evidence about the differential effects of interventions. BMC Med Res Methodol 2008;8:8.
15 Harris RP, Helfand M, Woolf SH, Lohr KN, Mulrow CD, Teutsch SM, et al. Current methods of the US Preventive Services Task Force: a review of the process. Am J Prev Med 2001;20(suppl 3):21-35S.
16 Baxter S, Killoran A, Kelly MP, Goyder E. Synthesising diverse evidence: the use of primary qualitative data analysis methods and logic models in public health reviews. Public Health 2010;124:99-106.
17 Evans T, Brown H. Road traffic crashes: operationalizing equity in the context of health sector reform. Inj Control Saf Promot 2003;10:11-2.

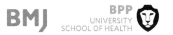

18 Tugwell P, Maxwell L, Welch V, Kristjansson E, Petticrew M, Wells G, et al. Is health equity considered in systematic reviews of the Cochrane Musculoskeletal Group? *Arthritis Rheum* 2008;59:1603-10.

19 Jackson N. *Systematic reviews of health promotion and public health interventions handbook* . Deakin University, Australian Department of Health and Aging, 2008. http://ph.cochrane.org/sites/ph.cochrane.org/files/uploads/HPPH_systematic_review_handbook.pdf.

20 Oliver S, Kavanagh J, Caird J, Lorenc T, Oliver K, Harden A, et al. *Health promotion, inequalities and young people's health. A systematic review of research*. EPPI-Centre, 2008. http://eppi.ioe.ac.uk/cms/LinkClick.px?fileticket=lsYdLJP8gBI%3d&tabid=2412&mid=4471&language=en-US.

21 Higgins JPT, Green S, eds. *Cochrane handbook for systematic reviews of interventions*. Version 5.0.1. 2008. www.cochrane-handbook.org.

22 Armstrong R, Waters E, Doyle J. Reviews in public health and health promotion. In: Higgins JPT, Green S, eds. *Cochrane handbook for systematic reviews of interventions*. Version 5.0.1. 2008. www.cochrane-handbook.org.

23 Friedli L. *Mental health, resilience and inequalities*. World Health Organization, 2009.

24 Korkeila J, Lehtinen V, Bijl R, Dalgard OS, Kovess V, Morgan A, et al. Establishing a set of mental health indicators for Europe. *Scand J Public Health* 2003;31:451-9.

25 Boers M, Brooks P, Strand CV, Tugwell P. The OMERACT filter for outcome measures in rheumatology. *J Rheumatol* 1998;25:198-9.

26 Lassere MN, Johnson KR, Boers M, Tugwell P, Brooks P, Simon L, et al. Definitions and validation criteria for biomarkers and surrogate endpoints: development and testing of a quantitative hierarchical levels of evidence schema. *J Rheumatol* 2007;34:607-15.

27 Gwatkin DR. How well do health programmes reach the poor? *Lancet* 2003;361:540-1.

28 Tugwell P, de Savigny D, Hawker G, Robinson V. Applying clinical epidemiological methods to health equity: the equity effectiveness loop. *BMJ* 2006;332:358-61.

29 Dans AL, Dans LF, Guyatt GH, Richardson S. Users' guides to the medical literature: XIV. How to decide on the applicability of clinical trial results to your patient. Evidence-Based Medicine Working Group. *JAMA* 1998;279:545-9.

30 Lagarde M, Haines A, Palmer N. The impact of conditional cash transfers on health outcomes and use of health services in low and middle income countries. *Cochrane Database Syst Rev* 2009;4:CD008137.

31 Moher D, Tetzlaff J, Tricco AC, Sampson M, Altman DG. Epidemiology and reporting characteristics of systematic reviews. *PLoS Med* 2007;4:e78.

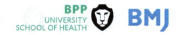

Prognosis and prognostic research: what, why, and how?

Karel G M Moons, professor of clinical epidemiology[1], Patrick Royston, senior statistician[2], Yvonne Vergouwe, assistant professor of clinical epidemiology[1], Diederick E Grobbee, professor of clinical epidemiology[1], Douglas G Altman, professor of statistics in medicine[3]

[1]Julius Centre for Health Sciences and Primary Care, University Medical Centre Utrecht, Utrecht, Netherlands

[2]MRC Clinical Trials Unit, London NW1 2DA

[3]Centre for Statistics in Medicine, University of Oxford, Oxford OX2 6UD

Correspondence to: K G M Moons
k.g.m.moons@umcutrecht.nl

Cite this as: BMJ 2009;338:b375

DOI: 10.1136/bmj.b375

http://www.bmj.com/content/338/bmj.b375

ABSTRACT

Doctors have little specific research to draw on when predicting outcome. In this first article in a series Karel Moons and colleagues explain why research into prognosis is important and how to design such research

This article is the first in a series of four aiming to provide an accessible overview of the principles and methods of prognostic researchHippocrates included prognosis as a principal concept of medicine.[1] Nevertheless, principles and methods of prognostic research have received limited attention, especially compared with therapeutic and aetiological research. This article is the first in a series of four aiming to provide an accessible overview of these principles and methods. Our focus is on prognostic studies aimed at predicting outcomes from multiple variables rather than on studies investigating whether a single variable (such as a tumour or other biomarker) may be prognostic. Here we consider the principles of prognosis and multivariable prognostic studies and the reasons for and settings in which multivariable prognostic models are developed and used. The other articles in the series will focus on the development of multivariable prognostic models,[2] their validation,[3] and the application and impact of prognostic models in practice.[4]

What is prognosis?

Prognosis simply means foreseeing, predicting, or estimating the probability or risk of future conditions; familiar examples are weather and economic forecasts. In medicine, prognosis commonly relates to the probability or risk of an individual developing a particular state of health (an outcome) over a specific time, based on his or her clinical and non-clinical profile. Outcomes are often specific events, such as death or complications, but they may also be quantities, such as disease progression, (changes in) pain, or quality of life.

In medical textbooks, however, prognosis commonly refers to the expected course of an illness. This terminology is too general and has limited utility in practice. Doctors do not predict the course of an illness but the course of an illness in a particular individual. Prognosis may be shaped

by a patient's age, sex, history, symptoms, signs, and other test results. Moreover, prognostication in medicine is not limited to those who are ill. Healthcare professionals, especially primary care doctors, regularly predict the future in healthy individuals—for example, using the Apgar score to determine the prognosis of newborns, cardiovascular risk profiles to predict heart disease in the general population, and prenatal testing to assess the risk that a pregnant woman will give birth to a baby with Down's syndrome.

Multivariable research

Given the variability among patients and in the aetiology, presentation, and treatment of diseases and other health states, a single predictor or variable rarely gives an adequate estimate of prognosis. Doctors—implicitly or explicitly—use multiple predictors to estimate a patient's prognosis. Prognostic studies therefore need to use a multivariable approach in design and analysis to determine the important predictors of the studied outcomes and to provide outcome probabilities for different combinations of predictors, or to provide tools to estimate such probabilities. These tools are commonly called prognostic models, prediction models, prediction rules, or risk scores.[5 6 7 8 9 10 11 12 13 14] They enable care providers to use combinations of predictor values to estimate an absolute risk or probability that an outcome will occur in an individual. A multivariable approach also enables researchers to investigate whether specific prognostic factors or markers that are, say, more invasive or costly to measure, have worthwhile added predictive value beyond cheap or simply obtained predictors—for example, from patient history or physical examination. Nonetheless, many prognostic studies still consider a single rather than multiple predictors.[15]

Use of prognostic models

Medical prognostication and prognostic models are used in various settings and for various reasons. The main reasons are to inform individuals about the future course of their illness (or their risk of developing illness) and to guide doctors and patients in joint decisions on further treatment, if any. For example, modifications of the Framingham cardiovascular risk score[16] are widely used in primary care to determine the indication for cholesterol lowering and antihypertensive drugs. Examples from secondary care include use of the Nottingham prognostic index to estimate the long term risk of cancer recurrence or death in breast cancer patients,[17] the acute physiology and chronic health evaluation (APACHE) score and simplified acute physiology score (SAPS) to predict hospital mortality in critically ill patients,[18 19] and models for predicting postoperative nausea and vomiting.[20 21]

Another reason for prognostication and use of prognostic models is to select relevant patients for therapeutic research. For example, researchers used a previously validated prognostic model to select women with an

SUMMARY POINTS

- Prognosis is estimating the risk of future outcomes in individuals based on their clinical and non-clinical characteristics
- Predicting outcomes is not synonymous with explaining their cause
- Prognostic studies require a multivariable approach to design and analysis
- The best design to address prognostic questions is a cohort study

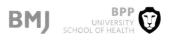

increased risk of developing cancer for a randomised trial of tamoxifen to prevent breast cancer.[22] Another randomised trial on the efficacy of radiotherapy after breast conserving resection used a prognostic model to select patients with a low risk of cancer recurrence.[23]

Prognostic models are also used to compare differences in performance between hospitals. For example, the clinical risk index for babies (CRIB) was originally developed to compare performance and mortality among neonatal intensive care units.[24] More recently Jarman et al developed a model to predict the hospital standardised mortality ratio to explain differences between English hospitals.[25]

Differences from aetiological research

Although there are clear similarities in the design and analysis of prognostic and aetiological studies, predicting outcomes is not synonymous with explaining their cause.[26][27] In aetiological research, the mission is to explain whether an outcome can reliably be attributed to a particular risk factor, with adjustment for other causal factors (confounders) using a multivariable approach. In prognostic research the mission is to use multiple variables to predict, as accurately as possible, the risk of future outcomes. Although a prognostic model may be used to provide insight into causality or pathophysiology of the studied outcome, that is neither an aim nor a requirement. All variables potentially associated with the outcome, not necessarily causally, can be considered in a prognostic study. Every causal factor is a predictor—albeit sometimes a weak one—but not every predictor is a cause. Nice examples of predictive but non-causal factors used in everyday practice are skin colour in the Apgar score and tumour markers as predictors of cancer progression or recurrence. Both are surrogates for obvious causal factors that are more difficult to measure.

Furthermore, to guide prognostication in individuals, analysis and reporting of prognostic studies should focus on absolute risk estimates of outcomes given combinations of predictor values. Relative risk estimates (eg odds ratio, risk ratio, or hazard ratio) have no direct meaning or relevance to prognostication in practice. In prediction research, relative risks are used only to obtain an absolute probability of the outcome for an individual, as we will show in our second article.[2] In contrast, aetiological and therapeutic studies commonly focus on relative risks—for example, the risk of an outcome in presence of a causal factor relative to the risk in its absence. Also, the calibration and discrimination of a multivariable model are highly relevant to prognostic research but meaningless in aetiological research.

How to study prognosis?

Building on previous guidelines[8][10][14][28][29] we distinguish three major steps in multivariable prognostic research that are also followed in the other articles in this series[2][3][4]: developing the prognostic model, validating its performance in new patients, and studying its clinical impact (box). We focus here on the non-statistical characteristics of a multivariable study aimed at developing a prognostic model. The statistical aspects of developing a model are covered in our second article.[2]

Objective

The main objective of a prognostic study is to determine the probability of the specified outcome with different combinations of predictors in a well defined population.

BOX 1 CONSECUTIVE PHASES IN MULTIVARIABLE PROGNOSTIC RESEARCH

- *Development studies*—Development of a multivariable prognostic model, including identification of the important predictors, assigning relative weights to each predictor, and estimating the model's predictive performance through calibration and discrimination and its potential for optimism using internal validation techniques, and, if necessary, adjusting the model for overfitting[2]
- *Validation studies*—Validating or testing the model's predictive performance (eg, calibration and discrimination) in new participants. This can be narrow (in participants from the same institution measured in the same manner by the same researchers though at a later time, or in another single institution by different researchers using perhaps slightly different definitions and data collection methods) or broad (participants obtained from various other institutions or using wider inclusion criteria)[3][4]
- *Impact studies*—Quantifying whether the use of a prognostic model by practising doctors truly improves their decision making and ultimately patient outcome, which can again be done narrowly or broadly.

Study sample

The study sample includes people at risk of developing the outcome of interest, defined by the presence of a particular condition (for example, an illness, undergoing surgery, or being pregnant).

Study design

The best design to answer prognostic questions is a cohort study. A prospective study is preferable as it enables optimal measurement of predictors and outcome (see below). Studies using cohorts already assembled for other reasons allow longer follow-up times but usually at the expense of poorer data. Unfortunately, the prognostic literature is dominated by retrospective studies. Case-control studies are sometimes used for prognostic analysis, but they do not automatically allow estimation of absolute risks because cases and controls are often sampled from a source population of unknown size. Since investigators are free to choose the ratio of cases and controls, the absolute outcome risks can be manipulated.[30] An exception is a case-control study nested in a cohort of known size.[31]

Data from randomised trials of treatment can also be used to study prognosis. When the treatment is ineffective (relative risk=1.0), the intervention and comparison group can simply be combined to study baseline prognosis. If the treatment is effective the groups can be combined, but the treatment variable should then be included as a separate predictor in the multivariable model. Here treatments are studied on their independent predictive effect and not on their therapeutic or preventive effects. However, prognostic models obtained from randomised trial data may have restricted generalisability because of strict eligibility criteria for the trial, low recruitment levels, or large numbers refusing consent.

Predictors

Candidate predictors can be obtained from patient demographics, clinical history, physical examination, disease characteristics, test results, and previous treatment. Prognostic studies may focus on a cohort of patients who

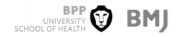

have not (yet) received prognosis modifying treatments—that is, to study the natural course or baseline prognosis of patients with that condition. They can also examine predictors of prognosis in patients who have received treatments.

Studied predictors should be clearly defined, standardised, and reproducible to enhance generalisability and application of study results to practice.[32] Predictors requiring subjective interpretation, such as imaging test results, are of particular concern in this context because there is a risk of studying the predictive ability of the observer rather than that of the predictors. Also, predictors should be measured using methods applicable—or potentially applicable—to daily practice. Specialised measurement techniques may yield optimistic predictions.

As discussed above, the prognostic value of treatments can also be studied, especially when randomised trials are used. However, caution is needed in including treatments as prognostic factors when data are observational. Indications for treatment and treatment administration are often not standardised in observational studies and confounding by indication could lead to bias and large variation in the (type of) administered treatments.[33] Moreover, in many circumstances the predictive effect of treatments is small compared with that of other important prognostic variables such as age, sex, and disease stage.

Finally, of course, studies should include only predictors that will be available at the time when the model is intended to be used.[34] If the aim is to predict a patient's prognosis at the time of diagnosis, for example, predictors that will not be known until actual treatment has started are of little value.

Outcome

Preferably, prognostic studies should focus on outcomes that are relevant to patients, such as occurrence or remission of disease, death, complications, tumour growth, pain, treatment response, or quality of life. Surrogate or intermediate outcomes, such as hospital stay or physiological measurements, are unhelpful unless they have a clear causal relation to relevant patient outcomes, such as CD4 counts instead of development of AIDS or death in HIV studies. The period over which the outcome is studied and the methods of measurement should be clearly defined. Finally, outcomes should be measured without knowledge of the predictors under study to prevent bias, particularly if measurement requires observer interpretation. Blinding is not necessary when the outcome is all cause mortality. But if the outcome is cause specific mortality, knowledge of the predictors might influence assessment of outcomes (and vice versa in retrospective studies where predictors are documented after the outcome was assessed).

Required number of patients

The multivariable character of prognostic research makes it difficult to estimate the required sample size. There are no straightforward methods for this. When the number of predictors is much larger than the number of outcome events, there is a risk of overestimating the predictive performance of the model. Ideally, prognostic studies require at least several hundred outcome events. Various studies have suggested that for each candidate predictor studied at least 10 events are required,[6][8][35][36] although a recent study showed that this number could be lower in certain circumstances.[37]

Validation and application of prognostic models

Formally developed and validated prognostic models are often used in weather forecasting and economics (with varying success), but not in medicine. There may be several reasons for this. Firstly, prognostic models are often too complex for daily use in clinical settings without computer support. The introduction of computerised patient records will clearly enhance not only the development and validation of models in research settings but also facilitate their application in routine care.[38][39] Secondly, because many prognostic models have not been validated in other populations, clinicians may (and perhaps should) not trust probabilities provided by these models.[14][40][41][42]

Finally, clinicians often do not know how to use predicted probabilities in their decision making. Validation studies are scarce, but even fewer models are tested for their ability to change clinicians' decisions, let alone to change patient outcome.[14] We support the view that no prediction model should be implemented in practice until, at a minimum, its performance has been validated in new individuals.[6][7][8][9][10][12][14][29][43][44] The third article in this series discusses why validation studies are important and how to design and interpret them.[3]

Validation studies are particularly important if a prediction model is to be used in individuals who were not represented in the development study—for example, when transporting a model from secondary to primary care or from adults to children, which seems a form of extrapolation rather than validation.[43][45] We will discuss this further in the fourth article in the series, as well as how to update existing models to other circumstances.[4]

We stress that prediction models are not meant to take over the job of the doctor.[7][40][41][46] They are intended to help doctors make decisions by providing more objective estimates of probability as a supplement to other relevant clinical information. Furthermore, they improve understanding of the determinants of the course and outcome of patients with a particular disease.

Funding: KGMM, YV, and DEG are supported by the Netherlands Organisation for Scientific Research (ZON-MW 917.46.360). PR is supported by the UK Medical Research Council (U.1228.06.001.00002.01). DGA is supported by Cancer Research UK.

Contributors: The four articles in the series were conceived and planned by DGA, KGMM, PR, and YV. KGMM wrote the first draft of this article. All the authors contributed to subsequent revisions.

Competing interests: None declared.

Provenance and peer review: Not commissioned; externally peer reviewed.

1   Hippocrates. On airs, waters and places. In: Adams F, ed. *The genuine works of Hippocrates* . Baltimore: Wilkins and Wilkins, 1939.
2   Royston P, Moons KG, Altman DG, Vergouwe Y. Prognosis and prognostic research: developing a prognostic model. *BMJ* 2009;338:b604.
3   Altman DG, Vergouwe Y, Royston P, Moons KG. Prognosis and prognostic research: Validating a prognostic model. *BMJ* 2009;338:b605.
4   Moons KG, Altman DG, Vergouwe Y, Royston P. Prognosis and prognostic research: Application and impact of prognostic models in clinical practice. *BMJ* 2009;338:b606.
5   Laupacis A, Wells G, Richardson WS, Tugwell P. Users' guides to the medical literature. V. How to use an article about prognosis. *JAMA* 1994;272:234-7.
6   Harrell FE, Lee KL, Mark DB. Multivariable prognostic models: issues in developing models, evaluating assumptions and adequacy, and measuring and reducing errors. *Stat Med* 1996;15:361-87.
7   Braitman LE, Davidoff F. Predicting clinical states in individual patients. *Ann Intern Med* 1996;125:406-12.
8   Laupacis A, Sekar N, Stiell IG. Clinical prediction rules. A review and suggested modifications of methodological standards. *JAMA* 1997;277:488-94.
9   Randolph AG, Guyatt GH, Calvin JE, Doig DVM, Richardson WS. Understanding articles describing clinical prediction tools. *Crit Care Med* 1998;26:1603-12.

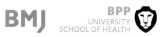

10 Altman DG, Royston P. What do we mean by validating a prognostic model? *Stat Med* 2000;19:453-73.

11 Concato J. Challenges in prognostic analysis. *Cancer* 2001;91:1607-14.

12 Steyerberg EW, Borsboom GJ, van Houwelingen HC, Eijkemans MJ, Habbema JD. Validation and updating of predictive logistic regression models: a study on sample size and shrinkage. *Stat Med* 2004;23:2567-86.

13 McShane LM, Altman DG, Sauerbrei W, Taube SE, Gion M, Clark GM. Reporting recommendations for tumour marker prognostic studies (REMARK). *Br J Cancer* 2005;93:387-91.

14 Reilly BM, Evans AT. Translating clinical research into clinical practice: impact of using prediction rules to make decisions. *Ann Intern Med* 2006;144:201-9.

15 Riley RD, Abrams KR, Sutton AJ, Lambert PC, Jones DR, Heney D, et al. Reporting of prognostic markers: current problems and development of guidelines for evidence-based practice in the future. *Br J Cancer* 2003;88:1191-8.

16 Kannel WB, McGee D, Gordon T. A general cardiovascular risk profile: the Framingham study. *Am J Cardiol* 1976;38:46-51.

17 Galea MH, Blamey RW, Elston CE, Ellis IO. The Nottingham prognostic index in primary breast cancer. *Breast Cancer Res Treat* 1992;22:207-19.

18 Knaus WA, Wagner DP, Draper EA, Zimmerman JE, Bergner M, Bastos PG, et al. The APACHE III prognostic system. Risk prediction of hospital mortality for critically ill hospitalized adults. *Chest* 1991;100:1619-36.

19 Le Gall JR, Lemeshow S, Saulnier F. A new simplified acute physiology score (SAPS II) based on a European/North American multicenter study. *JAMA* 1993;270:2957-63.

20 Van den Bosch JE, Moons KG, Bonsel GJ, Kalkman CJ. Does measurement of preoperative anxiety have added value for predicting postoperative nausea and vomiting? *Anesth Analg* 2005;100:1525-32.

21 Apfel CC, Laara E, Koivuranta M, Greim CA, Roewer N. A simplified risk score for predicting postoperative nausea and vomiting: conclusions from cross-validations between two centers. *Anesthesiol* 1999;91:693-700.

22 Fisher B, Costantino JP, Wickerham DL, Redmond CK, Kavanah M, Cronin WM, et al. Tamoxifen for prevention of breast cancer: report of the national surgical adjuvant breast and bowel project P-1 study. *J Natl Cancer Inst* 1998;90:1371-88.

23 Winzer KJ, Sauer R, Sauerbrei W, Schneller E, Jaeger W, Braun M, et al. Radiation therapy after breast-conserving surgery; first results of a randomised clinical trial in patients with low risk of recurrence. *Eur J Cancer* 2004;40:998-1005.

24 Cockburn F CR, Gamsu HR, Greenough A, Hopkins A, International Neonatal Network. The CRIB (clinical risk index for babies) score: a tool assessing initial neonatal risk and comparing performance of neonatal intensive care units. *Lancet* 1993;342:193-8.

25 Jarman B, Gault S, Alves B, Hider A, Dolan S, Cook A, et al. Explaining differences in English hospital death rates using routinely collected data. *BMJ* 1999;318:1515-20.

26 Moons KG, Grobbee DE. Clinical epidemiology: an introduction. In: Vaccaro AR, ed. *Orthopedic Knowledge Update: 8* . Rosemont: American Academy of Orthopaedic Surgeons, 2005:109-18.

27 Brotman DJ, Walker E, Lauer MS, O'Brien RG. In search of fewer independent risk factors. *Arch Intern Med* 2005;165:138-45.

28 Wasson JH, Sox HC, Neff RK, Goldman L. Clinical prediction rules. Applications and methodological standards. *N Engl J Med* 1985;313:793-9.

29 McGinn TG, Guyatt GH, Wyer PC, Naylor CD, Stiell IG, Richardson WS. Users' guides to the medical literature: XXII: how to use articles about clinical decision rules. *JAMA* 2000;284:79-84.

30 Moons KG, van Klei W, Kalkman CJ. Preoperative risk factors of intraoperative hypothermia in major surgery under general anesthesia. *Anesth Analg* 2003;96:1843-4.

31 Biesheuvel CJ, Vergouwe Y, Oudega R, Hoes AW, Grobbee DE, Moons KG. Rehabilitation of the nested case-control design in diagnostic research. *BMC Med Res Methodol* 2008;8:48.

32 Simon R, Altman DG. Statistical aspects of prognostic factor studies in oncology. *Br J Cancer* 1994;69:979-85.

33 Grobbee DE. Confounding and indication for treatment in evaluation of drug treatment for hypertension. *BMJ* 1997;315:1151-4.

34 Walraven vC, Davis D, Forster AJ, Wells GA. Time-dependent bias was common in survival analyses published in leading clinical journals. *J Clin Epidemiol* 2004;57:672-82.

35 Concato J, Peduzzi P, Holford TR, Feinstein AR. Importance of events per independent variable in proportional hazards analysis. I. Background, goals, and general strategy. *J Clin Epidemiol* 1995;48:1495-501.

36 Peduzzi P, Concato J, Feinstein AR, Holford TR. Importance of events per independent variable in proportional hazards regression analysis. II. Accuracy and precision of regression estimates. *J Clin Epidemiol* 1995;48:1503-10.

37 Vittinghoff E, McCulloch CE. Relaxing the rule of ten events per variable in logistic and Cox regression. *Am J Epidemiol* 2007;165:710-8.

38 James BC. Making it easy to do it right. *N Engl J Med* 2001;345:991-3.

39 Kawamoto K, Houlihan CA, Balas EA, Lobach DF. Improving clinical practice using clinical decision support systems: a systematic review of trials to identify features critical to success. *BMJ* 2005;330:765.

40 Concato J, Feinstein AR, Holford TR. The risk of determining risk with multivariable models. *Ann Intern Med* 1993;118:201-10.

41 Christensen E. Prognostic models including the Child-Pugh, MELD and Mayo risk scores—where are we and where should we go? *J Hepatol* 2004;41:344-50.

42 Wyatt JC, Altman DG. Prognostic models: clinical useful or quickly forgotten? *BMJ* 1995;311:1539-41.

43 Justice AC, Covinsky KE, Berlin JA. Assessing the generalizability of prognostic information. *Ann Intern Med* 1999;130:515-24.

44 Bleeker SE, Moll HA, Steyerberg EW, Donders AR, Derksen-Lubsen G, Grobbee DE, et al. External validation is necessary in prediction research: a clinical example. *J Clin Epidemiol* 2003;56:826-32.

45 Knottnerus JA. Between iatrotropic stimulus and interiatric referral: the domain of primary care research. *J Clin Epidemiol* 2002;55:1201-6.

46 Feinstein AR. Clinical Judgment revisited: the distraction of quantitative models. *Ann Intern Med* 1994;120:799-805.

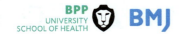

Prognosis and prognostic research: Developing a prognostic model

Patrick Royston, professor of statistics[1], Karel G M Moons, professor of clinical epidemiology[2], Douglas G Altman, professor of statistics in medicine[3], Yvonne Vergouwe, assistant professor of clinical epidemiology[2]

[1]MRC Clinical Trials Unit, London NW1 2DA

[2]Julius Centre for Health Sciences and Primary Care, University Medical Centre Utrecht, Utrecht, Netherlands

[3]Centre for Statistics in Medicine, University of Oxford, Oxford OX2 6UD

Correspondence to: P Royston pr@ctu.mrc.ac.uk

Cite this as: BMJ 2009;338:b604

DOI: 10.1136/bmj.b604

http://www.bmj.com/content/338/bmj.b604

ABSTRACT

In the second article in their series, Patrick Royston and colleagues describe different approaches to building clinical prognostic models

This article is the second in a series of four aiming to provide an accessible overview of the principles and methods of prognostic researchThe first article in this series reviewed why prognosis is important and how it is practised in different medical settings.[1] We also highlighted the difference between multivariable models used in aetiological research and those used in prognostic research and outlined the design characteristics for studies developing a prognostic model. In this article we focus on developing a multivariable prognostic model. We illustrate the statistical issues using a logistic regression model to predict the risk of a specific event. The principles largely apply to all multivariable regression methods, including models for continuous outcomes and for time to event outcomes.

The goal is to construct an accurate and discriminating prediction model from multiple variables. Models may be a complicated function of the predictors, as in weather forecasting, but in clinical applications considerations of practicality and face validity usually suggest a simple, interpretable model (as in box 1).

Surprisingly, there is no widely agreed approach to building a multivariable prognostic model from a set of candidate predictors. Katz gave a readable introduction to multivariable models,[3] and technical details are also widely available.[4 5 6] We concentrate here on a few fairly standard modelling approaches and also consider how to handle continuous predictors, such as age.

Preliminaries

We assume here that the available data are sufficiently accurate for prognosis and adequately represent the population of interest. Before starting to develop a multivariable prediction model, numerous decisions must be made that affect the model and therefore the conclusions of the research. These include:

- Selecting clinically relevant candidate predictors for possible inclusion in the model

SUMMARY POINTS

- Models with multiple variables can be developed to give accurate and discriminating predictions
- In clinical practice simpler models are more practicable
- There is no consensus on the ideal method for developing a model
- Methods to develop simple, interpretable models are described and compared

- Evaluating the quality of the data and judging what to do about missing values
- Data handling decisions
- Choosing a strategy for selecting the important variables in the final model
- Deciding how to model continuous variables
- Selecting measure(s) of model performance[5] or predictive accuracy.

Other considerations include assessing the robustness of the model to influential observations and outliers, studying possible interaction between predictors, deciding whether and how to adjust the final model for over-fitting (so called shrinkage),[5] and exploring the stability (reproducibility) of a model.[7]

Selecting candidate predictors

Studies often measure more predictors than can sensibly be used in a model, and pruning is required. Predictors already reported as prognostic would normally be candidates. Predictors that are highly correlated with others contribute little independent information and may be excluded beforehand.[5] However, predictors that are not significant in univariable analysis should not be excluded as candidates.[8 9 10]

Evaluating data quality

There are no secure rules for evaluating the quality of data. Judgment is required. In principle, data used for developing a prognostic model should be fit for purpose. Measurements of candidate predictors and outcomes should be comparable across clinicians or study centres. Predictors known to have considerable measurement error may be unsuitable because this dilutes their prognostic information.

Modern statistical techniques (such as multiple imputation) can handle data sets with missing values.[11] [12] However, all approaches make critical but essentially untestable assumptions about how the data went missing. The likely influence on the results increases with the amount of data that are missing. Missing data are seldom completely random. They are usually related, directly or indirectly, to other subject or disease characteristics, including the outcome under study. Thus exclusion of all individuals with a missing value leads not only to loss of statistical power but often to incorrect estimates of the predictive power of the model and specific predictors.[11] A complete case analysis may be sensible when few observations (say <5%) are missing.[5] If a candidate predictor has a lot of missing data it may be excluded because the problem is likely to recur.

Data handling decisions

Often, new variables need to be created (for example, diastolic and systolic blood pressure may be combined to give mean arterial pressure). For ordered categorical variables, such as stage of disease, collapsing of categories

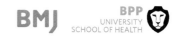

BOX 1 EXAMPLE OF A PROGNOSTIC MODEL

Risk score from a logistic regression model to predict the risk of postoperative nausea or vomiting (PONV) within the first 24 hours after surgery[2]:

Risk score= −2.28+(1.27×female sex)+(0.65×history of PONV or motion sickness)+(0.72×non-smoking)+(0.78×postoperative opioid use)

where all variables are coded 0 for no or 1 for yes.

The value −2.28 is called the intercept and the other numbers are the estimated regression coefficients for the predictors, which indicate their mutually adjusted relative contribution to the outcome risk. The regression coefficients are log(odds ratios) for a change of 1 unit in the corresponding predictor.

The predicted risk (or probability) of PONV=$1/(1+e^{-\text{risk score}})$.

Table 1 Selected predictors of 12 month survival for patients with kidney cancer. Estimated mutually adjusted regression coefficient (standard error) for three multivariable models obtained using different strategies to select variables (see text)

Predictor*	Full model	Akaike information criterion	5% significance level
WHO performance status 1 (versus 0)	0.62 (0.30)	0.55 (0.29)	0.50 (0.2)
WHO performance status 2 (versus 0)	1.69 (0.42)	1.62 (0.41)	1.55 (0.40)
Haemoglobin (g/l)	−0.45 (0.08)	−0.44 (0.08)	−0.39 (0.08)
White cell count (×10⁹/l)	0.12 (0.05)	0.13 (0.05)	0.13 (0.05)
Transformed time from diagnosis of metastatic disease to randomisation†	−0.29 (0.10)	−0.30 (0.10)	−0.27 (0.09)
Interferon treatment	−0.61 (0.27)	−0.61 (0.26)	−0.58 (0.26)
Nephrectomy	0.39 (0.29)	0.44 (0.28)	—
Female sex	−0.57 (0.29)	−0.56 (0.28)	—
Lung metastasis	−0.36 (0.28)	—	—
Age (per 10 year)	−0.07 (0.13)	—	—
Multiple sites of metastasis	−0.09 (0.36)	—	—
Intercept	6.54 (1.63)	5.70 (1.29)	4.99 (1.22)
C index	0.80 (0.02)	0.80 (0.02)	0.79 (0.02)

*We assumed linear effects of continuous predictors. Details of the distribution of each candidate predictor have been omitted to save space.
Binary variables are coded 0 for no, 1 for yes.
†Log(days from metastasis to randomisation + 1).

or a judicious choice of coding may be required. We advise against turning continuous predictors into dichotomies.[13] Keeping variables continuous is preferable since much more predictive information is retained.[14] [15]

Selecting variables

No consensus exists on the best method for selecting variables. There are two main strategies, each with variants.

In the full model approach all the candidate variables are included in the model. This model is claimed to avoid overfitting and selection bias and provide correct standard errors and P values.[5] However, as many important preliminary choices must be made and it is often impractical to include all candidates, the full model is not always easy to define.

The backward elimination approach starts with all the candidate variables. A nominal significance level, often 5%, is chosen in advance. A sequence of hypothesis tests is applied to determine whether a given variable should be removed from the model. Backward elimination is preferable to forward selection (whereby the model is built up from the best candidate predictor).[16] The choice of significance level has a major effect on the number of variables selected. A 1% level almost always results in a model with fewer variables than a 5% level. Significance levels of 10% or 15% can result in inclusion of some unimportant variables, as can the full model approach. (A variant is the Akaike information criterion,[17] a measure of model fit that includes a penalty against large models and hence attempts to reduce overfitting. For a single predictor, the criterion equates to selection at 15.7% significance.[17])

Selection of predictors by significance testing, particularly at conventional significance levels, is known to produce selection bias and optimism as a result of overfitting, meaning that the model is (too) closely adapted to the data.[5] [9] [17] Selection bias means that a regression coefficient is overestimated, because the corresponding predictor is more likely to be significant if its estimated effect is larger (perhaps by chance) rather than smaller. Overfitting leads to worse prediction in independent data; it is more likely to occur in small data sets or with weakly predictive variables. Note, however, that selected predictor variables with very small P values (say, <0.001) are much less prone to selection bias and overfitting than weak predictors with P values near the nominal significance level. Commonly, prognostic data sets include a few strong predictors and several weaker ones.

Modelling continuous predictors

Handling continuous predictors in multivariable models is important. It is unwise to assume linearity as it can lead to misinterpretation of the influence of a predictor and to inaccurate predictions in new patients.[14] See box 2 for further comments on how to handle continuous predictors in prognostic modelling.

Assessing performance

The performance of a logistic regression model may be assessed in terms of calibration and discrimination. Calibration can be investigated by plotting the observed proportions of events against the predicted risks for groups defined by ranges of individual predicted risks; a common approach is to use 10 risk groups of equal size. Ideally, if the observed proportions of events and predicted probabilities agree over the whole range of probabilities, the plot shows a 45° line (that is, the slope is 1). This plot can be accompanied by the Hosmer-Lemeshow test,[19] although the test has limited power to assess poor calibration. The overall observed and predicted event probabilities are by definition equal for the sample used to develop the model. This is not guaranteed when the model's performance is evaluated on a different sample in a validation study. As we will discuss in the next article,[18] it is more difficult to get a model to perform well in an independent sample than in the development sample.

Various statistics can summarise discrimination between individuals with and without the outcome event. The area under the receiver operating curve,[10] [20] or the equivalent c (concordance) index, is the chance that given two patients, one who will develop an event and the other who will not, the model will assign a higher probability of an event to the former. The c index for a prognostic model is typically between about 0.6 and 0.85 (higher values are seen in diagnostic settings[21]). Another measure is R^2, which for logistic regression assesses the explained variation in risk and is the square of the correlation between the observed outcome (0 or 1) and the predicted risk.[22]

Example of prognostic model for survival with kidney cancer

Between 1992 and 1997, 350 patients with metastatic renal carcinoma entered a randomised trial comparing interferon alfa with medroxyprogesterone acetate at 31 centres in the UK.[23] Here we develop a prognostic model for the (binary) outcome of death in the first year versus survived 12

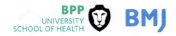

BOX 2 MODELLING CONTINUOUS PREDICTORS

Simple predictor transformations intended to detect and model non-linearity can be systematically identified using, for example, fractional polynomials, a generalisation of conventional polynomials (linear, quadratic, etc).[6] [27] Power transformations of a predictor beyond squares and cubes, including reciprocals, logarithms, and square roots are allowed. These transformations contain a single term, but to enhance flexibility can be extended to two term models (eg, terms in $\log x$ and x^2). Fractional polynomial functions can successfully model non-linear relationships found in prognostic studies. The multivariable fractional polynomial procedure is an extension to multivariable models including at least one continuous predictor,[4] [27] and combines backward elimination of weaker predictors with transformation of continuous predictors.

Restricted cubic splines are an alternative approach to modelling continuous predictors.[5] Their main advantage is their flexibility for representing a wide range of perhaps complex curve shapes. Drawbacks are the frequent occurrence of wiggles in fitted curves that may be unreal and open to misinterpretation[28] [29] and the absence of a simple description of the fitted curve.

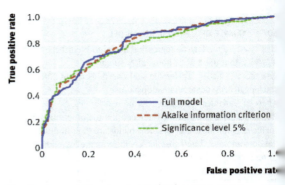

Fig 1 Receiver operating characteristic (ROC) curves for three multivariable models of survival with kidney cancer.

Table 2 Multivariable model for 12 month survival in the kidney cancer data, based on multivariable fractional polynomials for continuous predictors and selection of variables at the 5% significance level

Predictor*	Coefficient (SE)
WHO performance status 1 (versus 0)	0.55 (0.29)
WHO performance status 2 (versus 0)	1.67 (0.41)
$1/(haemoglobin/10)^2$	3.86 (0.73)
Time from diagnosis of metastatic disease to randomisation (years)	−0.55 (0.23)
Interferon treatment	−0.64 (0.26)
Intercept	−2.21 (0.52)
C index	0.78 (0.02)

Predicted risks can be calculated from the following standard formula (as in box 1): risk score = −2.21+0.55 (if WHO performance status =1)+1.67 (if WHO performance status =2)+3.86/(haemoglobin/10)^2 −0.55×(time from diagnosis of metastatic disease to randomisation)−0.64 (if on interferon treatment). Predicted risk =1/(1 + e$^{-risk score}$).

*Binary variables are coded 0 for no or 1 for yes.

months or more. Of 347 patients with follow-up information, 218 (63%) died in the first year.

We took the following preliminary decisions before building the model:

- We chose 14 candidate predictors, including treatment, that had been reported to be prognostic
- Four predictors with more than 10% missing data were eliminated. Table 1 shows the 10 remaining candidate predictors (11 variables).
- WHO performance status (0, 1, 2) was modelled as a single entity with two dummy variables
- For illustration, we selected the significant predictors in the model using backward elimination with the Akaike information criterion[17] and using 0.05 as the significance level. We compared the results with the full model (all 10 predictors)
- Because of its skew distribution, time to metastasis was transformed to approximate normality by adding 1 day and taking logarithms. All other continuous predictors were initially modelled as linear
- For each model, we calculated the c index and receiver operating curves and assessed calibration using the Hosmer-Lemeshow test.

Table 1 shows the full model and the two reduced models selected by backward elimination using the Akaike information criterion and 5% significance. Positive regression coefficients indicate an increased risk of death over 12 months. None of the three models failed the Hosmer-Lemeshow goodness of fit test (all P>0.4).

Two important points emerge. Firstly, larger significance levels gave models with more predictors. Secondly, reducing the size of the model by reducing the significance level hardly affected the c index. Figure 1 shows the similar receiver operating curves for the three models. We note, however, that the c index has been criticised for its inability to detect meaningful differences.[24] As often happens, a few

predictors were strongly influential and the remainder were relatively weak. Removing the weaker predictors had little effect on the c index.

An important goal of a prognostic model is to classify patients into risk groups. As an example, we can use as a cut-off value a risk score of 1.4 with the full model (vertical line, fig 2) which corresponds to a predicted risk of 80%. Patients with estimated risks above the cut-off value are predicted to die within 12 months, and those with risks below the cut-off to survive 12 months. The resulting false positive rate is 10% (specificity 90%) and the true positive rate (sensitivity) is 46%. The combination of false and true positive rates is shown in the receiver operating curve (fig 1) and more indirectly in the distribution of risk scores in fig 2. The overlap in risk scores between those who died or survived 12 months is considerable, showing that the interpretation of the c index of 0.8 (table 1) is not straightforward.[24]

Continuous predictors were next handled with the multivariable fractional polynomial procedure (see box 2) using backward elimination at the 5% significance level. Only one continuous predictor (haemoglobin) showed significant non-linearity, and the transformation 1/haemoglobin[2] was indicated. That variable was selected in the final model and white cell count was eliminated (table 2).

Figure 3 shows the association between haemoglobin concentration and 12 month mortality, when haemoglobin is included in the model in different ways. The model with haemoglobin as a 10 group categorical variable, although noisy, agreed much better with the model including the fractional polynomial form of haemoglobin than the other models. Low haemoglobin concentration seems to be more hazardous than the linear function suggested.

In this example, details of the model varied according to modelling choices but performance was quite similar across the different modelling methods. Although the fractional polynomial model described the association between haemoglobin and 12 month mortality better than the linear function, the gain in discrimination was limited. This may be explained by the small number of patients with low haemoglobin concentrations.

Discussion

We have illustrated several important aspects of developing a multivariable prognostic model with empirical data. Although there is no clear consensus on the best method of model building, the importance of having an adequate sample size and high quality data is widely agreed. Model building from small data sets requires particular care.[5] [9] [10] A model's performance is likely to be overestimated when it is developed and assessed on the same dataset.

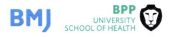

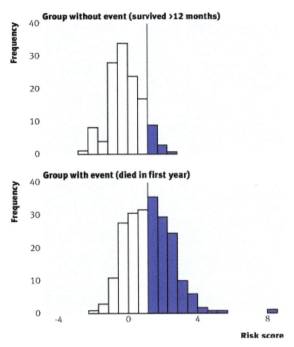

Fig 2 Distribution of risk scores from full model for patients who survived at least 12 months or died within 12 months. The vertical line represents a risk score of 1.4, corresponding to an estimated death risk of 80%. The specificity (90%) is the proportion of patients in the upper panel whose risk is below 1.4. The sensitivity (46%) is the proportion of patients in the lower panel whose risk score is above 1.4

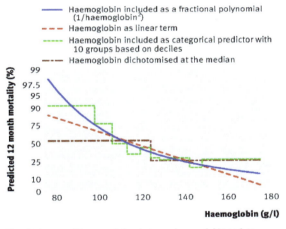

Fig 3 Estimates of the association between haemoglobin and 12 month mortality in the kidney cancer data, adjusted for the variables in the Akaike information criterion derived model (table 1). The vertical scale is linear in the log odds of mortality and is therefore non-linear in relation to mortality.

The problem is greatest with small sample sizes, many candidate predictors, and weakly influential predictors.[5 9 10] The amount of optimism in the model can be assessed and corrected by internal validation techniques.[5]

Developing a model is a complex process, so readers of a report of a new prognostic model need to know sufficient details of the data handling and modelling methods.[25] All candidate predictors and those included in the final model and their explicit coding should be carefully reported. All regression coefficients should be reported (including the intercept) to allow readers to calculate risk predictions for their own patients.

The predictive performance or accuracy of a model may be adversely affected by poor methodological choices or weaknesses in the data. But even with a high quality model there may simply be too much unexplained variation to generate accurate predictions. A critical requirement of a multivariable model is thus transportability, or external validity—that is, confirmation that the model performs as expected in new but similar patients.[26] We consider these issues in the next two articles of this series.[18 21]

Funding: PR is supported by the UK Medical Research Council (U1228.06.001.00002.01). KGMM and YV are supported by the Netherlands Organization for Scientific Research (ZON-MW 917.46.360). DGA is supported by Cancer Research UK.

Contributors: The four articles in the series were conceived and planned by DGA, KGMM, PR, and YV. PR wrote the first draft of this article. All the authors contributed to subsequent revisions. PR is the guarantor.

Competing interests: None declared.

1   Moons KGM, Royston P, Vergouwe Y, Grobbee DE, Altman DG. Prognosis and prognostic research: What, why and how? *BMJ* 2009;339:b375.
2   Van den Bosch JE, Kalkman CJ, Vergouwe Y, Van Klei WA, Bonsel GJ, Grobbee DE, et al. Assessing the applicability of scoring systems for predicting postoperative nausea and vomiting. *Anaesthesia* 2005;60:323-31.
3   Katz MH. Multivariable analysis: a primer for readers of medical research. *Ann Intern Med* 2003;138:644-50.
4   Royston P, Sauerbrei W. Building multivariable regression models with continuous covariates in clinical epidemiology—with an emphasis on fractional polynomials. *Methods Inf Med* 2005;44:561-71.
5   Harrell FE Jr. *Regression modeling strategies with applications to linear models, logistic regression, and survival analysis* . New York: Springer, 2001.
6   Royston P, Sauerbrei W. *Multivariable model-building: a pragmatic approach to regression analysis based on fractional polynomials for modelling continuous variables* . Chichester: John Wiley, 2008.
7   Austin PC, Tu JV. Bootstrap methods for developing predictive models. *Am Stat* 2004;58:131-7.
8   Sun GW, Shook TL, Kay GL. Inappropriate use of bivariable analysis to screen risk factors for use in multivariable analysis. *J Clin Epidemiol* 1996;49:907-16.
9   Steyerberg EW, Eijkemans MJ, Harrell FE Jr, Habbema JD. Prognostic modeling with logistic regression analysis: in search of a sensible strategy in small data sets. *Med Decis Making* 2001;21:45-56.
10 Harrell FE Jr, Lee KL, Mark DB. Multivariable prognostic models: issues in developing models, evaluating assumptions and adequacy, and measuring and reducing errors. *Stat Med* 1996;15:361-87.
11 Donders AR, van der Heijden GJ, Stijnen T, Moons KG. Review: a gentle introduction to imputation of missing values. *J Clin Epidemiol* 2006;59:1087-91.
12 Little RJA, Rubin DB. *Statistical analysis with missing data* . 2nd ed. New York: John Wiley, 2002.
13 Altman DG, Royston P. The cost of dichotomising continuous variables. *BMJ* 2006;332:1080.
14 Royston P, Altman DG, Sauerbrei W. Dichotomizing continuous predictors in multiple regression: a bad idea. *Stat Med* 2006;25:127-41.
15 Blettner M, Sauerbrei W. Influence of model-building strategies on the results of a case-control study. *Stat Med* 1993;12:1325-38.
16 Mantel N. Why stepdown procedures in variable selection? *Technometrics* 1970;12:621-5.
17 Sauerbrei W. The use of resampling methods to simplify regression models in medical statistics. *Appl Stat* 1999;48:313-29.
18 Altman DG, Vergouwe Y, Royston P, Moons KGM. Validating a prognostic model. *BMJ* 2009;338:b605.
19 Hosmer DW, Lemeshow S. *Applied logistic regression* . 2nd ed. New York: Wiley, 2000.
20 Hanley JA, McNeil BJ. The meaning and use of the area under a receiver operating characteristic (ROC) curve. *Radiology* 1982;143:29-36.
21 Moons KGM, Altman DG, Vergouwe Y, Royston P. Prognosis and prognostic research: application and impact of prediction models in clinical practice. *BMJ* 2009;338:b606.
22 DeMaris A. Explained variance in logistic regression. A Monte Carlo study of proposed measures. *Sociol Methods Res* 2002;31:27-74.
23 Ritchie A, Griffiths G, Parmar M, Fossa SD, Selby PJ, Cornbleet MA, et al. Interferon-alpha and survival in metastatic renal carcinoma: early results of a randomised controlled trial. *Lancet* 1999;353:14-7.
24 Pencina MJ, D'Agostino RB Sr, D'Agostino RB Jr, Vasan RS. Evaluating the added predictive ability of a new marker: from area under the ROC curve to reclassification and beyond. *Stat Med* 2008;27:157-72.
25 Hernandez AV, Vergouwe Y, Steyerberg EW. Reporting of predictive logistic models should be based on evidence-based guidelines. *Chest* 2003;124:2034-5.
26 Altman DG, Royston P. What do we mean by validating a prognostic model? *Stat Med* 2000;19:453-73.
27 Sauerbrei W, Royston P. Building multivariable prognostic and diagnostic models: transformation of the predictors by using fractional polynomials. *J R Stat Soc Series A* 1999;162:71-94.

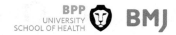

28 Rosenberg PS, Katki H, Swanson CA, Brown LM, Wacholder S, Hoover RN. Quantifying epidemiologic risk factors using non-parametric regression: model selection remains the greatest challenge. *Stat Med* 2003;22:3369-81.

29 Boucher KM, Slattery ML, Berry TD, Quesenberry C, Anderson K. Statistical methods in epidemiology: a comparison of statistical methods to analyze dose-response and trend analysis in epidemiologic studies. *J Clin Epidemiol* 1998;51:1223-33.

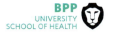

Prognosis and prognostic research: validating a prognostic model

Douglas G Altman, professor of statistics in medicine[1], Yvonne Vergouwe, assistant professor of clinical epidemiology[2], Patrick Royston, senior statistician[3], Karel G M Moons, professor of clinical epidemiology[2]

Centre for Statistics in Medicine, University of Oxford, Oxford OX2 6UD

Julius Centre for Health Sciences and Primary Care, University Medical Centre Utrecht, Utrecht, Netherlands

MRC Clinical Trials Unit, London W1 2DA

Correspondence to: D G Altman doug.altman@csm.ox.ac.uk

Cite this as: BMJ 2009;338:b605

DOI: 10.1136/bmj.b605

http://www.bmj.com/content/338/bmj.b605

ABSTRACT

Prognostic models are of little clinical value unless they are shown to work in other samples. Douglas Altman and colleagues describe how to validate models and discuss some of the problems

This article is the third in a series of four aiming to provide an accessible overview of the principles and methods of prognostic researchPrognostic models, like the one we developed in the previous article in this series,[1] yield scores to enable the prediction of the risk of future events in individual patients or groups and the stratification of patients by these risks.[2] A good model may allow the reasonably reliable classification of patients into risk groups with different prognoses. To show that a prognostic model is valuable, however, it is not sufficient to show that it successfully predicts outcome in the initial development data. We need evidence that the model performs well for other groups of patients.[1][3] In this article, we discuss how to evaluate the performance of a prognostic model in new data.[4][5]

Why prognostic models may not predict well

Various statistical or clinical factors may lead a prognostic model to perform poorly when applied to other patients.[4][6] The model's predictions may not be reproducible because of deficiencies in the design or modelling methods used in the study to derive the model, if the model was overfitted, or if an important predictor is absent from the model (which may be hard to know).[1] Poor performance in new patients can also arise from differences between the setting of patients in the new and derivation samples, including differences in healthcare systems, methods of measurement, and patient characteristics. We consider those issues in the final article in the series.[7]

Design of a validation study

The main ways to assess or validate the performance of a prognostic model on a new dataset are to compare observed and predicted event rates for groups of patients (calibration) and to quantify the model's ability to distinguish between patients who do or do not experience the event of interest (discrimination).[8][9] A model's performance can be assessed using new data from the same source as the derivation sample, but a true evaluation of generalisability (also called transportability) requires evaluation on data from elsewhere. We consider in turn three increasingly stringent validation strategies.[4]

Internal validation—A common approach is to split the dataset randomly into two parts (often 2:1), develop the model using the first portion (often called the "training" set), and assess its predictive accuracy on the second portion. This approach will tend to give optimistic results because the two datasets are very similar. Non-random splitting (for example, by centre) may be preferable as it reduces the similarity of the two sets of patients.[1][4] If the available data are limited, the model can be developed on the whole dataset and techniques of data re-use, such as cross validation and bootstrapping, applied to assess performance.[1] Internal validation is helpful, but it cannot provide information about the model's performance elsewhere.

Temporal validation—An alternative is to evaluate the performance of a model on subsequent patients from the same centre(s).[6][10] Temporal validation is no different in principle from splitting a single dataset by time. There will clearly be many similarities between the two sets of patients and between the clinical and laboratory techniques used in evaluating them. However, temporal validation is a prospective evaluation of a model, independent of the original data and development process. Temporal validation can be considered external in time and thus intermediate between internal validation and external validation.

External validation—Neither internal nor temporal validation examines the generalisability of the model, for which it is necessary to use new data collected from an appropriate (similar) patient population in a different centre. The data can be retrospective data and so external validation is possible for prediction models that need long follow-up to gather enough outcome events. Clearly, the second dataset must include data on all the variables in the model. Fundamental design issues for external validation, such as sample selection and sample size, have received limited attention.[11]

Comparing predictions with observations

Proper validation requires that we use the fully specified existing prognostic model (that is, both the selected variables and their coefficients) to predict outcomes for the patients in the second dataset and then compare these predictions with the patients' actual outcomes. This analysis uses each individual's event probability calculated from their risk score from the first model.[1]

Both calibration and discrimination should be evaluated.[1] Calibration can be assessed by plotting the observed proportions of events against the predicted probabilities for

Why prognostic models may not predict well

SUMMARY POINTS

• Unvalidated models should not be used in clinical practice

• When validating a prognostic model, calibration and discrimination should be evaluated

• Validation should be done on a different data from that used to develop the model, preferably from patients in other centres

• Models may not perform well in practice because of deficiencies in the development methods or because the new sample is too different from the original

groups defined by ranges of predicted risk, as discussed in the previous article.[1] This plot can be accompanied by the Hosmer-Lemeshow test,[12] although the test has limited statistical power to assess poor calibration and is oversensitive for very large samples. For grouped data, as in the examples below, a χ^2 test can be used to compare observed and predicted numbers of events. It may also be helpful to compare observed and predicted outcomes in groups defined by key patient variables, such as diagnostic or demographic subgroups. Discrimination may be summarised by the c index (area under the receiver-operator curve) or R^2.[1]

The figure shows a typical example of a poorly calibrated model.[13] The line fitting the data is very different from the diagonal line representing perfect calibration. A slope much smaller than 1 indicates that the range of observed risks is much smaller than the range of predicted risks. The poor discriminative ability of the model was shown by a low c index of 0.63 (95% confidence interval 0.60 to 0.66) in the validation sample compared with 0.75 (0.71 to 0.79) in the development sample.[13]

It may be helpful to prespecify acceptable performance of a model in terms of calibration and discrimination. If this performance is achieved, the model may be suitable for clinical use. It is, however, unclear how to determine what is acceptable, especially as prognostic assessments will still be necessary and even moderately performing models are likely to do better than clinicians' own assessments.[14 15]

Case studies
We illustrate the above ideas with four case studies with various performance characteristics.

Predicting operative mortality of patients having cardiac surgery
The European system for cardiac operative risk evaluation (EuroSCORE) was developed using data from eight European countries to predict operative mortality of patients having cardiac surgery.[16] The score combines nine patient factors and eight cardiac factors; it has been successfully validated in other European cohorts. Yap and colleagues examined the performance of EuroSCORE in an Australian cohort that was different from the derivation cohort, with a generally higher risk of death.[17] For example, 41% of the Australian cohort were aged over 70 compared to 27% in the European cohort, and there were 15% v 10% with recent myocardial infarction. Yet the observed mortality in the Australian cohort was consistently much lower than that predicted by the EuroSCORE model (table 1). Observed mortality for three risk groups was only half the predicted mortality. The calibration of the model in these new patients was thus poor, although it retained discrimination in the new population.

There are various possible explanations for this poor performance including different epidemiology of ischaemic heart disease and differences in access to health care. Also, the EuroSCORE model was based on data from 1995 and may not reflect current cardiac surgical practice even in Europe. In such a case, however, it is easy to recalibrate the original model so that calibration and predictions become accurate in the new population, while preserving discrimination.[18] [19] However, this updated model might require further validation. We will discuss this further in the next article.[7]

Predicting postoperative mortality after colorectal surgery
A prospective study recruited 1421 consecutive patients having colorectal surgery for cancer or diverticular disease from 81 centres in France in 2002.[20] A multiple logistic regression analysis on a large number of factors identified four that were significantly predictive of postoperative mortality. All were binary, although two (age and weight) were originally continuous. The investigators found that the number of the four factors present was a strong predictor of mortality (table 2).

The model development can be criticised: four variables were selected from numerous candidates, the number of deaths was small, continuous variables were dichotomised and the authors replaced the regression model by a simple count of factors present, neglecting the relative weights (regression coefficients) of the four predictors. Nevertheless, when this risk score was tested in a new series of 1049 patients recruited from 41 centres in 2004,[21] the mortality across the score categories (a kind of calibration) was similar to that in the original study (table 2). Both datasets show a strong risk gradient with good discrimination, but for one category the observed and predicted event probabilities are quite different. This example shows the difficulty of judging how well a model validates.

Predicting failure of non-invasive positive pressure ventilation
Non-invasive positive pressure ventilation may reduce mortality in patients with exacerbation of chronic obstructive pulmonary disease, but it fails in some patients. A prognostic model was developed to try to identify patients at high risk of failure of ventilation, both at admission and after two hours. Using data from 1033 patients admitted to 14 different units, researchers used stepwise logistic regression to develop a model comprising four continuous variables (APACHE II score, Glasgow coma scale, pH, and respiratory rate) each grouped into two or three categories.[22] The model for failure after two hours of ventilation had a c index of 0.88. Predicted probabilities of events varied widely from 3% to 99% for different combinations of variables.

The same researchers validated their model using data from an independent sample of 145 patients admitted to three units—it is unclear whether these were among the original 14 units. The Hosmer-Lemeshow test showed no significant difference (P>0.9) between observed and expected numbers of failures, and the c index of 0.83 was similar to that observed in the original sample. The high discrimination suggests that the model could help decide clinical management of patients. However, the size of their validation sample may be inadequate to support strong inferences.

Predicting complications of acute cough in preschool children
To reduce clinical uncertainty concerning preschool children presenting to primary care with acute cough, Hay and colleagues derived a clinical prediction rule for complications.[23] They used logistic regression to examine several potential predictors and produced a simple classification using two binary variables (fever and chest signs) to create four risk groups. Risk of complications varied from 6% with neither symptom to 40% with both (table 3). The c index was 0.68.

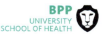

Table 1 Predicted and observed mortality by EuroSCORE risk level for Australian patients having coronary artery bypass grafting[17]

EuroSCORE	No of deaths/patients	Observed mortality (%) (95% CI)	Predicted mortality (%) (95% CI)
0-2 (low risk)	8/1955	0.41 (0.18 to 0.80)	1.03 (0.99 to 1.06)
3-5 (medium risk)	17/1996	0.85 (0.50 to 1.36)	3.90 (3.87 to 3.94)
≥6 (high risk)	87/1641	5.30 (4.27 to 6.50)	8.52 (8.39 to 8.65)
Total	112/5592	2.00 (1.65 to 2.40)	4.25 (4.16 to 4.34)

Table 2 Mortality after colorectal surgery in relation to number of risk factors present in two cohorts[20][21]

No of risk factors	Initial cohort		Validation cohort	
	No of deaths/patients	Mortality (%)	No of deaths/patients	Mortality (%)
0	3/580	0.5	2/424	0.5
1	11/557	2.0	6/366	1.6
2	20/223	9.0	11/153	7.2
3	9/56	16.1	22/47	46.8
4	5/10	50.0	7/10	70.0
Total	48/1426	3.3	48/1000	4.8

Table 3 Number (percentage) of preschool children developing complications after presenting to primary care with acute cough in relation to signs at presentation

Signs present	Initial cohort	Validation cohort
Neither sign	10/153 (6)	13/95 (14)
Chest signs only	6/33 (18)	4/29 (14)
Fever only	5/18 (28)	1/11 (9)
Both signs	2/5 (40)	0/8 (0)
Total	23/209 (11)	18/143 (13)

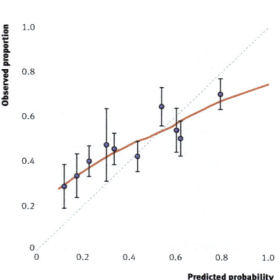

Fig Calibration plot for a scoring system for predicting postoperative nausea and vomiting.[13] Circles indicate the observed frequency of events per tenth of predicted risk, with vertical lines representing 95% confidence intervals. The solid line shows the relation between observed outcomes and predicted risks

Unfortunately, evaluation of the model in a second dataset failed to confirm the value of this classification (table 3).[24] The authors suggested several explanations, including the possibility that doctors might preferentially have treated symptomatic patients with antibiotics. It may simply be that the primary data included too few children who developed complications to allow reliable modelling.

Discussion

Validation studies are necessary because performance in the original data may well be optimistic,[6] but temporal and (especially) external validation studies are scarce.[25]

It seems to be widely believed that the statistical significance of predictors in a multivariable model shows the usefulness of a prediction model. Also, when evaluating a model with new data authors seem to want to calculate P values and conclude that the validation is satisfactory if there is no significant difference between, say, observed and predicted event rates, for example based on the Hosmer-Lemeshow test. Neither view is correct—P values do not provide a satisfactory answer.

Rather, in a validation study we evaluate whether the performance of the model on the new data (its calibration and, especially, discrimination) matches, or comes close to, the performance in the data on which it was developed. But even if the performance is less good, the model may still be clinically useful.[4] The assessment of usefulness of a model thus requires clinical judgment and depends on context.

A model is "a snapshot in place and time, not fundamental truth."[26] If the case mix in the validation sample differs greatly from that of the derivation sample the model may fail, although it may be possible to improve the model by simple recalibration, as in the EuroSCORE example above, or even by including new variable(s) that relate to the different case mix and are found to be prognostic in the new sample.[27] For example, the range of patients' ages in the

derivation and validation samples might differ markedly, so that age might not be recognised in the derivation set as an important prognostic factor. In addition, performance of a model may change over time and re-evaluation may be indicated after some years. We consider these possibilities further in the next article.[7]

Simplicity of models and reliability of measurements are important criteria in developing clinically useful prognostic models.[2][28] Experience shows that more complex models tend to give overoptimistic predictions, especially when extensive variable selection has been performed,[29] but there are notable exceptions.

As the aim of most prognostic studies is to create clinically valuable risk scores or indexes, the definition of risk groups should ideally be driven mainly by clinical rather than statistical criteria. If a clinician would leave untreated a patient with at least a 90% chance of surviving five years, would apply aggressive therapy if the prognosis was 30% survival or less, and would use standard therapy in intermediate cases, then three prognostic groups seem sensible. Validation of the model would investigate whether the observed proportions of events were similar in groups of patients from other settings and whether separation in outcome across those groups was maintained.

Few prognostic models are routinely used in clinical practice, probably because most have not been externally validated.[25][28] To be considered useful, a risk score should be clinically credible, accurate (well calibrated with good discriminative ability), have generality (be externally validated), and, ideally, be shown to be clinically effective—that is, provide useful additional information to clinicians that improves therapeutic decision making and thus patient outcome.[25][28] It is crucial to quantify the performance of a prognostic model on a new series of patients, ideally in a different location, before applying the model in daily practice to guide patient care. Although still rare, temporal and external validation studies do seem to be becoming more common.

DGA is supported by Cancer Research UK. KGMM and YV are supported by the Netherlands Organization for Scientific Research (ZON-MW 917.46.360). PR is supported by the UK Medical Research

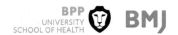

Council. We thank Yves Panis and Alastair Hay for clarifying some details of the case studies.

Contributors: The articles in the series were conceived and planned by DGA, KGMM, PR and YV. DGA wrote the first draft of this paper. All the authors contributed to subsequent revisions. DGA is the guarantor.

Competing interests: None declared.

Provenance and peer review: Not commissioned; externally peer reviewed.

1   Royston P, Moons KGM, Altman DG, Vergouwe Y. Prognosis and prognostic research: developing a prognostic model. *BMJ* 2009;338:b604.
2   Moons KGM, Royston P, Vergouwe Y, Grobbee DE, Altman DG. Prognosis and prognostic research: what, why and how? *BMJ* 2009;338:b375.
3   Bleeker SE, Moll HA, Steyerberg EW, Donders AR, Derksen-Lubsen G, Grobbee DE, et al. External validation is necessary in prediction research: a clinical example. *J Clin Epidemiol* 2003;56:826-32.
4   Altman DG, Royston P. What do we mean by validating a prognostic model? *Stat Med* 2000;19:453-73.
5   Altman DG, Royston P. Evaluating the performance of prognostic models. In: Rothwell P, ed. *Treating individuals: from randomised trials and systematic reviews to personalised medicine in routine practice* . Edinburgh: Lancet, 2007:213-29.
6   Justice AC, Covinsky KE, Berlin JA. Assessing the generalizability of prognostic information. *Ann Intern Med* 1999;130:515-24.
7   Moons KGM, Altman DG, Vergouwe Y, Royston P. Prognosis and prognostic research: application and impact of prediction models in clinical practice. *BMJ* 2009;338:b606.
8   Harrell FE Jr, Lee KL, Mark DB. Multivariable prognostic models: issues in developing models, evaluating assumptions and adequacy, and measuring and reducing errors. *Stat Med* 1996;15:361-87.
9   Mackillop WJ, Quirt CF. Measuring the accuracy of prognostic judgments in oncology. *J Clin Epidemiol* 1997;50:21-9.
10   Miller ME, Hui SL, Tierney WM. Validation techniques for logistic regression models. *Stat Med* 1991;10:1213-26.
11   Vergouwe Y, Steyerberg EW, Eijkemans MJC, Habbema JDF. Substantial effective sample sizes were required for external validation studies of predictive logistic regression models. *J Clin Epidemiol* 2005;58:475-83.
12   Hosmer DW, Lemeshow S. *Applied logistic regression* . 2nd ed. New York: Wiley, 2000.
13   Van den Bosch JE, Kalkman CJ, Vergouwe Y, Van Klei WA, Bonsel GJ, Grobbee DE, et al. Assessing the applicability of scoring systems for predicting postoperative nausea and vomiting. *Anaesthesia* 2005;60:323-31.
14   Ivanov J, Borger MA, David TE, Cohen G, Walton N, Naylor CD. Predictive accuracy study: comparing a statistical model to clinicians' estimates of outcomes after coronary bypass surgery. *Ann Thorac Surg* 2000;70:162-8.
15   Loeb M, Walter SD, McGeer A, Simor AE, McArthur MA, Norman G. A comparison of model-building strategies for lower respiratory tract infection in long-term care. *J Clin Epidemiol* 1999;52:1239-48.
16   Nashef SA, Roques F, Michel P, Gauducheau E, Lemeshow S, Salamon R. European system for cardiac operative risk evaluation (EuroSCORE). *Eur J Cardiothorac Surg* 1999;16:9-13.
17   Yap CH, Reid C, Yii M, Rowland MA, Mohajeri M, Skillington PD, et al. Validation of the EuroSCORE model in Australia. *Eur J Cardiothorac Surg* 2006;29:441-6.
18   Van Houwelingen HC, Thorogood J. Construction, validation and updating of a prognostic model for kidney graft survival. *Stat Med* 1995;14:1999-2008.
19   Steyerberg EW, Borsboom GJJM, Van Houwelingen HC, Eijkemans MJC, Habbema JDF. Validation and updating of predictive logistic regression models: a study on sample size and shrinkage. *Stat Med* 2004;23:2567-86.
20   Alves A, Panis Y, Mathieu P, Mantion G, Kwiatkowski F, Slim K. Postoperative mortality and morbidity in French patients undergoing colorectal surgery: results of a prospective multicenter study. *Arch Surg* 2005;140:278-83.
21   Alves A, Panis Y, Mantion G, Slim K, Kwiatkowski F, Vicaut E. The AFC score: validation of a 4-item predicting score of postoperative mortality after colorectal resection for cancer or diverticulitis: results of a prospective multicenter study in 1049 patients. *Ann Surg* 2007;246:91-6.
22   Confalonieri M, Garuti G, Cattaruzza MS, Osborn JF, Antonelli M, Conti G, et al. A chart of failure risk for noninvasive ventilation in patients with COPD exacerbation. *Eur Respir J* 2005;25:348-55.
23   Hay AD, Fahey T, Peters TJ, Wilson A. Predicting complications from acute cough in pre-school children in primary care: a prospective cohort study. *Br J Gen Pract* 2004;54:9-14.
24   Hay AD, Gorst C, Montgomery A, Peters TJ, Fahey T. Validation of a clinical rule to predict complications of acute cough in preschool children: a prospective study in primary care. *Br J Gen Pract* 2007;57:530-7.
25   Reilly BM, Evans AT. Translating clinical research into clinical practice: impact of using prediction rules to make decisions. *Ann Intern Med* 2006;144:201-9.
26   Iezzoni LI. Statistically derived predictive models. Caveat emptor. *J Gen Intern Med* 1999;14:388-9.
27   Hubacek J, Galbraith PD, Gao M, Humphries K, Graham MM, Knudtson ML, et al. External validation of a percutaneous coronary intervention mortality prediction model in patients with acute coronary syndromes. *Am Heart J* 2006;151:308-15.
28   Wyatt JC, Altman DG. Commentary: Prognostic models: clinically useful or quickly forgotten? *BMJ* 1995;311:1539-41.
29   Sauerbrei W. The use of resampling methods to simplify regression models in medical statistics. *Appl Stat* 1999;48:313-29.

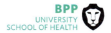

Prognosis and prognostic research: application and impact of prognostic models in clinical practice

Karel G M Moons, professor of clinical epidemiology[1], Douglas G Altman, professor of statistics in medicine[2], Yvonne Vergouwe, assistant professor of clinical epidemiology[1], Patrick Royston, senior statistician[3]

Julius Centre for Health Sciences and Primary Care, University Medical Centre Utrecht, Utrecht, Netherlands

Centre for Statistics in Medicine, University of Oxford, Oxford OX2 6UD

MRC Clinical Trials Unit, London NW1 2DA

Correspondence to: K G M Moons k.g.m.moons@umcutrecht.nl

Cite this as: BMJ 2009;338:b606

DOI: 10.1136/bmj.b606

http://www.bmj.com/content/338/bmj.b606

ABSTRACT

An accurate prognostic model is of no benefit if it is not generalisable or doesn't change behaviour. In the last article in their series Karel Moons and colleagues discuss how to determine the practical value of models

This article is the last in a series of four aiming to provide an accessible overview of the principles and methods of prognostic researchPrognostic models are developed to be applied in new patients, who may come from different centres, countries, or times. Hence, new patients are commonly referred to as different from but similar to the patients used to develop the models.[1][2][3][4] But what exactly does this mean? When can a new patient population be considered similar (enough) to the development population to justify validation and eventually application of a model? We have already considered the design, development, and validation of prognostic research and models.[5][6][7] In the final article of our series, we discuss common limitations to the application and generalisation of prognostic models and what evidence beyond validation is needed before practitioners can confidently apply a model to their patients. These issues also apply to prediction models with a diagnostic outcome (presence of a disease).

Limitations to application

Extrapolation versus validation

Most prediction models are developed in secondary care, and it is common to want to apply them to primary care.[1][8][9][10] The predictive performance of secondary care models is usually decreased when they are validated in a primary care setting.[1][9] One example is the diagnostic model to predict deep vein thrombosis, which had a negative predictive value of 97% (95% confidence interval 95% to 99%) and sensitivity 90% (83% to 96%) in Canadian secondary care patients.[11]

When the model was validated in Dutch primary care patients, the negative predictive value was only 88% (85% to 91%) and sensitivity 79% (74% to 84%).[12] The question arises whether primary and secondary care populations can indeed be considered to be different but similar.

A change in setting clearly results in a different case mix, which commonly affects the generalisability of prognostic models.[4][9][13][14] Case mix is here defined as the distribution of the outcome and predictive factors whether included in the model or not. Primary care doctors often selectively refer patients to specialists. Secondary care patients can thus largely be considered to be a subpopulation of primary care patients, commonly with a narrower range of patient characteristics, a larger fraction of patients in later disease stages, and worse outcomes.[9] Consequently, application of a secondary care model in general practice requires extrapolation. This view suggests that applying a primary care model to secondary care would have a limited effect on predictive performance, although this requires further research.

Another common generalisation, or rather extrapolation, is from adults to children. Various prognostic models have been developed to predict the risk of postoperative nausea and vomiting in adults scheduled for surgery under general anaesthesia. When validated in children, the models' predictive ability was substantially decreased.[15] The researchers considered children as a different population and developed and validated a separate model for children that included other predictors.[16] In contrast, the Intensive Care National Audit and Research Centre model to predict outcome in critical care was initially developed with data from adults but also has good accuracy in children.[17]

In general, models will be more generalisable when the ranges of predictor values in the new population are within the ranges seen in the development population. The above examples show that we cannot assume that prediction models can simply be generalised from one population or setting to another, although it may be possible. Therefore, accuracy of any prediction model should always be tested in a formal validation study (see third article in this series[7]).

Adequate prediction versus application

Just because a model is well used does not mean it has adequate prediction. For example, the Framingham risk model discriminates only reasonably in certain (sub) populations, with a receiver-operating characteristic (ROC) curve area of little over 0.70.[18] The model is nevertheless widely used. The same applies to various intensive care prediction models—for example, the APACHE scores and the simplified acute physiology scores (SAPS).[19][20] A likely reason is the relevance of the outcomes that these rules predict:

SUMMARY POINTS

- Prognostic models generalise best to populations that have similar ranges of predictor values to those in the development population
- When a prognostic model performs less well in a new population, using the new data to modify the model should first be considered rather than directly developing a new model
- Application of prognostic models requires unambiguous definitions of predictors and outcomes and reproducible measurements using methods available in clinical practice
- Impact studies quantify the effect of using a prognostic model on physicians' behaviour, patient outcome, or cost effectiveness of care compared with usual care without the model
- Impact studies require different design, outcome, analysis, and reporting from validation studies

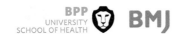

risk of cardiovascular disease (Framingham) and mortality in critically illness (APACHE, SAPS). Another reason for the wide use of such models is their face validity, such that doctors trust these models to guide their practice rather than their own experience.

Whether the predictive accuracy of a model in new patients is adequate is also a matter of judgment and depends on available alternatives.[21] For instance, a prognostic model to predict the probability of spontaneous ongoing pregnancy in couples with unexplained subfertility has good calibration but rather low discriminative ability (ROC area even below 0.70) but remains the best model available.[22] Hence, the model was used to identify couples with intermediate probability of spontaneous ongoing pregnancy for a clinical trial.[23]

Finally, the role of prognostic models and prognostic factors in clinical practice still depends on circumstances. A positive family history of subarachnoid haemorrhage increases the risk of subarachnoid haemorrhage 5.5 times, but only 10% of cases of subarachnoid haemorrhage occur in people with a family history. Thus screening for subarachnoid haemorrhage in people with a family history is not recommended as it will identify relatively too few cases.[24]

Usability

Constraints on the usability of the prognostic model can also limit the application. Application of prognostic models requires unambiguous definitions of predictors and reproducible measurements using methods available in clinical practice. For example, one of the predictors in the deep vein thrombosis model described above is "alternative diagnosis just as likely as deep vein thrombosis."[11] General practitioners may be less experienced in properly coding this predictor for a patient, leading to misclassification that potentially compromises the rule's predictive performance. Another example of an ambiguous predictor definition is "history of nausea and vomiting after previous anaesthesia" in the prognostic model for postoperative nausea and vomiting.[25] A negative answer could mean that the patient has had anaesthesia before but not experienced symptoms or that the patient has never had anaesthesia. Also, children will have had previous anaesthesia less often than adults. As a consequence, this predictor may have a different effect in children.

Similarly, the definition of the outcome variable may vary across populations. Occurrence of neurological sequelae after childhood bacterial meningitis was defined in a development population as mild cases (for example, hearing loss), severe cases (for example, deafness), or dead.[26] The prognostic model was validated in a population that included children with mainly mild neurological sequelae. The model showed poor performance in the validation population, possibly because of the different distribution of outcomes.[27] In addition, the follow-up time differed between the two populations (the maximum duration of follow-up was 3.3 years in the development population and 10 years in the validation population).

Changes over time

As we discussed in the first article in this series,[5] changes in practice over time can limit the application of prognostic models. Improvements in diagnostic tests, biomarker measurement, or treatments may change the prognosis of patients. For example, spiral computed tomography can better visualise the pulmonary circulation than older computed tomography.[28] As a consequence, a patient with pulmonary embolism detected by spiral computed tomography and treated accordingly may have a better prognosis on average than a patient with an embolism detected by conventional computed tomography.

Changes over time may even lead to the situation that prognostic models are no longer used to estimate outcome risks and to influence patient management. For example, the suggestion that everyone older than 55 is given a "polypill" to reduce the risk of cardiovascular diseases[29] may make models to predict these diseases redundant.

Evidence beyond validation studies

Adjusting and updating prognostic models to improve performance

Newly collected data from prediction research are often used to develop a new prognostic model rather than to validate existing models.[2 3 7 14] For example, there are over 60 models to predict outcome after breast cancer[30] and about 25 models to predict long term outcome in patients with neurological trauma.[31] If researchers do perform a formal validation study of a published model and find poor performance, they often then re-estimate the associations of the predictors with the outcome in their own data. Sometimes even the entire selection of important predictors is repeated. This is unfortunate, since predictive information captured in developing the original model is neglected. Furthermore, validation studies commonly include fewer patients than development studies, making the new model more subject to overfitting and thus even less generalisable than the original model.[4 14]

When a prognostic model performs less well in another population, adjusting the model using the new data should first be considered to determine whether it will improve the performance in that population.[4 13 14] The adjusted model is then based on both the development and validation data, further improving its stability and generalisability. Such adjustment of prognostic models is called updating. Updating methods vary from simple recalibration to more extensive methods referred to as model revision.[4 13 14] Recalibration includes adjustment of the intercept of the model and overall adjustment of the associations (relative weights) of the predictors with the outcome. Model revision includes adjustment of individual predictor-outcome associations and addition of new predictors. Interestingly, simple recalibration methods are often sufficient.[4 14] The extent to which this process of model validation and adjustment has to be pursued before clinical application, will depend on the context. General rules are as yet unavailable.

Impact of prognostic models

Prognostic models are developed to provide objective estimates of outcome probabilities to complement clinical intuition and guidelines.[5 8 10 21] The underlying assumption is that accurately estimated probabilities improve doctors' decision making and consequently patient outcome. The effect of a previously developed, validated, and (if needed) updated prognostic model on behaviour and patient outcomes should be studied separately in so called impact studies (box).

Validation and impact studies differ in their design, study outcome, statistical analysis, and reporting (table). A validation study ideally uses a prospective cohort design

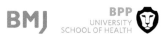

and does not require a control group.[7] For each patient, predictors and outcome are documented, and the rule's predictive performance is quantified.

By contrast, impact studies quantify the effect of using a prognostic model on doctors' behaviour, patient outcome, or cost effectiveness of care compared with not using such model (table). They require a control group of healthcare professionals who provide usual care. The preferred design is a randomised trial.[3] If behaviour changes of professionals is the main outcome, a randomised study without follow-up of patients would suffice. Follow-up is required if patient outcome or cost effectiveness is assessed. However, since changes in outcome depend on changes in doctors' behaviour, it may be sensible to start with a randomised study assessing the model's impact on therapeutic decisions, especially when long follow-up times are needed to assess patient outcome. The same applies to diagnostic procedures[32] and therapeutic interventions for which effects are realised by changing behaviour and decisions—for example, exercise therapy to reduce body mass index.

Impact studies may use an assistive approach—simply providing the model's predicted probabilities of an outcome between 0% and 100%—or a decisive approach that explicitly suggests decisions for each probability category.[3] [33] The assistive approach clearly leaves room for intuition and judgment, but a decisive approach may have greater effect.[3] [34] [35] Introduction of computerised patient records that automatically give predictions for individual subjects, enhances implementation and thus impact analysis of prognostic models in routine care.[35] [36]

Randomising individual patients in an impact study may result in learning effects because the same doctor will alternately apply and not apply the model to subsequent patients, reducing the contrast between both randomised groups. Randomisation of doctors (clusters) is preferable, although this requires more patients.[37] Randomising centres is often the best method as it avoids exchange of experiences between doctors within a single centre.

An alternative design is a before and after study with the same doctors or centres, as was used to evaluate the effect of the Ottawa ankle rule on physicians' behaviour and cost effectiveness of care.[38] [39] A disadvantage of this design is the sensitivity to temporal changes in therapeutic approaches. Although impact studies are scarce, are a few good examples exist.[40] [41] [42]

CONSECUTIVE STAGES TO PRODUCE A USABLE MULTIVARIABLE PROGNOSTIC MODEL

- *Development studies*[5] [6]—Development of a multivariable prognostic model, including identification of the important predictors, assigning the relative weights to each predictor, and estimating the model's predictive performance (eg, calibration and discrimination) adjusted if necessary for overfitting
- *Validation studies*[7]—Validating or testing the model's predictive performance in new subjects, preferably from different centres, with a different case mix or using (slightly) different definitions and measurements of predictors and outcomes
- *Impact studies*—Quantifying whether use of a prognostic model in daily practice improves decision making and, ultimately, patient outcome using a comparative design

When to apply a prognostic model?

Do all prognostic models require a three step assessment (box) before they are used in daily care? Does a model that has shown adequate prediction for its intended use in validation studies—adequately predicting the outcome—still require an impact analysis using a large, multicentre cluster randomised study? The answers depend on the rate of (acceptable) false positives and false negative predictions and their consequences for patient management and outcome. For models with (near) perfect discrimination and calibration in several validation studies the answer may be no, though such success is rare. An example is a model to predict the differential diagnosis of acute meningitis. It showed an area under the ROC curve of 0.97 in the development population[43] and of 0.98 in two validation populations.[44] [45]

For models with less perfect performance, only an impact analysis can determine whether use of the model is better than usual care. Impact studies also provide the opportunity to study factors that may affect implementation of a prognostic model in daily care, including the acceptability of the prognostic model to clinicians and ease of use.

An intermediate step using decision modelling techniques or Markov chain models can be helpful. These evaluate the potential consequences of using the prognostic model in terms of subsequent therapeutic decisions and patient outcome.[46] If such analysis does not indicate any potential for improved patient outcome, a formal impact study would not be warranted.

Concluding remarks

Many prognostic models are developed but few have their predictive performance validated in new patients, let alone an evaluation of their impact on decision making and patient outcome.[3] [47] [48] Thus it seems right that few such models are actually used in practice. Recent methodological advances enable the adjustment of prognostic models to local circumstances to give improved generalisability. With these innovations, correctly developed and evaluated prediction models may become more common.

Many questions remain unresolved. How much validation, and perhaps adjustment, is needed before an impact study is justified? Is it feasible for a single model to apply to all patient subgroups, across all levels of care and countries? These issues require further research. Finally, we reiterate that unvalidated models should not be used in clinical practice, and more impact studies are needed to

Comparison of characteristics of validation study and impact study for prognostic models

Characteristic	Validation study[7]	Impact study
Control group	No	Yes. Index group includes doctors exposed to or using the prognostic model; control group is usual care (without using the model)
Design	Prospective cohort (preferred); retrospective cohort	Cluster randomisation (preferred); before and after
Outcome	Usually occurrence of event (eg, death, complication, treatment response) after a certain time or follow-up period	(Change in) doctors' decisions or behaviour
		Patient outcome (eg, events, pain, quality of life)
		Cost effectiveness of care
Follow-up	Yes	No, if outcome is doctors' decisions or behaviour
		Yes, if outcome is patient outcome or cost effectiveness of care
Statistical analysis and reporting	Model's calibration and discrimination	Comparison of outcome between index and control group—eg, using relative risks, odds ratios, or difference in means
	Defining particular risk groups by introducing thresholds	
	Improving or updating a model (if needed)	

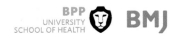

determine whether a prognostic or diagnostic model should be implemented in daily practice.

KGMM and YV are supported by the Netherlands Organization for Scientific Research (ZON-MW 917.46.360). PR is supported by the UK Medical Research Council. DGA is supported by Cancer Research UK.

Contributors: This series was conceived and planned by DGA, KGMM, PR, and YV. KGMM wrote the first draft of this paper. All the authors contributed to subsequent revisions. KGMM is guarantor.

Competing interests: None declared.

Provenance and peer review: Not commissioned; externally peer reviewed.

1 Justice AC, Covinsky KE, Berlin JA. Assessing the generalizability of prognostic information. *Ann Intern Med* 1999;130:515-24.
2 Altman DG, Royston P. What do we mean by validating a prognostic model? *Stat Med* 2000;19:453-73.
3 Reilly BM, Evans AT. Translating clinical research into clinical practice: impact of using prediction rules to make decisions. *Ann Intern Med* 2006;144:201-9.
4 Steyerberg EW, Borsboom GJ, van Houwelingen HC, Eijkemans MJ, Habbema JD. Validation and updating of predictive logistic regression models: a study on sample size and shrinkage. *Stat Med* 2004;23:2567-86.
5 Moons K, Royston P, Vergouwe Y, Grobbee D, Altman D. Prognosis and prognostic research: what, why and how? *BMJ* 2008;b375.
6 Royston P, Moons K, Altman D, Vergouwe Y. Prognosis and prognostic research: developing a prognostic model. *BMJ* 2008;b604.
7 Altman DG, Vergouwe Y, Royston P, Moons KG. Prognosis and prognostic research: validating a prognostic model. *BMJ* 2008;b605.
8 McGinn TG, Guyatt GH, Wyer PC, Naylor CD, Stiell IG, Richardson WS. Users' guides to the medical literature: XXII: how to use articles about clinical decision rules. *JAMA* 2000;284:79-84.
9 Knottnerus JA. Between iatrotropic stimulus and interiatric referral: the domain of primary care research. *J Clin Epidemiol* 2002;55:1201-6.
10 Laupacis A, Sekar N, Stiell IG. Clinical prediction rules. A review and suggested modifications of methodological standards. *JAMA* 1997;277:488-94.
11 Wells PS, Anderson DR, Bormanis J, Guy F, Mitchell M, Gray L, et al. Value of assessment of pretest probability of deep-vein thrombosis in clinical management. *Lancet* 1997;350:1795-8.
12 Oudega R, Hoes AW, Moons KG. The Wells rule does not adequately rule out deep venous thrombosis in primary care patients. *Ann Intern Med* 2005;143:100-7.
13 Van Houwelingen JC. Validation, calibration, revision and combination of prognostic survival models. *Stat Med* 2000;19:3401-15.
14 Janssen KJM, Moons KGM, Kalkman CJ, Grobbee DE, Vergouwe Y. Updating methods improved the performance of a clinical prediction model in new patients. *J Clin Epidemiol* 2008;61:76-86.
15 Eberhart LH, Morin AM, Guber D, Kretz FJ, Schauffelen A, Treiber H, et al. Applicability of risk scores for postoperative nausea and vomiting in adults to paediatric patients. *Br J Anaesth* 2004;93:386-92.
16 Eberhart LH, Geldner G, Kranke P, Morin AM, Schauffelen A, Treiber H, et al. The development and validation of a risk score to predict the probability of postoperative vomiting in pediatric patients. *Anesth Analg* 2004;99:1630-7.
17 Harrison DA, Rowan KM. Outcome prediction in critical care: the ICNARC model. *Curr Opin Crit Care* 2008;14:506-12.
18 Liao Y, McGee DL, Cooper RS, Sutkowski MB. How generalizable are coronary risk prediction models? Comparison of Framingham and two national cohorts. *Am Heart J* 1999;137:837-45.
19 Knaus WA, Wagner DP, Draper EA, Zimmerman JE, Bergner M, Bastos PG, et al. The APACHE III prognostic system. Risk prediction of hospital mortality for critically ill hospitalized adults. *Chest* 1991;100:1619-36.
20 Le Gall JR, Lemeshow S, Saulnier F. A new simplified acute physiology score (SAPS II) based on a European/North American multicenter study. *JAMA* 1993;270:2957-63.
21 Wyatt JC, Altman DG. Prognostic models: clinically useful or quickly forgotten? *BMJ* 1995;311:1539-41.
22 Hunault CC, Habbema JD, Eijkemans MJ, Collins JA, Evers JL, te Velde ER. Two new prediction rules for spontaneous pregnancy leading to live birth among subfertile couples, based on the synthesis of three previous models. *Hum Reprod* 2004;19:2019-26.
23 Steures P, van der Steeg JW, Hompes PG, Habbema JD, Eijkemans MJ, Broekmans FJ, et al. Intrauterine insemination with controlled ovarian hyperstimulation versus expectant management for couples with unexplained subfertility and an intermediate prognosis: a randomised clinical trial. *Lancet* 2006;368:216-21.
24 Rinkel GJ. Intracranial aneurysm screening: indications and advice for practice. *Lancet Neurol* 2005;4:122-8.
25 Van de Bosch J, Moons KGM, Bonsel GJ, Kalkman CJ. Does measurement of preoperative anxiety have added value in the prediction of postoperative nausea and vomiting? *Anesth Analg* 2005;100:1525-32.
26 Oostenbrink R, Moons KGM, Derksen-Lubsen G, Grobbee DE, Moll HA. Early prediction of neurological sequelae or death after bacterial meningitis. *Acta Paediatr* 2002;91:391-8.
27 Biesheuvel CJ, Koomen I, Vergouwe Y, Van Furth M, Oostenbrink R, Moll HA, et al. Validating and updating a prediction rule for neurological sequelae after childhood bacterial meningitis. *Scand J Infect Dis* 2006;38:19-26.
28 Holbert JM, Costello P, Federle MP. Role of spiral computed tomography in the diagnosis of pulmonary embolism in the emergency department. *Ann Emerg Med* 1999;33:520-8.
29 Wald NJ, Law MR. A strategy to reduce cardiovascular disease by more than 80%. *BMJ* 2003;326:1419.
30 Altman D. Prognostic models: a methodological framework and review of models for breast cancer. In: Lyman GH, Burstein HJ, eds. *Breast cancer. Translational therapeutic strategies* . New York: Informa Healtcare, 2007:11-25.
31 Perel P, Edwards P, Wentz R, Roberts I. Systematic review of prognostic models in traumatic brain injury. *BMC Med Inform Decis Mak* 2006;6:38.
32 Deeks JJ. Assessing outcomes following tests. In: Price CP, Christenson RH, eds. *Evidence-based laboratory medicine: principles, practice, and outcomes* . 2nd ed. Washington: AACC Press, 2007:95-111.
33 Gordon-Lubitz RJ. Risk communication: problems of presentation and understanding. *JAMA* 2003;289:95.
34 Michie S, Johnston M. Changing clinical behaviour by making guidelines specific. *BMJ* 2004;328:343-5.
35 Kawamoto K, Houlihan CA, Balas EA, Lobach DF. Improving clinical practice using clinical decision support systems: a systematic review of trials to identify features critical to success. *BMJ* 2005;330:765.
36 James BC. Making it easy to do it right. *N Engl J Med* 2001;345:991-3.
37 Campbell MK, Elbourne DR, Altman DG. CONSORT statement: extension to cluster randomised trials. *BMJ* 2004;328:702-8.
38 Stiell I, Wells G, Laupacis A, Brison R, Verbeek R, Vandemheen K, et al. Multicentre trial to introduce the Ottawa ankle rules for use of radiography in acute ankle injuries. *BMJ* 1995;311:594-7.
39 Cameron C, Naylor CD. No impact from active dissemination of the Ottawa ankle rules: further evidence of the need for local implementation of practice guidelines. *CMAJ* 1999;160:1165-8.
40 Foy R. A randomised controlled trial of a tailored multifaceted strategy to promote implementation of a clinical guideline on induced abortion care. *BJOG* 2004;111:726-33.
41 Meyer G, Kopke S, Bender R, Muhlhauser I. Predicting the risk of falling—efficacy of a risk assessment tool compared to nurses' judgement: a cluster-randomised controlled trial. *BMC Geriatr* 2005;5:14.
42 Marrie TJ, Lau CY, Wheeler SL, Wong CJ, Vandervoort MK, Feagan BG. A controlled trial of a critical pathway for treatment of community-acquired pneumonia. *JAMA* 2000;283:749-55.
43 Spanos A, Harrell FE Jr, Durack DT. Differential diagnosis of acute meningitis. An analysis of the predictive value of initial observations. *JAMA* 1989;262:2700-7.
44 McKinney WP, Heudebert GR, Harper SA, Young MJ, McIntire DD. Validation of a clinical prediction rule for the differential diagnosis of acute meningitis. *J Gen Intern Med* 1994;9:8-12.
45 Hoen B, Viel JF, Paquot C, Gerard A, Canton P. Multivariate approach to differential diagnosis of acute meningitis. *Eur J Clin Microbiol Infect Dis* 1995;14:267-74.
46 Steyerberg EW, Keizer HJ, Habbema JD. Prediction models for the histology of residual masses after chemotherapy for metastatic testicular cancer. *Int J Cancer* 1999;83:856-9.
47 Graham ID, Stiell IG, Laupacis A, McAuley L, Howell M, Clancy M, et al. Awareness and use of the Ottawa ankle and knee rules in 5 countries: can publication alone be enough to change practice? *Ann Emerg Med* 2001;37:259-66.
48 Cabana MD, Rand CS, Powe NR, Wu AW, Wilson MH, Abboud PA, et al. Why don't physicians follow clinical practice guidelines? A framework for improvement. *JAMA* 1999;282:1458-65.

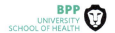

Ten steps towards improving prognosis research

Harry Hemingway, professor of clinical epidemiology[1], Richard D Riley, senior lecturer in medical statistics[2], Douglas G Altman, professor[3]

University College London, London C1 6BT

epartment of Public Health, Epidemiology and Biostatistics, University of Birmingham, Birmingham B15 2TT

Centre for Statistics in Medicine, Oxford

Correspondence to: h.hemingway@ucl.ac.uk

Cite this as: BMJ 2009;339:b4184

DOI: 10.1136/bmj.b4184

http://www.bmj.com/content/339/bmj.b4184

ABSTRACT

Prognosis research should be a basic science in translational medicine, but methodological problems mean systematic reviews are unable to reach firm conclusions. **Harry Hemingway and colleagues** recommend action to improve the quality

Stemming the tide of low quality, low impact, prognosis research is an urgent priority for the medical and research community. Diverting currently wasted research resources into high quality prognosis research will require major changes, one of which is the implicit collusion between researchers, medical journal editors, and conference organisers: "If you agree to inflate the importance of your research, we will agree to showcase it." We outline challenges facing prognosis research, and possible next steps, drawing on recent evidence from different clinical specialties and study designs.

Problems with prognosis research

Prognosis research has been defined as the study of relations between occurrences of outcomes and predictors in defined populations of people with disease.[1] It encompasses (ideally) prospective, observational research evaluating three broad questions—causes of disease progression, prediction of risk in individuals, and individual response to treatment. High quality prognosis research results in better understanding of disease progression, offers improved opportunities for mitigating that progression, and allows more reliable communication of outcome risk to patients.[1][2] Prognosis research should be a basic science in translational medicine.

Analysing 168 reports, Malats and colleagues concluded that "after 10 years of research [including over 10000 patients], evidence is not sufficient to conclude whether changes in P53 act as markers of outcome in patients with bladder cancer."[3] This is not an isolated example. Such concerns have been identified in systematic reviews of different types of prognostic biomarkers[4][5] and across different clinical specialties and major global burdens of disease including cancer,[6] coronary disease,[7] stroke,[8] trauma,[9] and musculoskeletal disorders.[10][11] Although some systematic reviews and meta-analyses of prognostic studies

SUMMARY POINTS

- The quality of much prognosis research is poor
- Systematic reviews can often reach only limited conclusions because of variation in methods, poor reporting, and publication bias
- Ten steps towards improving prognosis research are outlined
- Study and protocol registration and guidelines for reporting are urgently required

do reach clear conclusions, not all pay attention to the quality of the primary studies.[12][13]

It is inconceivable that 168 randomised controlled trials could fail to reach an answer on the effectiveness of an intervention. Why does the scientific community generate, and apparently tolerate, prognosis research with such limitations? Here we identify 10 areas where specific actions (table) might make investments in prognosis research more effective (in terms of generating reliable new knowledge with benefits for patient outcomes) and more efficient (less redundant or misleading research).

Purpose

In the absence of an accepted classification used across clinical specialties, we need to clarify the goals of prognosis research and thereby provide a framework with which to assess progress. Standard nomenclature is urgently needed. Broadly, three aims can be recognised:

- Identification of single biomarkers that have independent associations with outcome (relating to the causal pathway)
- Development of multivariable risk prediction models (risk score or prognostic index) that predict an individual's outcome, and
- Identification of biomarkers that predict response to treatment (treatment-covariate interactions or predictive factors).

Such a taxonomy could identify different goals at different stages in the translation of emerging putative prognostic biomarkers from the laboratory to the bedside. For example, early prognostic studies may aim at discovering possible prognostic biomarkers and will tolerate false positive results; later studies may evaluate the probability that such biomarkers are useful (in risk prediction models) and seek to minimise false positive results.[14] Existing systematic reviews of prognostic biomarkers suggest that current prognosis research concentrates on the first goal. For example, in a systematic review of the prognostic value of C reactive protein on the prognosis of stable coronary disease,[7] only three of the 77 studies reported a measure of its ability to discriminate risk in individuals.

A greater appreciation of the distinction between the three goals is required. For instance, it is wrong to assume that a biomarker that is (causally) related to incidence of disease (aetiology) is necessarily (causally) related to progression (prognosis). For example, body mass index is associated in aetiological studies with onset of coronary disease but not with subsequent fatal and non-fatal events among people with coronary disease.[15] Risk prediction models are easy to produce, hard to validate,[16] and harder still to implement in clinical practice. And, thus far, evidence of impact on decision making or prognosis is nearly always lacking.[17] The next generation of such models needs to tackle these problems.

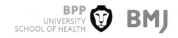

Table 1 Ten challenges facing prognostic research

Stage in research process	Challenge	Proposed solution
Purpose	Lack of agreed research goals	Develop a taxonomy of the goals and types of prognostic research; agree nomenclature
Funding	Lack of strategic framework for funding	Identify research priorities among adequately sized de novo prospective studies, enriching existing collections, including registries, and meta-analysis of individual participant data
Protocols	Protocols are rarely available (published or unpublished) and may rarely exist	Encourage the publication of protocols outlining the prognostic questions and biomarkers to be assessed; data quality and statistical analysis plan; and prespecified outcomes of interest. Improving the quality of primary prognostic research by emulating, where appropriate, the design standards expected of a high quality randomised trial
Predictors	Novel high cost biomarkers more researched than available clinical information	Better prognostic understanding of the available clinical information is required (including information from the history, examination, blood, imaging and other investigations, and markers of quality of care); clarify the strength of evidence required for prognostic biomarkers to be considered "established" or "useful"
Outcomes	Patient reported outcomes (symptoms, functional status, quality of life) neglected; primary outcomes often not defined	Better integration of patient relevant outcomes (including those reported by patients) into prognostic research; definition of primary outcomes in protocol
Methods	Current methodological standards are poor	Catch up with trial methodology (where appropriate), and develop methods that are particular to prognostic research
Publication	Small, positive studies bias the literature	Systematically identify the extent of, and reasons for, publication bias in prognostic research and encourage methods to prevent it, including prospective study registration, increasing study size, and adherence to reporting guidelines
Reporting	No reporting standards generic across clinical disciplines and types of prognostic research, so authors omit important information, and inflate importance of conclusions	Develop generic standards for reporting prognosis research studies (potentially using the REMARK guidelines as a starting point); encourage journals and authors to adhere to these standards
Synthesis	High quality systematic reviews that reach a robust, useful conclusion are uncommon	As well as improving quality of primary studies, develop better systematic review methods; easier identification of prognostic research; and facilitate of access to individual participant data
Impact	Unclear effectiveness of prognosis research in translational medicine and clinical decision making	Develop metrics for assessing the effectiveness and cost effectiveness of doing more prognostic research and using prognostic information to change clinical decisions and patient outcomes

Funding

Prognosis research has attracted much less funding than diagnostic and therapeutic research. As a crude marker of this, a search of the website of the US National Institutes of Health, globally one of the largest funding bodies, returns about 132 000 hits for the term "diagnostic," 76 000 for "trial," and only 4000 for "prognostic." Indeed one reason for the large number of small, poor quality prognostic studies may be that many are conducted without peer reviewed external sources of funding. A "what's in the freezer?" approach has been too common,[18] in which the investigator apparently argues: given the data we already have, what abstract can be produced to allow a junior colleague to present at a conference. For example, in cancer biomarker studies, Kyzas and colleagues suggest "investigators may tend to conduct opportunistic studies on the basis of specimen availability rather than on thoughtful design."[19] Such an approach perpetuates poor quality research.

Funders need a strategic framework to guide investment across complementary study designs. This will enable them to judge when it is best to set up bespoke investigator-led prognostic cohorts, to add biomarker or other measurements to existing clinical cohort collections (including registry data), to exploit linkages between different electronic health records (such as in primary care and disease registries), or to stimulate meta-analysis of data on individual participants.[20]

Protocols

All research on humans should have a protocol,[21] [22] yet many current prognosis research studies seem not to be protocol driven. Most prognostic studies are retrospective

in the sense that the investigator decides which analyses to do after the data have been collected. Just four of the 77 studies in the C reactive protein systematic review referred to a previously written study protocol.[7] Thus the reader does not know whether the analyses were part of the rationale for entering patients into the study or were prespecified in a statistical analysis plan and there is large potential for selective and biased reporting. It should become mandatory for prognosis research to have a registered study protocol outlining the aims and detailing the methods of data collection and statistical analysis that will be used.[23] Study registration and publication of analytical and study protocols should also help improve the quality of studies.

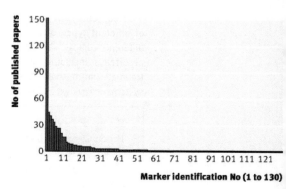

Fig 1 Mile wide inch deep focus of research shown by systematic review of studies of genetic and other circulating biomarkers for recurrence or death from neuroblastoma.[24] 130 different biomarkers were studied with a median of one study per marker

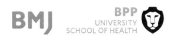

Predictors

Given the wide range of factors that may influence prognosis—the social and healthcare environment, psychosocial factors, health behaviours, and biological factors—why is the focus of prognosis research so uneven? The "mile wide, inch deep" focus on circulating biomarkers is illustrated in a systematic review of 130 different factors in neuroblastoma in which the median number of publications per biomarker was 1 (fig 1).[24] By contrast, the prognostic importance of history, examination, and simple investigations has been relatively neglected.[25] For example, whereas meta-analyses have examined the relation between alcohol consumption in initially healthy populations and subsequent death from coronary disease,[26] there has been little research into the relation between alcohol and prognosis among people with cardiovascular disease,[27] and no meta-analyses. This is a clinically important question because doctors need evidence on which to base advice to patients and a framework to evaluate new prognostic biomarkers in the context of existing knowledge. There is a need for clarity over the strength of evidence required for prognostic biomarkers to be considered "established" or "useful."

Outcomes

Most prognosis research in cancer and cardiovascular disease fails to report suffering from symptoms, functional status, and quality of life. Mortality may not be the most important outcome to the patient, nor is it necessarily a good proxy for other outcomes. Patient values are a constituent, not a contingent, property of a full understanding of prognosis. Assessments of the impact of a particular disease on a patient's life vary widely among patients, and are commonly discordant with the severity assessed by doctors.[28]

As most prognostic studies examine multiple outcomes, selective reporting, where only those outcomes found to be statistically or clinically significant are reported, is a concern. Selective reporting is a problem in cancer prognostic studies,[29] but is likely to be prevalent in other fields too. This problem underscores the need for study and protocol registration, with pre-specification of the primary outcomes of interest.

Methods

Prognosis research must catch up with the standards of high quality randomised trials or observational aetiological research, in terms of design, conduct, analysis, and reporting.[20] Many studies are simply too small to provide reliable evidence—for example, a meta-analysis of 47 studies among patients with Barrett's oesophagus reported

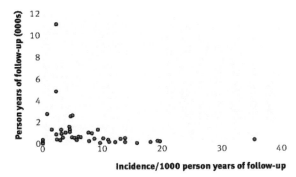

Fig 2 Systematic review of 47 studies investigating incidence of oesophageal cancer in patients with Barrett's oesophagus found that most were too small to provide reliable evidence.[30] Larger studies tended to show lower incidence of cancer

a total of just 209 incident cases of oesophageal cancer (fig 2).[30] Prognosis research needs to be seen as a distinct field in order to foster scientifically justified, rather than idiosyncratic, methods. For example, in cancer research continuous biomarkers are almost always dichotomised, whereas in cardiovascular research this is much less common.

Hayden and colleagues list six stages in the design, conduct, and analysis of prognosis studies where bias may operate,[31] but most primary studies inadequately protect against these threats to validity.[10]

Publication

A prudent default position would be to assume that prognosis research is seriously afflicted by publication bias, until there is evidence to the contrary. Evaluating 1575 articles on different prognostic biomarkers for cancer, Kyzas and colleagues found that almost all report significant results,[6] signalling a major problem of publication bias. The C reactive protein systematic review found that publication bias was so large that different methods to adjust for its effect either substantially attenuated, or abolished, the apparent association between C reactive protein and outcome.[7] Study and protocol registration would help with this problem because it would make it easier to identify unpublished studies.

Reporting

Authors of prognosis research articles often omit key details, outcomes, and analyses and inflate the importance of their findings.[32] Currently there are no generic reporting guidelines for prognosis research, which means that journal editors, peer reviewers, authors, and readers do not have a framework for distinguishing reliable observations from the merely new. An important start has been made by the REMARK guidelines for biomarkers in cancer,[33] though lack of adherence to these guidelines has recently been noted.[34] Prognostic studies share many methodological features with healthy population studies, but require reporting of additional items, such as the initial medical condition, its stage, and duration since onset; the translational clinical question examined; absolute risks; and the clinical outcomes that are more varied than the singular end points used in aetiological studies.

Importantly, there are currently no reporting standards for risk prediction scores,[9] nor any central register where clinicians and researchers can access and compare these rapidly expanding technologies.[35] We propose that reporting guidelines are developed that span the scope of prognosis research (perhaps using REMARK as a starting point). As a related but distinct exercise a checklist of quality criteria should be developed.

Synthesis

Given the concerns about the quality of primary prognosis research, efforts at evidence synthesis should be viewed with caution. Evaluating 17 systematic reviews in the prognosis of low back pain, Hayden and colleagues concluded that "because of the methodological shortcomings . . . there remains uncertainty about the reliability of conclusions regarding prognostic factors."[10] Such a conclusion is common for systematic reviews of prognostic studies. The Cochrane Collaboration Prognosis Methods Group, established in 2008, aims to facilitate and improve the quality of systematic reviews of prognosis research.[36]

Developments are required at multiple stages, starting with improvements in primary studies and working towards improving methodology for synthesis. Remarkably, electronic searches of publications on PubMed cannot distinguish studies among people with disease from studies among healthy people who go on to develop disease. We therefore need a standardised nomenclature for describing the results of studies. The term prognosis is used variably, with at least three meanings: any outcome study including those in initially healthy populations; synonymous with mortality; and as risk prediction (or prognostication).

When high quality primary research studies exist, meta-analysis of individual participant data [20] is the most reliable method synthesis and is achievable.[20] [37] [38] An emerging challenge is the synthesis of different types of evidence relating to one prognosis research question. For example, studies assessing whether a new prognostic biomarker is causally related to disease progression use different, and potentially complementary, methods for dealing with confounding (observational study designs use statistical adjustment and genetic study designs use mendelian randomisation).[39]

Impact of research

However well prognosis research comes to protect against this range of biases, the "so what?" question demands answering. Prognosis research is not having the effect it should have both at early stages in the translational spectrum (for example, on informing the design and development of drug or other targets for patient management) or at later stages supporting clinical decision making (for example, in facilitating individualised or stratified medicine). Since 1991 there have been 102 risk prediction models reported for traumatic brain injury in 53 articles; in only five articles were models externally validated, and none has been widely implemented in clinical practice (fig 3.[9] From the perspective of a clinician and a patient, effectiveness means altered clinical decisions and consequent patient outcomes.[17] The psychosocial effect of prognostic information on patients and their families also warrants consideration in such effectiveness criteria.

From the perspective of a policy maker the impact of prognosis research should be made explicit in a cost effectiveness framework. For example, a recent study showed the value of cost effectiveness decision models for evaluating different prognostic risk scores to prioritise the waiting list for coronary surgery.[40] From the perspective of a research funder, the cost of investing in new prognosis

research and the impact of the resulting reduction in scientific uncertainty can be formally modelled.[41] [42]

Conclusion

Prognosis research across multiple disease areas faces challenges at each stage of the research process. We acknowledge that our backgrounds (in cardiovascular epidemiology and cancer biostatistics) both inform, and limit, our views. A systematic comparison of the state of the art of prognosis research across several clinical conditions would clarify the need for action and help prioritise our proposed 10 steps. Progress in prognosis research should be empirically demonstrated. One marker of progress is the emphasis that prognosis research commands in evidence based medicine; an influential book currently includes only 14 pages out of a total of 809.[43] This needs to change.

Contributors: Discussions among the authors were facilitated by John Scadding and David Misselbrook (Royal Society of Medicine) and Trish Groves (BMJ). Each author contributed examples and critically commented on the text. HH wrote the first draft and is the guarantor.

Competing interests: None declared.

Provenance and peer review: Not commissioned; externally peer reviewed.

1   Hemingway H. Prognosis research: why is Dr Lydgate still waiting? J Clin Epidemiol 2006;59:1229-38.
2   Moons KG, Royston P, Vergouwe Y, Grobbee DE, Altman DG. Prognosis and prognostic research: what, why, and how? BMJ 2009;338:b375.
3   Malats N, Bustos A, Nascimento CM, Fernandez F, Rivas M, Puente D, et al. P53 as a prognostic marker for bladder cancer: a meta-analysis and review. Lancet Oncol 2005;6:678-86.
4   Ntzani EE, Ioannidis JP. Predictive ability of DNA microarrays for cancer outcomes and correlates: an empirical assessment. Lancet 2003;362:1439-44.
5   Nicholson A, Kuper H, Hemingway H. Depression as an aetiologic and prognostic factor in coronary heart disease: a meta-analysis of 6362 events among 146 538 participants in 54 observational studies. Eur Heart J 2006;27:2763-74.
6   Kyzas PA, Denaxa-Kyza D, Ioannidis JP. Almost all articles on cancer prognostic markers report statistically significant results. Eur J Cancer 2007;43:2559-79.
7   Hemingway H, Henriksson M, Chen R, Damant J Fitzpatrick N, Abrams K, et al. The effectiveness and cost effectiveness of biomarkers for the prioritisation of patients awaiting coronary revascularisation: a systematic review and decision model. Health Technol Assess (in press).
8   Whiteley W, Chong WL, Sengupta A, Sandercock P. Blood markers for the prognosis of ischemic stroke: a systematic review. Stroke 2009;40:e380-9.
9   Perel P, Edwards P, Wentz R, Roberts I. Systematic review of prognostic models in traumatic brain injury. BMC Med Inform Decis Mak 2006;6:38.
10 Hayden JA, Chou R, Hogg-Johnson S, Bombardier C. Systematic reviews of low back pain prognosis had variable methods and results-guidance for future prognosis reviews. J Clin Epidemiol 2009;62:781-96.
11 Pengel LH, Herbert RD, Maher CG, Refshauge KM. Acute low back pain: systematic review of its prognosis. BMJ 2003;327:323.
12 Williams MD, Harris R, Dayan CM, Evans J, Gallacher J, Ben-Shlomo Y. Thyroid function and the natural history of depression: findings from the Caerphilly Prospective Study (CaPS) and a meta-analysis. Clin Endocrinol (Oxf) 2009;70:484-92.
13 Zandbergen EG, de Haan RJ, Hijdra A. Systematic review of prediction of poor outcome in anoxic-ischaemic coma with biochemical markers of brain damage. Intensive Care Med 2001;27:1661-7.
14 Hayden JA, Cote P, Steenstra IA, Bombardier C. Identifying phases of investigation helps planning, appraising, and applying the results of explanatory prognosis studies. J Clin Epidemiol 2008;61:552-60.
15 Romero-Corral A, Montori VM, Somers VK, Korinek J, Thomas RJ, Allison TG, et al. Association of bodyweight with total mortality and with cardiovascular events in coronary artery disease: a systematic review of cohort studies. Lancet 2006;368:666-78.
16 Altman DG, Royston P. What do we mean by validating a prognostic model? Stat Med 2000;19:453-73.
17 Reilly BM, Evans AT. Translating clinical research into clinical practice: impact of using prediction rules to make decisions. Ann Intern Med 2006;144:201-9.
18 Schmitz-Drager BJ, Goebell PJ, Ebert T, Fradet Y. p53 immunohistochemistry as a prognostic marker in bladder cancer. Playground for urology scientists? Eur Urol 2000;38:691-9.
19 Kyzas PA, Denaxa-Kyza D, Ioannidis JP. Quality of reporting of cancer prognostic marker studies: association with reported prognostic effect. J Natl Cancer Inst 2007;99:236-43.

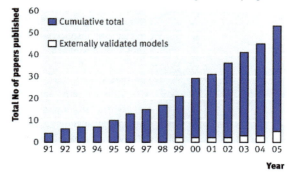

Fig 3 Illustration of lack of clinical impact of some prognostic research. Systematic review identified 53 papers on 102 risk prediction models for death and disability in patients with traumatic brain injury published during 1991-2005, but only five were externally validated and none of the models is used in clinical practice[9]

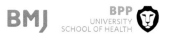

20 Riley RD, Sauerbrei W, Altman DG. Prognostic markers in cancer: the evolution of evidence from single studies to meta-analysis, and beyond. *Br J Cancer* 2009;100:1219-29.

21 World Medical Association. Declaration of Helsinki. WMA, 2008.

22 Council for International Organizations of Medical Sciences. International ethical guidelines for biomedical research involving human subjects. 2nd ed. Geneva: WHO, 2002.

23 Rifai N, Altman DG, Bossuyt PM. Reporting bias in diagnostic and prognostic studies: time for action. *Clin Chem* 2008;54:1101-3.

24 Riley RD, Burchill SA, Abrams KR, Heney D, Lambert PC, Jones DR, et al. A systematic review and evaluation of the use of tumour markers in paediatric oncology: Ewing's sarcoma and neuroblastoma. *Health Technol Assess* 2003;7:1-162.

25 Sutcliffe P, Hummel S, Simpson E, Young T, Rees A, Wilkinson A, et al. Use of classical and novel biomarkers as prognostic risk factors for localised prostate cancer: a systematic review. *Health Technol Assess* 2009;13:1-242.

26 Corrao G, Rubbiati L, Bagnardi V, Zambon A, Poikolainen K. Alcohol and coronary heart disease: a meta-analysis. *Addiction* 2000;95:1505-23.

27 Muntwyler J, Hennekens CH, Buring JE, Gaziano JM. Mortality and light to moderate alcohol consumption after myocardial infarction. *Lancet* 1998;352:1882-5.

28 Nease RF Jr, Kneeland T, O'Connor GT, Sumner W, Lumpkins C, Shaw L, et al. Variation in patient utilities for outcomes of the management of chronic stable angina. Implications for clinical practice guidelines. *JAMA* 1995;273):1185-90.

29 Kyzas PA, Loizou KT, Ioannidis JP. Selective reporting biases in cancer prognostic factor studies. *J Natl Cancer Inst* 2005;97:1043-55.

30 Yousef F, Cardwell C, Cantwell MM, Galway K, Johnston BT, Murray L. The incidence of esophageal cancer and high-grade dysplasia in Barrett's esophagus: a systematic review and meta-analysis. *Am J Epidemiol* 2008;168:237-49.

31 Hayden JA, Cote P, Bombardier C. Evaluation of the quality of prognosis studies in systematic reviews. *Ann Intern Med* 2006;144:427-37.

32 Riley RD, Abrams KR, Sutton AJ, Lambert PC, Jones DR, Heney D, et al. Reporting of prognostic markers: current problems and development of guidelines for evidence-based practice in the future. *Br J Cancer* 2003;88:1191-8.

33 McShane LM, Altman DG, Sauerbrei W, Taube SE, Gion M, Clark GM. Reporting recommendations for tumor marker prognostic studies (REMARK). *J Natl Cancer Inst* 2005;97:1180-4.

34 Gould Rothberg BE, Bracken MB, Rimm DL. Tissue biomarkers for prognosis in cutaneous melanoma: a systematic review and meta-analysis. *J Natl Cancer Inst* 2009;101:452-74.

35 Hlatky MA, Greenland P, Arnett DK, Ballantyne CM, Criqui MH, Elkind MS, et al. Criteria for evaluation of novel markers of cardiovascular risk: a scientific statement from the American Heart Association. *Circulation* 2009;119:2408-16.

36 Riley RD, Ridley G, Williams K, Altman DG, Hayden J, de Vet HC. Prognosis research: toward evidence-based results and a Cochrane methods group. *J Clin Epidemiol* 2007;60:863-5.

37 Thakkinstian A, Dmitrienko S, Gerbase-Delima M, McDaniel DO, Inigo P, Chow KM, et al. Association between cytokine gene polymorphisms and outcomes in renal transplantation: a meta-analysis of individual patient data. *Nephrol Dial Transplant* 2008;23:3017-23.

38 Look MP, van Putten WL, Duffy MJ, Harbeck N, Christensen IJ, Thomssen C, et al. Pooled analysis of prognostic impact of urokinase-type plasminogen activator and its inhibitor PAI-1 in 8377 breast cancer patients. *J Natl Cancer Inst* 2002;94:116-28.

39 Kuper H, Nicholson A, Kivimaki M, Hemingway H, et al. Evaluating the causal relevance of diverse risk markers: horizontal systematic review. *BMJ* 2009;339:b4265.

40 Henriksson M, Palmer S, Chen R, Damant J, Fitzpatrick N, Abrams KR, et al. Assessing the cost-effectiveness of prognostic biomarkers: a case study in prioritising patients waiting for coronary artery surgery. *BMJ* (in press).

41 Fenwick E, Claxton K, Sculpher M. The value of implementation and the value of information: combined and uneven development. *Med Decis Making* 2008;28:21-32.

42 Claxton K, Ginnelly L, Sculpher M, Philips Z, Palmer S. A pilot study on the use of decision theory and value of information analysis as part of the NHS health technology assessment programme. *Health Technol Assess* 2004;8(31):1-103, iii.

43 Guyatt G, Rennie D, Meade M, Cook D. *Users' guides to the medical literature: a manual for evidence-based clinical practice* . 2nd ed. AMA Press, 2008.

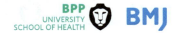

Prognosis research strategy (PROGRESS) 1: A framework for researching clinical outcomes

Harry Hemingway, professor of clinical epidemiology[1], Peter Croft, professor of epidemiology[2], Pablo Perel, clinical senior lecturer[3], Jill A Hayden, assistant professor[4], Keith Abrams, professor of medical statistics[5], Adam Timmis, professor of clinical cardiology[6], Andrew Briggs, Lindsay chair in health policy & economic evaluation[7], Ruzan Udumyan, research assistant[1], Karel G M Moons, professor of clinical epidemiology[8], Ewout W Steyerberg, professor of medical decision making[9], Ian Roberts, professor of epidemiology and public health[3], Sara Schroter, senior researcher[10], Douglas G Altman, professor of statistics in medicine[11], Richard D Riley, senior lecturer in medical statistics[12], for the PROGRESS Group

[1]Department of Epidemiology and Public Health, University College London, London WC1E 7HB, UK

[2]Arthritis Research UK Primary Care Centre, Keele University, Keele ST5 5BG, UK

[3]London School of Hygiene & Tropical Medicine, London WC1E 7HT

[4]Department of Community Health and Epidemiology, Dalhousie University, Halifax, Nova Scotia, Canada B3H 1V7

[5]Centre for Biostatistics & Genetic Epidemiology, Department of Health Sciences, School of Medicine, University of Leicester, Leicester LE1 7RH, UK

[6]London Chest Hospital, London E2 9JX

[7]Health Economics & Health Technology Assessment, Centre for Population & Health Sciences, University of Glasgow, Glasgow G12 8RZ, UK

[8]Julius Center for Health Sciences and Primary Care, UMC Utrecht, Utrecht, Netherlands

[9]Department of Public Health, Erasmus MC, Rotterdam, Netherlands

[10]BMJ, BMA House, London WC1H 9JR

[11]Centre for Statistics in Medicine, University of Oxford, Oxford OX2 6UD, UK

[12]School of Health and Population Sciences, University of Birmingham, Birmingham B15 2TT, UK

Correspondence to: H Hemingway
h.hemingway@ucl.ac.uk

Cite this as: BMJ 2013;346:e5595

DOI: 10.1136/bmj.e5595

http://www.bmj.com/content/346/bmj.e5595

ABSTRACT

Understanding and improving the prognosis of a disease or health condition is a priority in clinical research and practice. In this article, the authors introduce a framework of four interrelated themes in prognosis research, describe the importance of the first of these themes (understanding future outcomes in relation to current diagnostic and treatment practices), and introduce recommendations for the field of prognosis research

In clinical medicine, the term prognosis refers to the risk of future health outcomes in people with a given disease or health condition. Prognosis research is thus the investigation of the relations between future outcomes (endpoints) among people with a given baseline health state (startpoint) in order to improve health (see supplementary figure on bmj.com). The study of prognosis has never been more important, as globally more people are living with one or more disease or health impairing condition than at any previous time.[1] For this reason, governments across the world are increasing their interest in the outcomes of healthcare currently provided for people with disease.[2] Similarly, research funders and researchers are increasingly focused on translating new interventions and technologies from the laboratory to clinical practice and then healthcare policy in order to establish and implement new standards of high quality care and improve patient outcomes.

Prognosis research findings should thus be integral to clinical decision making, healthcare policy, and discovering and evaluating new approaches to patient management. However, there is a concerning gap between the potential and actual impact of prognosis research on health. Prognosis research studies too often fall a long way short of the high standards required in other fields, such as therapeutic trials and genetic epidemiology.

In the PROGnosis RESearch Strategy (PROGRESS) series (www.progress-partnership.org), we propose a framework of four distinct but inter-related prognosis research themes: (1) The course of health related conditions in the context of the nature and quality of current care (fundamental prognosis research) (2) Specific factors (such as biomarkers) that are associated with prognosis (prognostic factor research)[3] (3) The development, validation, and impact of statistical models that predict individual risk of a future outcome (prognostic model research)[4]

SUMMARY POINTS

- The PROGRESS series (www.progress-partnership.org) sets out a framework of four interlinked prognosis research themes and provides examples from several disease fields to show why evidence from prognosis research is crucial to inform all points in the translation of biomedical and health related research into better patient outcomes. Recommendations are made in each of the four papers to improve current research standards
- What is prognosis research? Prognosis research seeks to understand and improve future outcomes in people with a given disease or health condition. However, there is increasing evidence that prognosis research standards need to be improved
- Why is prognosis research important? More people now live with disease and conditions that impair health than at any other time in history; prognosis research provides crucial evidence for translating findings from the laboratory to humans, and from clinical research to clinical practice
- This first article introduces the framework of four interlinked prognosis research themes and then focuses on the first of the themes—fundamental prognosis research, studies that aim to describe and explain future outcomes in relation to current diagnostic and treatment practices, often in relation to quality of care
- Fundamental prognosis research provides evidence informing healthcare and public health policy, the design and interpretation of randomised trials, and the impact of diagnostic tests on future outcome. It can inform new definitions of disease, may identify unanticipated benefits or harms of interventions, and clarify where new interventions are required to improve prognosis
- The other papers in the series are:
- PROGRESS 2: PLoS Med 2013, doi:10.1371.journal/pmed.1001380
- PROGRESS 3: PLoS Med 2013, doi:10.1371.journal/pmed.1001381
- PROGRESS 4: BMJ 2013, doi:10.1136/bmj.e5793

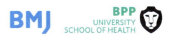

(4) The use of prognostic information to help tailor treatment decisions to an individual or group of individuals with similar characteristics (stratified medicine research).[5]

Figure 1 illustrates these four prognosis research areas for women with breast cancer (startpoint) and the endpoint of death or disease-free survival. Part (a) shows country variations in age adjusted, five year survival (fundamental prognosis research)[6]; part (b) shows survival curves according to the value of extracellular domain of human epidermal growth factor receptor 2 (HER2 ECD), which is identified to be prognostic of disease outcome (prognostic factor research)[7]; part (c) shows the use of multiple clinical variables within a statistical model to estimate individual risk of a particular endpoint (prognostic model research)[8]; and part (d) shows why a positive oestrogen receptor status is used to identify those who will benefit from tamoxifen therapy (stratified medicine research).[9]

The overarching aim of the PROGRESS series is to explain how each of these four prognosis research themes provides important evidence that can be used at multiple (translational) pathways toward improving clinical outcomes—from the discovery of new interventions, through to their evaluation and implementation in the clinical management of individual patients, and to examining the impact of interventions and healthcare policies on patient outcomes. This contrasts with previous reviews of prognosis research which consider impact at one end of the translational spectrum (such as clinical decision making) or on just one type of prognosis question (such as prognostic models[10]). Whereas previous reviews focus on one specific disease area (such as cancer),[11] [12] we include examples from cancer, cardiovascular disease, musculoskeletal disorders, trauma, and other conditions. Our series describes the current challenges and opportunities in the field and makes

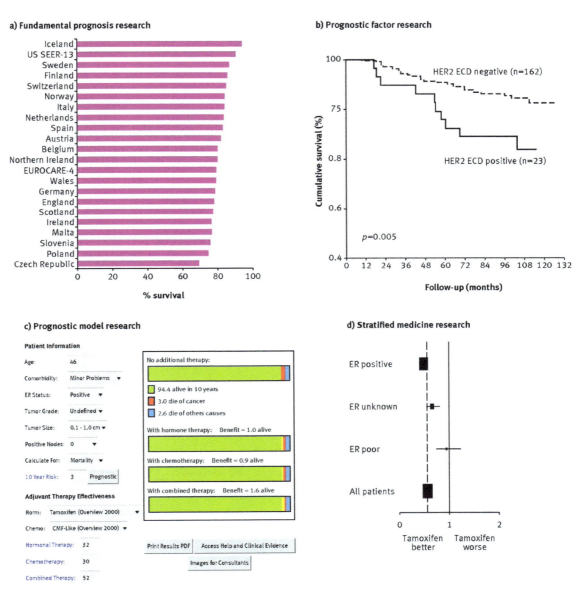

Fig 1 Framework of four different types of prognosis research question, illustrated for breast cancer. a) Fundamental prognosis research: variations between countries in age adjusted, five year survival (with permission from Cancer Research UK[6]). b) Prognostic factor research: survival curves showing that patients with "positive" values (>8.9 ng/mL) of the extracellular domain of human epidermal growth factor receptor 2 (HER2 ECD) have a worse survival than those with negative values (≤8.9 ng/mL), and thus HER ECD is a potential prognostic factor (from Tsai et al[7]). c) Prognostic model research: use of multiple clinical variables in a model to estimate risk of endpoint, and then combined with evidence of treatment effectiveness to inform clinical decisions (ER=oestrogen receptor) (from Adjuvant! Online[8]). d) Stratified medicine research: predictors of differential treatment response identified in randomised trials, showing that the benefit of tamoxifen is confined to those with positive oestrogen receptor (ER) status (based on data from Early Breast Cancer Trialists Collaborative Group[9])

recommendations for necessary improvements to move toward a clearer map for prognosis research that ultimately improves patient outcomes (summarised in supplementary table 1 on bmj.com).

An important place to start is with research that aims to examine the outcomes of a disease or health condition in the context of current clinical practice, and this we term fundamental prognosis research. In this first article we consider what this entails, explain its importance in pathways toward improving patient outcomes, and outline a set of recommendations with the aim of improving the quality and impact across all of the inter-related themes in prognosis research and which will be expanded in the other articles in our series.

What is fundamental prognosis research?

Before carrying out research into novel prognostic factors, prognostic models, or stratified medicine it is necessary to carry out research describing and explaining future outcomes in people with a disease or health condition in relation to current diagnostic and treatment practices. There is a close relation between the questions "What is the prognosis of people with this condition?" and "What are the outcomes of the care which people receive for this condition?" In order to improve the quality of healthcare, evidence is required on how the specific patterns of care received (such as investigation, treatment, support), and their variations (such as underuse, overuse, misuse) have an impact on future endpoints.[13] Such research has a broad remit. It spans, for example, investigations into societal influences (inequitable variations in care and outcome among older people, women, the socially disadvantaged, and ethnic minorities),[14] [15] patient safety, unanticipated harms and benefits from treatments, and screening research. Prognosis in the absence of care—which is sometimes termed natural history—is an important parameter for judging the potential impact of screening for asymptomatic disease (such as mammography for breast cancer), as well as for case detection of symptomatic undiagnosed or unpresented conditions such as back pain or angina.[16] [17]

These relations may be expressed as an absolute risk (or rate) of one or more type of endpoint among groups of people who share demographic and clinical characteristics; some refer to this as an average prognosis in a particular group of interest, or as a baseline risk. Here the research provides initial answers to the question "What is the prognosis of people with a given disease?" For example, on average about 15% of people aged 65 years or older, admitted in 2006 in the US died within 30 days of admission to hospital with a heart attack compared with an average of 19% in 1995.[18] Such a change in the average mortality rate is illustrated in figure 2. This shows the decreasing prognostic burden of heart attack and motivates inquiry into new approaches to understand and reduce this risk further. This clinical scenario also exemplifies that "the prognosis" of a disease or condition is a somewhat misleading expression: what is observed is prognosis of people in particular clinical contexts, defined by current clinical approaches in diagnosing, characterising, and managing patients with a symptom or disease.

Such prognosis research is also concerned with describing and understanding the variations around the average course.[19] [20] These variations may occur between individual patients or between patients clustered, for example, within surgeons, hospitals, or regions. The acute myocardial infarction example above demonstrates striking variations between hospitals in prognosis, and similar variations are seen in traumatic brain injury and other conditions.[18] [21] Indeed, for most hospitals the national average is a poor guide to the mortality of their patients (fig 2).

Stephen J Gould, the evolutionary biologist, having survived 20 years after being told the median survival of his abdominal mesothelioma was eight months, famously remarked, "the median isn't the message."[22] Describing and explaining the sources of variability in prognosis is a theme throughout our PROGRESS framework.[3] [4] [5] Fundamental prognosis research may help explain Gould's long survival in terms of the demographic and clinical context (for example, his high educational status and the quality of care received), whereas research into emerging prognostic factors may examine psychological, behavioural, or biomarker factors associated with improved outcome (see paper 2 in our series[3]), or the extent to which his survival was predictable from statistical models of individual risk prediction (paper 3 in our series[4]), or whether particular treatments had a larger beneficial effect for him than for others (paper 4 in our series[5]).

Importance of fundamental prognosis research in the pathways toward improved health outcomes

Healthcare professionals, people with a disease or health condition, funders, and policy makers require valid, reliable evidence about the outcomes of diseases and health conditions in order to make decisions. Here we review the potential impact of such evidence across translational pathways in healthcare, starting from the applied, healthcare delivery end (far right of pathways schema shown at bottom of figs 2, 3, and 4) and working back to discovery and new approaches (far left of schema).

Importance for public health policy

Public health policy makers need estimates of average prognosis to model the population burden of diseases and assess the relative contribution of healthcare delivery among those with disease (secondary prevention) and without disease (primary prevention). For example, the

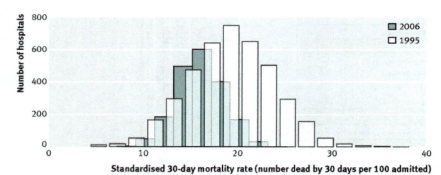

Standardised 30-day mortality rate (number dead by 30 days per 100 admitted)

Position along translational pathways toward improved outcomes

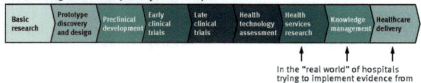

In the "real world" of hospitals trying to implement evidence from randomised trials, what outcomes are achieved?
Knowledge management is involved partly because the evidence comes from hospital admission data

Fig 2 Example of use of fundamental prognosis research to examine variations in outcomes from medical care: inter-hospital variation in mortality per 100 population within 30 days of admission with acute myocardial infarction (created using fictional data for illustration purposes, but based on the findings of Krumholz et al[18])

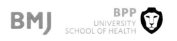

public health objective of reducing overall coronary heart disease mortality (a conflation of incidence of non-fatal coronary disease and subsequent death) has been helped by modelling the impact of population interventions aimed at early detection and primary and secondary prevention.[23] [24] [25] Such models use an average prognosis of heart attack survival from the date of diagnosis among age and sex strata to attribute quality adjusted life years (and health service costs of managing the disease) which would be saved with successful prevention.

By contrast with the improvements over time in the prognosis of coronary disease, for people with low back pain there is little evidence that the average prognosis (based on symptom relief[26] [27]) has changed over the past 20 years, nor does it differ between countries with different healthcare systems.[28] This suggests that healthcare itself is not a major influence on average symptomatic outcome in people with back pain. However, when considering the outcome of sickness absence, there are dramatic variations over time and between countries—suggesting the importance of the broader public health context of working patterns and benefit payments for chronic illness.[29]

Importance for comparative effectiveness and health services research

Insights into health and healthcare policy may come from comparing the prognosis of specific conditions over time and place in order to assess the comparative effectiveness of systems of care.[30] [31] For example, figure 1 shows that the five year survival from breast cancer in 2000-03 varies widely from country to country (from about 70% in the Czech Republic to 90% in Iceland). The UK seems to have worse cancer survival than most other European countries,[32] and the latter have worse survival for some cancers than the US. Such international comparisons of average prognosis provide a motivation for researchers to uncover explanations and for healthcare policy makers to improve the quality of care and deliver better health outcomes.[2] Policy makers seeking to improve national cancer outcomes may consider a range of interventions, including: early detection (such as mammography screening), population-wide guidance (such as encouraging self examination),[33] [34] centralisation of services, and systematic implementation of cost effective therapies. Ecological comparisons of country-level factors (such as smoking prevalence or number of specialists per capita population) can be related to outcomes. Such research may generate hypotheses for prognostic factor research (see paper 2 in our series[3]) as well as helping to formulate service and policy development.

Fundamental prognosis research is vital in addressing the "second gap" in translation,[35] in which evidence from randomised trials of effective treatments may fail to be implemented in usual clinical practice (far right of translational pathway toward improved clinical outcomes). For example, the between hospital variations in outcome from acute myocardial infarction (fig 2) may, in part, stem from differing use of evidence based therapies. These findings have profound implications for healthcare policy. It demonstrates a "normal distribution" of mortality between hospitals; over time the whole distribution of hospital mortality improves and shifts to the left and the variation between hospitals in outcomes narrows. The policy implication is that improvements in the quality of care in the population of all hospitals may have contributed to the observed shift in the average prognosis. Thus the evidence

did not support a contrasting policy alternative of focusing on the identification of, and remedial action in, outlying poor performers.[36] Here prognosis research is contributing evidence about health services and is managing knowledge generated from electronic health records. Such evidence[35] informs policy choices which are themselves highly unlikely to be subjected to randomised trials.[37]

Importance for health technology assessment of imaging and other tests

A key target for translational research is the development of new clinical imaging and molecular markers which may identify patient phenotypes in such a way as to lead to improved outcomes. Such new technologies may change the spectrum of diagnosed disease, and the question is whether prognosis is the same as with the use of standard tests and whether the balance of benefit and harm of treatment remains the same. For example, for decades exercise electrocardiography has been used in the characterisation of patients with stable chest pain, and recent guidelines recommend the use of an emerging technology, non-invasive computed tomographic coronary angiography, in some patients.[38] Since event powered randomised trials of imaging remain rare, fundamental prognosis research provides an important method of health technology assessment.[39]

Importance for trials and decision models

Estimates of average prognosis are also crucial for the rationale, design, interpretation, and impact modelling of trials of an intervention to improve prognosis. For example, prognosis research among people with angina shows that 50% of people with existing therapies have recurrent or persistent symptoms,[40] suggesting the need for trials of new interventions. Reliable estimates of prognosis inform the estimates of likely accrual of endpoints in the trial arms (such as expected proportion experiencing an event by a particular time), and hence facilitate statistical sample size calculations. They also contribute to the interpretation in terms of generalisability of clinical trial results, as one can compare the average prognosis of patients in the trial without treatment with the average prognosis in particular populations.

Importantly, in order to translate relative treatment effects (such as relative risks or hazard ratios) back to the absolute scale, one needs to know the average prognosis (baseline risk) in the untreated group. One can then talk in terms of the reduction in probability of a poor outcome (risk difference), which leads to clinically informative measures such as the number needed to treat in order to save one patient from a particular poor outcome. Absolute effects are used within decision models and cost effectiveness analyses, which are highly influential to decision makers such as the National Institute of Health and Clinical Excellence (NICE). Such models combine parameters of average prognosis along with estimates of treatment effects and costs. Conclusions from these models are often particularly sensitive to the accuracy of the data on average prognosis among those without the specific treatment of interest.

Importance for new approaches, mechanisms, and targets for trials

Fundamental prognosis research may provide insights beyond evaluating the status quo of clinical care. Estimating the prospective associations between two diseases has

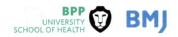

Study	Relative risk (95% CI)

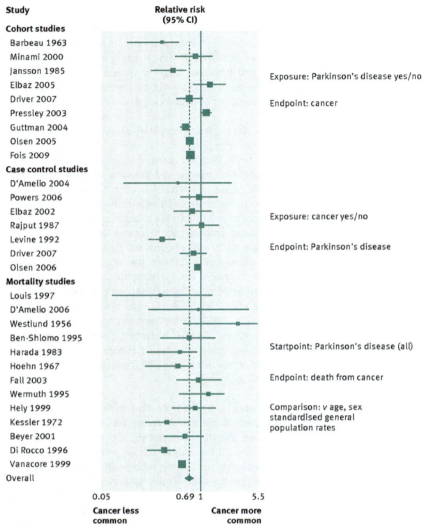

Cohort studies
Barbeau 1963
Minami 2000
Jansson 1985
Elbaz 2005 — Exposure: Parkinson's disease yes/no
Driver 2007
Pressley 2003 — Endpoint: cancer
Guttman 2004
Olsen 2005
Fois 2009

Case control studies
D'Amelio 2004
Powers 2006
Elbaz 2002
Rajput 1987 — Exposure: cancer yes/no
Levine 1992
Driver 2007 — Endpoint: Parkinson's disease
Olsen 2006

Mortality studies
Louis 1997
D'Amelio 2006
Westlund 1956
Ben-Shlomo 1995 — Startpoint: Parkinson's disease (all)
Harada 1983
Hoehn 1967 — Endpoint: death from cancer
Fall 2003
Wermuth 1995
Hely 1999 — Comparison: v age, sex standardised general population rates
Kessler 1972
Beyer 2001
Di Rocco 1996
Vanacore 1999
Overall

0.05   0.69 1   5.5
Cancer less common   **Cancer more common**

Position along translational pathways toward improved outcomes

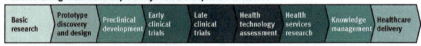

Basic research | Prototype discovery and design | Preclinical development | Early clinical trials | Late clinical trials | Health technology assessment | Health services research | Knowledge management | Healthcare delivery

↑
A possible protective effect of Parkinson's disease for cancer might suggest new biological pathways

Fig 3 Example of use of fundamental prognosis research to discover new associations between diseases: cancer among non-smoking people with Parkinson's disease (drawn using data from Bajaj et al[42]). Path element adapted from chart 7.1 in the Cooksey report (2006) http://bit.ly/Ro27rL (made available for use through the Open Government License)

with (as yet) unknown implications for developing new interventions. Consider the example of following up people with Parkinson's disease. The risk of cancer is not an endpoint that would conventionally be considered. However, a meta-analysis found that the risk of cancer was significantly reduced compared with people without Parkinson's disease (fig 3).[42] This raises the question whether specific characteristics of Parkinson's disease that explain this apparent protective effect can be identified, and whether this might lead to new intervention targets. There are probably many prognostic associations between two or more diseases that have yet to be uncovered. Some have proposed that approaches using all available clinical data (so called phenome-wide scans), agnostic to any prior theories about mechanism, might identify new associations between conditions.[43]

Importance for overcoming the limitations of diagnosis
The understanding of future outcome risk (prognosis) may be a more useful way of formulating clinical problems than pursuing diagnosis for several reasons. First, subjectively reported illness such as mental health problems and pain syndromes is often managed more with prognostic than diagnostic labels.[44] For example, a physician may reasonably say to a person presenting with back pain, "I do not know what is wrong, but I do know that this is the sort of back pain that is very likely to get better quickly." Evidence from prognosis research has helped to redefine low back pain. Spinal radiography and magnetic resonance imaging contribute little to understanding the average prognosis of most back pain,[16 45] but the duration of symptoms at presentation in primary care is strongly related to outcome. Figure 4 shows that the chance of reduced disability at one year is about 70% in those with a shorter duration (<3 years) of symptoms at presentation versus 40% in those with a longer duration.[26 29 46] Clinical practice guideline recommendations use symptom duration to guide management decisions.[47] Symptom duration is associated with clinical outcome and is thus a prognostic factor (see paper 2 in our series[3]), which has resulted in it being a standard component of the clinical evaluation of back pain.

Second, fundamental prognosis research can take a holistic view of all comorbidities that a person experiences, whereas diagnosis implies a focus on a single organ system or pathology. The prognosis of some cancers, traumatic brain injury, and back pain are importantly influenced by conditions not related to the tumour, brain, and spine respectively. Third, diagnosis implies a dichotomy (case v not at a single point in time), which may be a misleading basis for clinical decision making. For example, in many countries the decision to lower blood cholesterol is not based on a diagnosis of hypercholesterolaemia but on thresholds of continuous risk, determined by age, sex, smoking, blood pressure, and lipids (see paper 3 in our series[4]). Such observations have led to the radical proposition that the dichotomous, cross sectional snapshot of diagnostic practice may become redundant, as clinicians increasingly have access to continuous measures of future risk.[48 49]

Importance for discovering new diseases
Fundamental prognosis research drives definitions of the diseases for which interventions are sought.[50] Such research helps define our current view of what distinct clinical conditions exist and what role new clinical tests might have

led to startling discoveries that have stimulated the development of new interventions and new clinical trials that have ultimately changed clinical practice. For example, few foresaw that a prognostic consequence of *Helicobacter pylori* infection was peptic ulcer before the Nobel prize winning work that established the link and subsequent antibiotic trials.[41] Importantly, the outcomes of uncommon conditions may give insights into disease mechanisms of common conditions. For example, the increased risk of coronary outcomes among people with familial hypercholesterolaemia focused interest on the low density lipoprotein cholesterol pathways which are important in coronary disease experienced by people without this genetic disorder and contributed to the development of lipid lowering therapy.

Taking a broad view of prognostic outcomes may generate new knowledge at the start of translational pathways

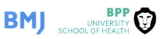

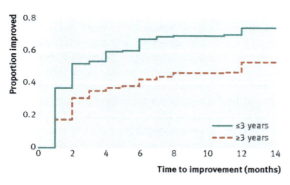

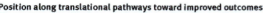

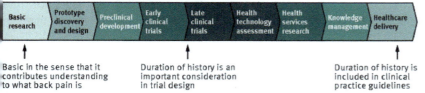

Basic in the sense that it contributes understanding to what back pain is

Duration of history is an important consideration in trial design

Duration of history is included in clinical practice guidelines

Fig 4 Example of use of fundamental prognosis research to define clinically relevant subgroups: duration of low back pain at presentation (<3 or ≥3 years) and the time to improvement of disability disease (drawn using data from Dunn et al[46]). Path element adapted from chart 7.1 in the Cooksey report (2006) http://bit.ly/Ro27rL (made available for use through the Open Government License)

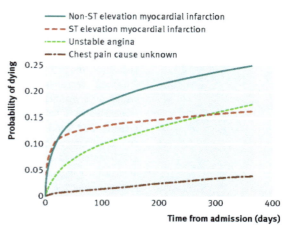

Fig 5 Example of use of fundamental prognosis research to distinguish clinically relevant groups: people admitted with suspected acute myocardial infarction (results based on an analysis of 180 000 patients in the Myocardial Ischaemia National Audit Project, A Timmis and H Hemingway personal communication)

in changing our classification of disease entities (nosology). The question "what is the prognosis of this condition?" is intimately related to the question "what is this condition?" For example, the entity of non-fatal myocardial infarction was identified only after many decades of clinical prognostic observation that symptoms of chest pain may precede death, replacing the view that the disease of myocardial infarction was inevitably and instantly fatal. More recently, prognosis research has helped to redefine non-fatal acute myocardial infarctions[51] based on the presence or absence of ST elevation, a predictor of differential response to therapy, and serum troponin measurement. Figure 5 shows that examination of survival patterns differentiates clinical phenotypes among people admitted with suspected non-fatal myocardial infarction. An example of a newly recognised genetic disorder discovered through prognostic observation is Brugada syndrome in which an ST elevation pattern on resting electrocardiogram is associated with sudden death.[52]

Recommendations for improving the quality and impact of prognosis research

For each of the four themes of prognosis research to achieve its potential for improving clinical outcomes, important challenges need to be addressed and opportunities seized in prognosis research as a whole. The research community needs to address serious flaws in the design, conduct, and reporting of prognosis studies and to recognise the clinical value of reliable prognostic evidence. In the PROGRESS series we thus make recommendations for progress in the field, and these are summarised in supplementary table 1 on bmj.com. Here we introduce recommendations that cut across the different research themes. In papers 2–4 in the PROGRESS series,[3] [4] [5] we discuss the other recommendations from supplementary table 1. These recommendations add to, and further specify, those which we have previously made in the BMJ.[53]

Fuelling changes in medicine and healthcare

As shown in the examples above, improvements in electronic health records, clinical imaging, and "omic" technologies (genotyping and phenotyping) are beginning to challenge current disease taxonomy, the focus of much healthcare policy on process (rather than clinical outcomes), and the clinical preoccupation with diagnosis (rather than risk). There should be a formative shift in clinical practice, healthcare policy, and translational research based on evidence from prognosis research—that is, the prospective relationships between the phenotypic, genomic, and environmental assessment of people with a given startpoint and subsequent endpoints (recommendation 1 in supplementary table 1). Over their life course, individuals develop multiple diseases (both distinct and related) that often do not respect the current organisation of medical research or practice. There should be new programmes of prognosis research that bridge multiple clinical specialties, health systems, pathological mechanisms, and biological systems and that put the whole patient across his or her "journey" as the central unit of concern (recommendation 2).

Electronic health records

The scope and impact of prognosis research and electronic health records research (in primary and secondary care, and in disease and procedure registries) are intimately related. There is increasing availability of electronic health records in primary[54] and secondary care, and disease and procedure registries. Particularly where such sources can be linked,[55] there is the possibility of examining the "patient journey" with repeated measures of risk and care in larger populations than are feasible with bespoke, investigator led studies. Population coverage, data quality, and the extent of blood, imaging, and other diagnostic data are all improving. But concerted efforts are required to harmonise data on startpoints, endpoints, and populations of interest in order to make temporal and international comparisons in prognosis. There should be new programmes of methodological and empirical prognosis research exploiting electronic health

123

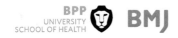

records to define, phenotype, and follow up people with different health related conditions (recommendation 3).

Visibility of the field

Prognosis research is currently fragmented and not visible as a distinct entity. Prognosis research should be recognised as a field of inquiry important in translational research and intrinsic to the practice of clinical medicine and development of healthcare policy (recommendation 4). Efforts should be made to establish prognosis research as a distinct branch of knowledge, with a set of scientific methods aimed at understanding and improving health. Evidence about prognosis is somewhat neglected; such as in medical textbooks, where the focus is on the effectiveness of therapies, with only brief details given on average prognosis,[56] sometimes as if therapies can be divorced from the context of clinical care.[57] [58]

Fundamental prognosis research should compare the prognosis of clinical cohorts with that of the healthy population (recommendation 5). Relative survival methods are commonly applied in cancer, but less often in other disease areas. Relative survival methods model the survival probability of people with a condition relative to the expected survival without the condition (obtained from national population life tables stratified by age, sex, calender year, and other covariates). By comparing the observed and expected survival, one can estimate the added risk of mortality due to having the condition rather than not having it (that is, measure how prognosis is modified by onset of a disease). Such methods help prognosis research prioritise which clinical cohorts require the most attention and most translational research (that is, identify those cohorts whose prognosis is most changed by disease onset).

The situation for cancer, where estimates of survival are readily available (such as Surveillance Epidemiology and End Results, SEER[59]) is exceptional. Knowledge management in prognosis seems somewhat chaotic in generation, dissemination, and accessibility. Difficulties in identifying and accessing information about prognosis, and evidence from prognosis research studies, hamper efforts to inform patients and evaluate the impact of translational efforts to improve outcomes. Evidence from prognosis research and information about prognosis should be systematically collated, made easily accessible, and updated (recommendation 6).

Teaching and training

Undergraduate and postgraduate training do not currently provide instruction in how to generate or use evidence from prognosis research. All healthcare professionals should be trained in the generation and use of prognosis research evidence; there should be an expansion of training and education opportunities for those interested in methodological aspects of prognosis research (recommendation 7).

Patient and public involvement

Questions of prognosis are among the most important to patients, but the level of patient and public involvement in prognosis research is low. Patient reported outcomes are important to clinical decision and policy making but are understudied. For example, people with angina might reasonably ask "will my symptoms get better?" yet a recent systematic review of 83 studies found none that reported symptomatic status as an endpoint (favouring acute coronary events instead).[60] Symptom status is acknowledged as a major determinant of the clinical decision to recommend revascularisation.[61] Prognosis research using person focused endpoints may yield unanticipated results. For example, people with rheumatoid arthritis may care more about fatigue than about the joint pain, on which doctors tend to focus.[62] Patients and the wider public should be more engaged in the goals and value of prognosis research, appropriate use of their clinical data, and better integration of patient reported outcome measures (recommendation 8).

Conclusion

In this first article in the PROGRESS series, we have introduced a framework of four themes in prognosis research, and outlined the importance of initial, fundamental prognosis research. This first theme is central to the practice of medicine; from basic understanding of the categories we choose to call disease through to understanding how variations in healthcare influence the risk of endpoints. As such, it has a broad array of uses for policy makers, patients, and clinical decision making and should be considered a core component of prognosis research. To maximise the impact of each interrelated theme of prognosis research,[3] [4] [5] we have begun outlining a set of recommendations to enhance the prognosis field, including better use of electronic health records, greater training and public involvement, and a wider appreciation of the clinical value of prognosis research findings.

We thank John Scadding, emeritus dean at the Royal Society of Medicine, for his support of the PROGRESS Group, contributions to discussions, and helpful comments on drafts of the manuscripts. We thank Ruzan Udumyan for assistance in drawing figures and preparing manuscripts. We thank Virginia Barbour and Trish Groves for contributing to the workshops and their support for the series. We thank Lucy Chappell (King's College London) for her valuable help as guest editor on the PROGRESS series.

Contributors: HH, RDR, SS, and DGA initiated the PROGRESS Group, organised the three workshops, coordinated the writing groups, and were the scientific writing editors for all the papers in the PROGRESS series. HH, RDR, and DGA are the guarantors for this paper. HH wrote the first version, and PC, PP, JAH, KA, AT, AB, KGMM, EWS, IR, SS, DGA, and RDR contributed to the conception of the paper and to the revising of draft versions and approved the final version. All members of PROGRESS Group contributed through workshops and discussions to the development of the article series.

Members of the PROGRESS Group: Keith Abrams (UK), Doug Altman (UK), Andrew Briggs (UK), Nils Brunner (Denmark), Peter Croft (UK), Jill Hayden (Canada), Aroon D Hingorani (UK), Harry Hemingway (UK), Panayiotis Kyzas (UK), Núria Malats (Spain), Karel Moons (Netherlands), George Peat (UK), Pablo Perel (UK), Richard Riley (UK), Ian Roberts (UK), Willi Sauerbrei (Germany), Sara Schroter (UK), Ewout Steyerberg (Netherlands), Adam Timmis (UK), Daniëlle van der Windt (UK).

Funding: This series had no explicit funding, but some of the authors were supported by research grants: PROGRESS is supported by a Partnership grant from the Medical Research Council (G0902393), involving University College London (HH, AH), Oxford University (DGA), Birmingham University (RDR), London School of Hygiene and Tropical Medicine (IR, PP), Keele University (PC, D van der Windt), and Queen Mary University London (ADT). DGA is supported by a programme grant from Cancer Research UK (C5529). HH is supported by grants from the UK National Institute for Health Research (RP-PG-0407-10314) and the Wellcome Trust (086091/Z/08/Z). The work of HH and AT is supported by the Health eResearch Centre Network (HERC-UK), funded by the Medical Research Council in partnership with Arthritis Research UK, the British Heart Foundation, Cancer Research UK, the Economic and Social Research Council, the Engineering and Physical Sciences Research Council, the National Institute of Health Research, the National Institute for Social Care and Health Research (Welsh Assembly Government), the Chief Scientist Office (Scottish Government Health Directorates) and the Wellcome Trust (the views expressed in this paper are those of the authors and not necessarily those of the NHS, the NIHR, or the Department of Health). RDR is supported by the MRC Midlands Hub for Trials Methodology Research. JAH is supported by a New Investigator Award from the Canadian Institutes of Health Research and a grant from the Nova Scotia Health

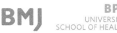

Research Foundation, and holds a Dalhousie University/CCRF research professorship. KGMM is supported by The Netherlands Organization for Scientific Research (ZON-MW 918.10.615 and 9120.8004). EWS was supported by The Netherlands Organization for Scientific Research (grant 9120.8004). PC holds a UK National Institute of Health Research Senior Investigator Award (NI-SI-0509-10183). KA holds a UK National Institute of Health Research Senior Investigator Award (NI-SI-0508-10061).

Competing interests: All authors have completed the ICMJE uniform disclosure form at www.icmje.org/coi_disclosure.pdf (available on request from the corresponding author) and declare: no support from any organisation for the submitted work; no financial relationships with any organisations that might have an interest in the submitted work in the previous three years, no other relationships or activities that could appear to have influenced the submitted work. SS is a full time employee of the BMJ Group but is not involved in deciding which manuscripts are accepted for publication.

Provenance and peer review: Not commissioned; externally peer reviewed. In order to disseminate the output widely, these papers are being published jointly between *BMJ* (PROGRESS papers 1 and 4) and *PLoS Medicine* (PROGRESS papers 2 and 3). As one of the authors is a member of staff at BMJ Group, the handling editor at the BMJ for the manuscripts was an external guest editor, Lucy Chappell (King's College London).

1   Mathers CD, Loncar D. Projections of global mortality and burden of disease from 2002 to 2030. *PLoS Med* 2006;3:e442.
2   Department of Health. *White paper. Equity and excellence: liberating the NHS* . Stationery Office, 2010.
3   Riley RD, Hayden JA, Steyerberg EW, Moons KGM, Abrams K, Kyzas PA, et al. Prognosis research strategy (PROGRESS) 2: Prognostic factor research. *PLoS Med* 2013, doi:10.1371.journal/pmed.1001380.
4   Steyerberg EW, Moons KGM, van der Windt DA, Hayden JA, Perel P, Schroter S, et al. Prognosis research strategy (PROGRESS) 3: Prognostic model research. *PLoS Med* 2013, doi:10.1371.journal/pmed.1001381.
5   Hingorani AD, van der Windt DA, Riely RD, Abrams K, Moons KGM, Steyerberg EW, et al. Prognosis research strategy (PROGRESS) 4: stratified medicine research. *BMJ* 2013;346:e5793.
6   Cancer Research UK. *CancerStats: cancer statistics for the UK* . Cancer Research UK, 2009. (Original data source: Verdecchia et al.Recent cancer survival in Europe: a 2000-02 period analysis of EUROCARE-4 data. Lancet Oncology 2007;8:784-96.)
7   Tsai H, Chen S, Chien H, Jan Y, Chao T, Chen M, et al. Relationships between serum HER2 ECD, TIMP-1 and clinical outcomes in Taiwanese breast cancer. *World J Surg Oncol* 2012;10:42.
8   Adjuvant! Online: Decision making tools for health care professionals. www.adjuvantonline.com/index.jsp.
9   Early Breast Cancer Trialists Collaborative Group. Tamoxifen for early breast cancer: an overview of the randomised trials. *Lancet* 1998;351:1451-67.
10   Moons KG, Royston P, Vergouwe Y, Grobbee DE, Altman DG. Prognosis and prognostic research: what, why, and how? *BMJ* 2009;338:b375.
11   Hlatky MA, Greenland P, Arnett DK, Ballantyne CM, Criqui MH, Elkind MS, et al. Criteria for evaluation of novel markers of cardiovascular risk: a scientific statement from the American Heart Association. *Circulation* 2009;119:2408-16.
12   McShane LM, Altman DG, Sauerbrei W, Taube SE, Gion M, Clark GM, et al. Reporting recommendations for tumor marker prognostic studies (REMARK). *J Natl Cancer Inst* 2005;97:1180-4.
13   Krumholz HM. Outcomes research: generating evidence for best practice and policies. *Circulation* 2008;118:309-18.
14   Nissen H, Rosnes JT, Brendehaug J, Kleiberg GH. Safety evaluation of sous vide-processed ready meals. *Lett Appl Microbiol* 2002;35:433-8.
15   Sipahi I, Debanne SM, Rowland DY, Simon DI, Fang JC. Angiotensin-receptor blockade and risk of cancer: meta-analysis of randomised controlled trials. *Lancet Oncol* 2010;11:627-36.
16   Chou R, Shekelle P. Will this patient develop persistent disabling low back pain? *JAMA* 2010;303:1295-302.
17   Hemingway H, Shipley M, Britton A, Page M, Macfarlane P, Marmot M. Prognosis of angina with and without a diagnosis: 11 year follow up in the Whitehall II prospective cohort study. *BMJ* 2003;327:895.
18   Krumholz HM, Wang Y, Chen J, Drye EE, Spertus JA, Ross JS, et al. Reduction in acute myocardial infarction mortality in the United States: risk-standardized mortality rates from 1995-2006. *JAMA* 2009;302:767-73.
19   Henderson R, Keiding N. Individual survival time prediction using statistical models. *J Med Ethics* 2005;31:703-6.
20   Royston P, Parmar MK, Altman DG. Visualizing length of survival in time-to-event studies: a complement to Kaplan-Meier plots. *J Natl Cancer Inst* 2008;100:92-7.
21   Lingsma HF, Roozenbeek B, Li B, Lu J, Weir J, Butcher I, et al. Large between-center differences in outcome after moderate and severe traumatic brain injury in the international mission on prognosis and clinical trial design in traumatic brain injury (IMPACT) study. *Neurosurgery* 2011;68:601-7.
22   CancerGuide: Statistics. The median isn't the message. http://cancerguide.org/median_not_msg.html (updated 2002).
23   Ford ES, Ajani UA, Croft JB, Critchley JA, Labarthe DR, Kottke TE, et al. Explaining the decrease in US deaths from coronary disease, 1980-2000. *N Engl J Med* 2007;356:2388-98.
24   Hunink MG, Goldman L, Tosteson AN, Mittleman MA, Goldman PA, Williams LW, et al. The recent decline in mortality from coronary heart disease, 1980-1990. The effect of secular trends in risk factors and treatment. *JAMA* 1997;277:535-42.
25   Weinstein MC, Coxson PG, Williams LW, Pass TM, Stason WB, Goldman L. Forecasting coronary heart disease incidence, mortality, and cost: the Coronary Heart Disease Policy Model. *Am J Public Health* 1987;77:1417-26.
26   Croft PR, Macfarlane GJ, Papageorgiou AC, Thomas E, Silman AJ. Outcome of low back pain in general practice: a prospective study. *BMJ* 1998;316:1356-9.
27   Von KM, Deyo RA, Cherkin D, Barlow W. Back pain in primary care. Outcomes at 1 year. *Spine* 1993;18:855-62.
28   Costa LC, Maher CG, McAuley JH, Hancock MJ, Herbert RD, Refshauge KM, et al. Prognosis for patients with chronic low back pain: inception cohort study. *BMJ* 2009;339:b3829.
29   Hestbaek L, Leboeuf-Yde C, Manniche C. Low back pain: what is the long-term course? A review of studies of general patient populations. *Eur Spine J* 2003;12:149-65.
30   De Silva MJ, Roberts I, Perel P, Edwards P, Kenward MG, Fernandes J, et al. Patient outcome after traumatic brain injury in high-, middle- and low-income countries: analysis of data on 8927 patients in 46 countries. *Int J Epidemiol* 2009;38:452-8.
31   Sox HC, Greenfield S. Comparative effectiveness research: a report from the Institute of Medicine. *Ann Intern Med* 2009;151:203-5.
32   Coleman MP, Quaresma M, Berrino F, Lutz JM, De AR, Capocaccia R, et al. Cancer survival in five continents: a worldwide population-based study (CONCORD). *Lancet Oncol* 2008;9:730-56.
33   Buchbinder R, Jolley D, Wyatt M. Population based intervention to change back pain beliefs and disability: three part evaluation. *BMJ* 2001;322:1516-20.
34   Buchbinder R, Jolley D. Population based intervention to change back pain beliefs: three year follow up population survey. *BMJ* 2004;328:321.
35   Sung NS, Crowley WF Jr, Genel M, Salber P, Sandy L, Sherwood LM, et al. Central challenges facing the national clinical research enterprise. *JAMA* 2003;289:1278-87.
36   Rose G. *The strategy of preventive medicine* . Oxford University Press, 1993.
37   Stukel TA, Fisher ES, Wennberg DE, Alter DA, Gottlieb DJ, Vermeulen MJ. Analysis of observational studies in the presence of treatment selection bias: effects of invasive cardiac management on AMI survival using propensity score and instrumental variable methods. *JAMA* 2007;297:278-85.
38   National Institute for Health and Clinical Excellence. Chest pain of recent onset: assessment and diagnosis of recent onset chest pain or discomfort of suspected cardiac origin (clinical guideline 95). www.nice.org.uk/guidance/CG95 (updated 2010).
39   Min JK, Shaw LJ, Devereux RB, Okin PM, Weinsaft JW, Russo DJ, et al. Prognostic value of multidetector coronary computed tomographic angiography for prediction of all-cause mortality. *J Am Coll Cardiol* 2007;50:1161-70.
40   Griffin SC, Barber JA, Manca A, Sculpher MJ, Thompson SG, Buxton MJ, et al. Cost effectiveness of clinically appropriate decisions on alternative treatments for angina pectoris: prospective observational study. *BMJ* 2007;334:624.
41   Malfertheiner P, Chan FK, McColl KE. Peptic ulcer disease. *Lancet* 2009;374:1449-61.
42   Bajaj A, Driver JA, Schernhammer ES. Parkinson's disease and cancer risk: a systematic review and meta-analysis. *Cancer Causes Control* 2010;21:697-707.
43   Hanauer DA, Rhodes DR, Chinnaiyan AM. Exploring clinical associations using '-omics' based enrichment analyses. *PLoS One* 2009;4:e5203.
44   Kroenke K, Harris L. Symptoms research: a fertile field. *Ann Intern Med* 2001;134(9 Pt 2):801-2.
45   Von Korff M, Miglioretti DL. A prognostic approach to defining chronic pain. *Pain* 2005;117:304-13.
46   Dunn KM, Croft PR. The importance of symptom duration in determining prognosis. *Pain* 2006;121:126-32.
47   O'Neill CJ, Spence A, Logan B, Suliburk JW, Soon PS, Learoyd DL, et al. Adrenal incidentalomas: risk of adrenocortical carcinoma and clinical outcomes. *J Surg Oncol* 2010;102:450-3.
48   Wiesemann C. The significance of prognosis for a theory of medical practice. *Theor Med Bioeth* 1998;19:253-61.
49   Vickers AJ, Basch E, Kattan MW. Against diagnosis. *Ann Intern Med* 2008;149:200-3.
50   Scadding JG. Diagnosis: the clinician and the computer. *Lancet* 1967;2:877-82.
51   Thygesen K, Alpert JS, White HD, Jaffe AS, Apple FS, Galvani M, et al. Universal definition of myocardial infarction. *Circulation* 2007;116:2634-53.
52   Probst V, Veltmann C, Eckardt L, Meregalli PG, Gaita F, Tan HL, et al. Long-term prognosis of patients diagnosed with Brugada syndrome: results from the FINGER Brugada Syndrome Registry. *Circulation* 2010;121:635-43.
53   Hemingway H, Riley RD, Altman DG. Ten steps towards improving prognosis research. *BMJ* 2009;339:b4184.
54   General Practice Research Database. www.gprd.com/home/default.asp (updated 2011).
55   Jernberg T, Attebring MF, Hambraeus K, Ivert T, James S, Jeppsson A, et al. The Swedish Web-system for enhancement and development

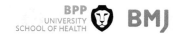

of evidence-based care in heart disease evaluated according to recommended therapies (SWEDEHEART). *Heart* 2010;96:1617-21.

56   Gospodarowicz M, Henson D, Hutter R, O'Sullivan B, Sobin L, Wittekind C. *Prognostic factors in cancer* . 2nd ed. John Wiley & Sons, 2001.

57   Guyatt G, Rennie D, Meade M, Cook D. *Users' guides to the medical literature: a manual for evidence-based clinical practice* . 2nd ed. AMA Press, 2008.

58   Laupacis A, Wells G, Richardson WS, Tugwell P. Users' guides to the medical literature. V. How to use an article about prognosis. Evidence-Based Medicine Working Group. *JAMA* 1994;272:234-7.

59   National Cancer Institute. Surveillance Epidemiology and End Results. http://seer.cancer.gov/ (updated 2012).

60   Hemingway H, Philipson P, Chen R, Fitzpatrick NK, Damant J, Shipley M, et al. Evaluating the quality of research into a single prognostic biomarker: a systematic review and meta-analysis of 83 studies of C-Reactive protein in stable coronary artery disease. *PLoS Med* 2010;7:e1000286.

61   Fox K, Garcia MA, Ardissino D, Buszman P, Camici PG, Crea F, et al. Guidelines on the management of stable angina pectoris: executive summary: the Task Force on the Management of Stable Angina Pectoris of the European Society of Cardiology. *Eur Heart J* 2006;27:1341-81.

62   Repping-Wuts H, Uitterhoeve R, van RP, van AT. Fatigue as experienced by patients with rheumatoid arthritis (RA): a qualitative study. Int J Nurs Stud 2008;45:995-1002.

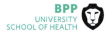

Prognosis research strategy (PROGRESS) 4: Stratified medicine research

Aroon D Hingorani, professor of genetic epidemiology[1], Daniëlle A van der Windt, professor in primary care epidemiology[2], Richard D Riley, senior lecturer in medical statistics[3], Keith Abrams, professor of medical statistics[4], Karel G M Moons, professor of clinical epidemiology[5], Ewout W Steyerberg, professor of medical decision making[6], Sara Schroter, senior researcher[7], Willi Sauerbrei, professor of medical biometry[8], Douglas G Altman, professor of statistics in medicine[9], Harry Hemingway, professor of clinical epidemiology[1], for the PROGRESS Group

[1] Department of Epidemiology and Public Health, University College London, London WC1E 7HB, UK

[2] Arthritis Research UK Primary Care Centre, Primary Care Sciences, Keele University, Keele ST5 5BG, UK

[3] School of Health and Population Sciences, University of Birmingham, Birmingham B15 2TT, UK

[4] Centre for Biostatistics & Genetic Epidemiology, Department of Health Sciences, School of Medicine, University of Leicester, Leicester LE1 7RH, UK

[5] Julius Center for Health Sciences and Primary Care, UMC Utrecht, Utrecht, Netherlands

[6] Department of Public Health, Erasmus MC, 3000 CA Rotterdam, Rotterdam, Netherlands

[7] BMJ, BMA House, London WC1H 9JR, UK

[8] Institute of Medical Biometry and Informatics, University Medical Center Freiburg, 79104 Freiburg, Germany

[9] Centre for Statistics in Medicine, University of Oxford, Oxford OX2 6UD, UK

Correspondence to: H Hemingway h.hemingway@ucl.ac.uk

Cite this as: BMJ 2013;346:e5793

DOI: 10.1136/bmj.e5793

http://www.bmj.com/content/346/bmj.e5793

ABSTRACT

In patients with a particular disease or health condition, stratified medicine seeks to identify those who will have the most clinical benefit or least harm from a specific treatment. In this article, the fourth in the PROGRESS series, the authors discuss why prognosis research should form a cornerstone of stratified medicine, especially in regard to the identification of factors that predict individual treatment response

A woman with newly diagnosed breast cancer is deciding on a course of therapy, guided by her physician. Evidence on the average prognosis[1] and effectiveness of therapeutic interventions is available from studies of large groups of patients with breast cancer in observational studies and randomised trials. But the patient and doctor are faced with making a decision in an individual case, where the prognosis and response to treatment may deviate from average. One way to select the optimal treatment is to consider a test that predicts treatment effect, such as the human epidermal growth factor receptor 2 (HER-2) status.[2] The use of HER-2 status in breast cancer management is an example of the translation of results from prognosis research toward improved patient outcomes. The prognosis of breast cancer patients is highly variable,[1] HER-2 was discovered as a prognostic factor,[3] which provided a specific target for an intervention (trastuzumab), which was then evaluated in trials which recruited women with HER-2 positive cancers (see fig 1). After the success of these trials in improving clinical outcome, trastuzumab is now given to the subgroup (stratum) of women who are HER-2 positive, but not to those testing negative;[4] this type of approach has been termed stratified medicine.

The aims of this fourth paper in our PROGRESS series (www.progress-partnership.org) are to describe the rationale for stratified medicine, and to explain why prognosis research is pivotal for this purpose; from identifying priority areas for stratification, to discovering candidate factors that may predict treatment response, through to trials and health technology assessment that examine the impact of stratified medicine approaches in healthcare. We identify current challenges and deficiencies in such research and make recommendations for improvement with examples across a variety of disease areas.

What is stratified medicine?

Stratified medicine refers to the targetting of treatments (including pharmacological and non-pharmacological interventions) according to the biological or risk characteristics shared by subgroups of patients. Stratified medicine is regarded as central to the progress of healthcare according to the leaders of the National Institutes of Health, and the Food and Drug Administration[6] among others.[7] In contrast with "all comer" or "empirical" medicine, stratified medicine seeks to target therapy and make the best decisions for groups of similar patients.[8] [9]

One approach to stratifying the use of treatments is to consider absolute risks. In the third article of our series[10] we described how prognostic models are used to estimate the absolute risk of an outcome for an individual. Those people with the highest absolute risk will derive the largest absolute benefit from a treatment (that is, the greatest reduction in probability of the outcome) when the treatment effect expressed in relative terms is the same for all patients. This is illustrated in the upper panel of fig 2, where the relative treatment effect on mortality risk is estimated as 0.75 for all patients but the reduction in absolute probability of death is 5% for low risk patients and 15% for high risk patients. In such situations treatments could be restricted (or "personalised") to those who will benefit the most. Examples in common clinical practice include the decision to give lipid lowering therapy to people above a certain threshold of cardiovascular risk estimated from a prognostic model,[11] the use of bisphosphonates for women over the age of 50 considered to have an increased risk of vertebral fractures, and the targeting of primary care management of back pain.[12]

By contrast, clinicians may also stratify medicine because the relative treatment effect is inconsistent across patients (fig 2, lower panel). In this situation, at least one individual patient measure is associated with changes in the treatment effect. In statistical terms there is an interaction between a patient-level variable and the effect of treatment on the outcome, and in biological terms there may be an underlying mechanism explaining the interaction. In this situation, a stratified medicine approach seeks to test patients for the presence of individual factors that are considered predictive of an improved treatment response (more benefit, less harm, or both), as in the aforementioned test for positive HER-2 status in breast cancer and the use of trastuzumab. Other examples in clinical use include imatinib in patients with chronic myeloid

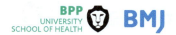

SUMMARY POINTS

- The PROGRESS series (www.progress-partnership.org) sets out a framework of four interlinked prognosis research themes and provides examples from several disease fields to show why evidence from prognosis research is crucial to inform all points in the translation of biomedical and health related research into better patient outcomes. Recommendations are made in each of the four papers to improve current research standards

- What is prognosis research? Prognosis research seeks to understand and improve future outcomes in people with a given disease or health condition. However, there is increasing evidence that prognosis research standards need to be improved

- Why is prognosis research important? More people now live with disease and conditions that impair health than at any other time in history; prognosis research provides crucial evidence for translating findings from the laboratory to humans, and from clinical research to clinical practice

- Stratified medicine involves tailoring therapeutic decisions for specific, often biologically distinct, individuals, the aim being to maximise benefit and reduce harm from treatment, or to rescue a treatment that fails to show overall benefit in unselected patients but does benefit specific patients

- Stratified medicine can use absolute risks. When a treatment effect measured on a relative scale (such as relative risk) is the same for all patients, those with the highest absolute risk will derive the largest absolute benefit from the treatment

- When the relative treatment effect is inconsistent across patients, stratified medicine can use tests which measure factors (such as biomarker levels or genotypes) that predict individual treatment response. However, the clinical use of such tests is currently small, and rigorous evidence of impact is sometimes lacking, with flaws in study design, analysis, and reporting leading to potentially spurious evidence either for or against a factor

- Research to identify factors that truly predict treatment effect could be improved by:

- Labelling exploratory analyses as exploratory, to minimise false positive findings

- Increasing statistical power by designing trials with adequate sample sizes, facilitating collaborations across research groups and meta-analyses of individual participant data from multiple trials, and by analysing continuous factors on their original scale

- Estimating, for a truly binary factor, the difference in relative treatment effect between positive and negative groups within randomised trials that include both factor positive and factor negative patients in both control and treatment groups

- Considering biological or other mechanisms for modification of treatment response, either to motivate new research or to support statistical evidence that a factor interacts with treatment

- Prognosis research in general should play a more central role in stratified medicine research: from identifying conditions with clinically important differences in absolute risk of outcome across patients, to identifying factors that predict individual treatment response, and to examining the cost and impact of implementing stratified medicine approaches in practice

- The other papers in the series are:

- PROGRESS 1: *BMJ* 2013, doi:10.1136/bmj.e5595

- PROGRESS 2: *PLoS Med* 2013, doi:10.1371.journal.pmed.1001380

- PROGRESS 3: *PLoS Med* 2013, doi:10.1371.journal.pmed.1001381

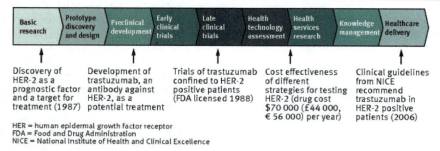

Discovery of HER-2 as a prognostic factor and a target for treatment (1987)

Development of trastuzumab, an antibody against HER-2, as a potential treatment

Trials of trastuzumab confined to HER-2 positive patients (FDA licensed 1988)

Cost effectiveness of different strategies for testing HER-2 (drug cost $70 000 (£44 000, € 56 000) per year)

Clinical guidelines from NICE recommend trastuzumab in HER-2 positive patients (2006)

HER = human epidermal growth factor receptor
FDA = Food and Drug Administration
NICE = National Institute of Health and Clinical Excellence

Fig 1 Example of stratified medicines research, with translation from discovery of human epidermal growth factor receptor 2 (HER-2) status as a prognostic factor for metastatic breast cancer[5] to development of trastuzumab treatment and use in clinical practice. Path element adapted from chart 7.1 in the Cooksey report (2006) (made available for use through the Open Government License)

leukaemia targeted to those with the BCR-ABL mutation[13] and gefitinib used to treat pulmonary adenocarcinoma in patients with epidermal growth factor receptor mutations.[14]

An example of identifying patients with greater risk of harms include the antiretroviral drug abacavir,[15] where HLA typing helps identify patients at high risk of abacavir toxicity. Thus a key part of stratified medicine research is to identify suitable tests for predicting treatment response from specific interventions.

The use of HER-2 status in breast cancer management illustrates how tests of differential treatment response are often thought of as binary factors: a biomarker is classed as positive or negative, or laboratory values are deemed low or high. Such dichotomisation facilitates clinical decision making and is used in most examples described in this paper. However, many tests have original values measured on an ordinal or a continuous scale. Similarly if prognostic

models[10] are considered as tests, they usually produce a continuous risk score for each individual; the same applies to gene signatures or related indices derived from high dimensional data. Statistically, there is more power and less potential for bias if such tests are evaluated on their original scale (see later[10]) rather than being dichotomised by means of a cut point[10]; categorisation may then be done after analysis to aid clinical strategies. For example, Flynn et al derived a prognostic model to identify patients with back pain who would respond well to manipulation rather than to other types of treatment such as exercise.[16] Some trials randomising patients to these treatments found that patients with positive scores from the model had greater relative and absolute benefits from manipulation than those with negative scores.[17][18]

Thus stratified medicine uses baseline information about a patient's likely response to treatment to tailor treatment decisions. This is different from stepped[19] or adaptive[20] models of care in which tailoring of treatment depends on the patient's actual response to previously offered treatment, with a sequence of interventions (which may differ in intensity, duration, cost, or complexity) being offered to those who have not responded sufficiently. Our focus here, though, is on the initial stratification of treatment based on the predicted (rather than actual) response to treatment.

Why is prognosis research important for stratified medicine?

Prognosis research is a fundamental component of stratified medicine because it contributes evidence at multiple stages in translation (see fig 1 as an example). We now consider each of these stages in turn.

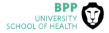

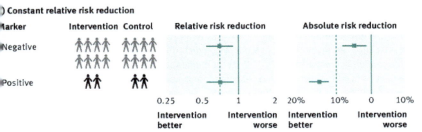

) Constant relative risk reduction

Marker	Intervention	Control	Relative risk reduction	Absolute risk reduction
Negative				
Positive				

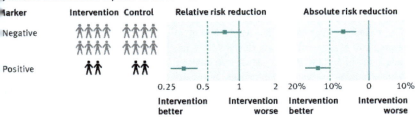

) Relative risk reduction depends on marker status

Marker	Intervention	Control	Relative risk reduction	Absolute risk reduction
Negative				
Positive				

Fig 2 Estimated treatment effect in subgroups defined according to (upper panel) risk from a prognostic model and (lower panel) a factor that predicts differential treatment response. The prevalence of positive factor and high risk is shown, arbitrarily, as 20%. The dotted vertical line shows the overall treatment effect, the centre of each box shows the effect estimate, and the horizontal lines show confidence intervals

Assessing priorities for stratified medicine

Targeting interventions at defined patient strata is likely to be more important in some disease-treatment combinations than in others, and prognosis research can help prioritise areas for research. Several questions arise. First, is there clinically important variation in prognosis across individuals?[1] For example, among people with symptomatic severe aortic stenosis, one year survival is poor and valve replacement or implementation is the default option. By contrast, among people with aortic regurgitation, one year survival is better, and so tools to help decide when and for which patients valve replacement would yield the greatest benefit, and incur the least harm, would be a substantial advance. Second, is the intervention in question associated with a substantial risk of harm or cost? Third, for drug interventions, is there robust evidence of important individual variation in metabolism or pharmacological effect? For example, it has been claimed that some individuals have "clinical aspirin resistance" if they sustain a cardiovascular event despite aspirin prophylaxis. However, because of the lack of an optimal assay of platelet function and the paucity of high quality epidemiological data, it is unclear to what extent this observation reflects true pharmacological resistance to aspirin, non-adherence to medication,[21] the expected reduction but not abolition of cardiovascular risk from aspirin treatment, or some combination of these factors.

Discovery and candidate approaches to developing new tests

Prognosis research is important to identify which factors to study as potential predictors of differential treatment response, which might lead to a new prototype test (left hand of translational pathway in fig 1). Prognostic factors, which were discussed in paper 2 of our series,[3] are characteristics associated with a particular outcome even in the absence of specific treatment. Prognostic factors with causal or mechanistically relevant effects are also potential predictors of differential treatment response. For example, among people with atrial fibrillation, age influences both response to warfarin and risk of stroke, and so is a both a prognostic factor[3] and a factor that predicts differential treatment response.

However, most prognostic factors do not also predict differential treatment response.[22] That is, they identify groups of patients with different absolute outcome risks, but not groups with different relative risks for a particular treatment. Conversely, a factor that predicts differential treatment response is not necessarily a prognostic factor. That is, some factors (such as those that influence the metabolism or elimination of a specific drug) may influence the response to treatment (that is, they modify relative risk) without affecting prognosis in the absence of treatment (that is, they do not change absolute risk). For example, the CYP2C9 and VKORC1 genotypes are associated with differential warfarin response but do not influence the risk of stroke in the absence of warfarin treatment.[23]

DNA based, genome-wide association studies (genomics) and mRNA based gene expression profiling (transcriptomics) of disease affected tissues are beginning to uncover new and, in some cases, unanticipated disease mechanisms and factors that potentially predict differential treatment response.

Evaluation in randomised trials

Once a factor potentially predicting differential treatment response has been identified the next step is to evaluate it, ideally as an a priori primary objective within a randomised trial of the specific therapy in question. Figure 2 illustrates such a comparison of outcomes in treated and control groups, separately among factor positive and factor negative individuals. However, few individual trials are large enough to assess reliably whether a factor is truly predictive of treatment response as a primary objective, so evidence may often appear gradually, from secondary analyses of existing randomised trials and then their meta-analysis. This process was used for examining whether tamoxifen treatment of breast cancer differed according to the oestrogen receptor status of the breast cancer.[24]

Evaluations of factors that may predict differential treatment response become more pressing when a drug fails in late stage trials after substantial research investment; there is then intense interest in moving from targeting all people to identifying those specific patients who may benefit. For example, gefitinib in advanced non-small cell lung cancer failed to show a survival benefit among all patients, and this stimulated exploratory analyses in relation to epidermal growth factor receptor status.[14] Even in trials that do show a positive average effect of a drug, there may still be some patients who hardly benefit from the drug, and it is clearly important to identify this subgroup.[25] However, it is notoriously difficult to identify genuine predictors of differential treatment from single trials, as such investigations are usually exploratory with high potential for type I and type II errors (see later).

Assessment of tests as a health technology

Even seemingly robust evidence for the existence of a factor that predicts differential treatment response does not guarantee that it will be effective when used as a test in clinical practice to inform therapeutic decisions. Consider the example of pharmacogenetic testing to guide warfarin dosing. Here the testing, not the drug, is the technology being evaluated. In a high quality meta-analysis of nine observational studies (2775 patients),[26] CYP2C9*2 and CYP2C9*3 alleles were associated with a requirement for a lower warfarin dose and an increased risk of bleeding.

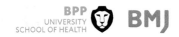

Despite this clear association, which is unlikely to have arisen by chance, a systematic review of three randomised controlled trials did not provide evidence in favour of warfarin dosing based on genetic information in comparison with standard clinical care with respect to bleeding rate or time spent in the therapeutic range.[27]

Cost effectiveness evaluations

Decision analytic models are important for the evaluation of the cost effectiveness of stratified therapeutic strategies.[28] [29] [30] These models require valid estimates of prognosis under different scenarios, based on treatment with and without knowledge of the predictor of differential treatment response. Such models are important for policy makers because they evaluate strategies which are unlikely to be evaluated within trials. For example, decision analysis comparing different strategies for assessing HER-2 status to decide on treating breast cancer with trastuzumab found that fluorescent in situ hybridisation testing for all patients, with one year of adjuvant treatment with trastuzumab for those who were positive, was associated with the longest quality adjusted survival, with an estimated cost per quality adjusted life year gained of €41 500 (£32 600, $51 200).[31] [32]

Healthcare policy and delivery

Health services research is required to examine variations in the uptake of using tests to predict differential treatment response,[33] the validity of these tests,[34] and variations in treatments based on test results. Prognosis research also examines endpoints in relation to these variations, allowing, for example, national estimates to be made of the number of endpoints averted by current levels of testing.[35]

Once incorporated in clinical practice guidelines[4] and usual clinical care, tests that predict differential treatment response may help define the disease and how it is characterised. This is termed "back translation." For example, in breast cancer, HER-2 and oestrogen receptor status are predictors of differential treatment response, and so their measurement is now integral to the definition of the disease upon diagnosis.

Premature implementation of stratified medicine approaches into clinical practice may be harmful if people who might otherwise benefit from treatment are denied access. For example, carriage of a variant of the KIF6 gene was associated with a higher risk of coronary heart disease events and a smaller reduction in event rate from statin treatment in a genetic substudy from a randomised trial.[36] It would have been premature to implement these findings; indeed, a later, larger meta-analysis of case-control studies of myocardial infarction casts doubt on the role of this variant in coronary heart disease and prediction of statin response,[37] arguing that statins should be used according to existing guidelines without any genetic testing.

Recommendations for improving prognosis research for stratified medicine

Several methodological challenges and current research deficiencies need to be addressed in this field. Currently we lack a systematic framework for guiding research on stratified medicine, and standards must be raised. Many of the recommendations highlighted across the PROGRESS series (see supplementary table on bmj.com) are relevant. For example, integrated standards of design, analysis,

and reporting should be developed across the stage of discovery, replication, and evaluation of factors that potentially predict differential treatment response[38] [39] [40] [41] [42] [43] (recommendation 10 in supplementary table). Here we highlight four key areas, with recommendations for improvement.

False negative findings (type II errors)

There are important problems with statistical analyses, which should be addressed by having a statistical analysis plan in the protocol and by a greater appreciation of the potential for type I and II errors that may lead to inappropriate conclusions (recommendation 13 in supplementary table).

Most randomised trials are not designed with the statistical power to detect a factor truly predictive of differential treatment effect, should it exist, and so may wrongly conclude that a particular factor is not useful as a predictive test when actually it is.[44] [45] To increase power and reduce the opportunity for false negatives, we recommend that meta-analyses based on individual participant data from multiple trials are facilitated (recommendation 17).[46] This approach was crucial in establishing the role of oestrogen receptor status for the targeting of tamoxifen treatment in breast cancer,[24] and researchers can support its greater use by initiating collaborative groups and data sharing.[46] Another cause of false negative findings is the aforementioned dichotomisation of continuous factors that may predict treatment response, which reduces power further. Statistical methods are available to screen a large number of continuous factors on their original scale and identify their potential interactions with treatment.[47] Identified interactions should be interpreted as hypothesis generating and replication sought in other studies, and meta-analyses. Results for all interactions and subgroups considered should be clearly reported regardless of their significance (recommendation 15), and guidelines for such reporting need development.

False positive findings (type I errors)

Subgroup analyses can provide valuable, albeit predominately exploratory information, about factors that potentially predict treatment response if they are performed in accordance with recommendations and guidelines[38] [48] (recommendation 13). However, inappropriate subgroup analysis of trial data can give spurious evidence for stratified medicine. Firstly, because of the large number of potential factors to consider, appropriate correction for multiple statistical testing is required to reduce the risk of false positives arising by chance.[45] [49] Alternatively, we recommend that such analyses should be recognised as exploratory and require replication using new data from related studies and in meta-analysis of individual participant data (recommendations 17 and 9).

Secondly, the choice and handling of endpoints can influence interpretation of evidence about whether a factor predicts treatment response. For example, in a field synopsis of pharmacogenetic studies, there was evidence of bias in which positive findings were more likely when examining surrogate markers of treatment effects rather than the more clinically relevant endpoints such as a disease complication or death.[50]

Thirdly, arbitrary or "data dredging" categorisation of continuous factors and continuous outcomes can easily bias findings toward a significant result, particularly if analyses are repeated for multiple cut-offs until a categorisation

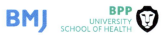

is found that provides the most significant P value.[51] Continuous factors should rather be analysed on their continuous scale to avoid this.

Fourthly, as Senn has argued, studies claiming to distinguish responders (say 70% of people) and non-responders (30%) after a single exposure to a drug are also consistent with an alternative explanation that 100% of patients respond 70% of the time, which would indicate the absence of differential response to treatment.[52]

Fifthly, a meta-analysis of summary data from trials may also give misleading positive results, and a meta-analysis of individual participant data is preferred. For example, fig 3 shows a meta-analysis of summary data from 10 trials suggesting women experience a greater and clinically important reduction in blood pressure from hypertension treatment than men. By contrast, in a meta-analysis of individual participant data from the same trials this apparent sex-treatment interaction was found to be small and not clinically important.[46 53] The discrepant findings were caused by study level confounding when looking at aggregated relationships across trials, rather than investigating patient level relationships within trials using individual participant data.

Away from trials, many consider molecular and microarray data are the key to stratified medicine, but so far the high expectations have not been met, and a more realistic view is important.[3] The large number of variables collected in a relatively small number of patients results in severe methodological problems,[3] and type I errors are again a particular concern.

Analyses restricted to just individuals testing positive for a factor, or just individuals receiving treatment
Robust trial designs to identify factors that truly predict differential treatment response should ideally involve the four groups of patients illustrated in the lower panel of fig 2 so that the difference in treatment effect between patients who are positive for the factor and those who are negative

can be estimated (recommendation 22). However, such a design is often not carried out.

Increasingly, drug trials are being undertaken exclusively among individuals who test positive for a potential (but unproved) factor that predicts differential treatment response (upper panel of fig 4). For example, a randomised trial of heart rate lowering drug ivabradine failed to show a benefit in primary outcome of events among people with stable coronary disease, but subgroup analysis suggested a benefit among those with higher heart rates.[3] The subsequent trial was confined to people with higher heart rates.

Emerging trial designs even propose the integration of drug evaluation with the discovery and evaluation of novel biomarker signatures in real time.[3 54 55] Such studies are sometimes referred to as enrichment trials because, by selecting people in whom the treatment effect is hypothesised to be large, they provide a mechanism for reducing the sample size of a trial. This is only a sensible approach as long as inferences are restricted to the selected patients in the trial. In particular, such trials cannot then compare outcomes between patients with positive and negative factor values, and so cannot assess whether the relative treatment effect (or differences in absolute risk) are indeed smaller in individuals with negative values for the factor, let alone the differences in absolute risk.

Of much more concern are observational analyses (either within or outside the framework of a trial) confined to just those who are treated, as then no comparison can be made with control patients and thus the treatment effect cannot be estimated. In this type of approach, to be able to conclude that a factor truly predicts treatment response, one must assume that the factor does not influence the outcome of interest in the absence of treatment (lower panel of fig 4). If the factor is associated with outcome in both treated and untreated individuals, then it may be a prognostic factor (as discussed in paper 2 of our series[3]) but not predictive of treatment response. Thus, the approach is more correctly interpreted as an evaluation of a prognostic factor among those who are treated, but this is often not recognised.

Biological reasoning and prioritisation of funding areas
Statistical evidence of an interaction between a particular factor and treatment response should ideally be explained by biological reasoning and by understanding the mechanism

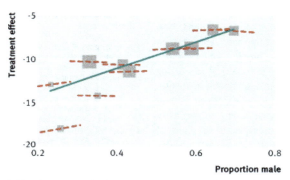

Is blood pressure reduction greater among women than men?

Meta-analysis of 10 trials using aggregate data suggested that women had 15.10 mm Hg (95% CI 8.78 to 21.41) greater lowering than men (gradient of solid line)

Meta-analysis of same trials using individual participant data (IPD) estimated that women had 0.89 mm Hg (0.07 to 1.30) greater lowering (average gradient of the dashed lines)

Bias in aggregate data analysis likely caused by study level confounding. IPD analysis is more reliable as it directly assesses patient level information, and so examines across patients within each trial rather than across trials

Each block represents a trial, and block size is inversely proportional to the standard error of the trial's treatment effect estimate

Fig 3 Example of spurious finding in meta-analysis of summary data refuted by meta-analysis of individual participant data: whether antihypertensive treatment has a greater effect in women than men (reproduced with permission from Riley et al[46 53])

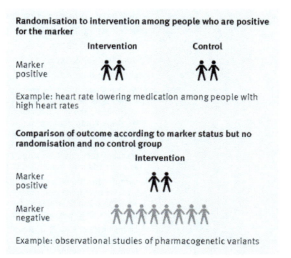

Example: observational studies of pharmacogenetic variants

Fig 4 Commonly used (but suboptimal) study designs in assessment of a factor that potentially predicts differential treatment response

by which response is modified. For instance, for drug interventions, clinicians and policy makers are more likely to believe that a factor truly modifies treatment response if there is a well reasoned biological mechanism in addition to statistical significance. Indeed, stratified medicine research may be entirely motivated by such a biological mechanism in the first place, and funders should prioritise stratified medicine investigations that have such plausibility. "Biological mechanism" should be interpreted in a broad sense here, since behavioural and sociocultural factors may be of equal importance (and have plausible mechanisms for their effects on health outcomes) to biologically measured factors and pathways.

There should be rigorous evaluation of the impact of "personalised medicine" approaches on health outcomes, including comparisons of approaches based on targeting intervention (with prognostic models or factors that predict differential treatment response) and "all comer" approaches (recommendation 23 in supplementary table). In certain situations subgroups with weaker treatment effects on relative risk may have the greater potential benefit in terms of absolute risk. Uncertainty about treatment effects is usually greater in low risk groups, and adequately powered prognosis research is required.

Funders and policy makers should also recognise that a treatment may benefit all patients even when there is a factor that predicts treatment response. In this situation, patients testing negative for the factor will still benefit from the treatment, and so treatment policies should not automatically exclude such patients.

Industry interest (drug, device, biomarker, information technology) in prognosis research including tests for stratified medicine (sometimes called "companion diagnostics"), drug safety, outcomes research and real world evidence is growing. Appropriate models of industry and publicly funded prognosis research should be developed which allow unbiased inference. (recommendation 24 in supplementary table).

Conclusions

In this article we have illustrated and described how prognosis research contributes important evidence in discovering, developing, evaluating, and implementing new approaches in stratified medicine, especially in identifying factors that truly predict differential treatment response. Such research faces many challenges, and often current study designs and statistical analyses are substandard. We have provided recommendations with the aim of accelerating the potential of prognosis research in this context, and these build on others presented throughout our PROGRESS series to improve the care, treatment, and clinical outcomes of individual patients.

We thank John Scadding, emeritus dean at the Royal Society of Medicine for his support of the PROGRESS Group, contributions to discussions, and helpful comments on drafts of the manuscripts. We thank Ruzan Udumyan for assistance in drawing figures and preparing manuscripts. We thank Virginia Barbour and Trish Groves for contributing to the workshops and their support for the series. We thank Lucy Chappell (King's College London) for her valuable help as guest editor on the PROGRESS series.

Contributors: HH, RDR, SS, and DGA initiated the PROGRESS Group, organised the three workshops, coordinated the writing groups, and were the scientific writing editors for all the papers in the PROGRESS series. HH, RDR, and DGA are the guarantors for this paper.

All members of PROGRESS Group contributed through workshops and discussions to the development of the article series. AH wrote the first version, and the other authors contributed to the conception of the paper and to revising earlier versions, and approved the final version. RDR revised the document in light of coauthor comments and restructured it to align with the other PROGRESS papers. All members of PROGRESS Group contributed through workshops and discussions to the development of the article series.

Members of the PROGRESS Group: Keith Abrams (UK), Doug Altman (UK), Andrew Briggs (UK), Nils Brunner (Denmark), Peter Croft (UK), Jill Hayden (Canada), Aroon D Hingorani (UK), Harry Hemingway (UK), Panayiotis Kyzas (UK), Núria Malats (Spain), Karel Moons (Netherlands), George Peat (UK), Pablo Perel (UK), Richard Riley (UK), Ian Roberts (UK), Willi Sauerbrei (Germany), Sara Schroter (UK), Ewout Steyerberg (Netherlands), Adam Timmis (UK), Daniëlle van der Windt (UK).

Funding: This series had no explicit funding, but some of the authors were supported by research grants: PROGRESS is supported by a Partnership grant from the Medical Research Council (G0902393), involving University College London (HH, AH), Oxford University (DGA), Birmingham University (RDR), London School of Hygiene and Tropical Medicine (I Roberts, P Perel), Keele University (P Croft, DAvdW), and Queen Mary University London (A Timmis). DGA is supported by a programme grant from Cancer Research UK (C5529). HH is supported by grants from the UK National Institute for Health Research (RP-PG-0407-10314) and the Wellcome Trust (086091/Z/08/Z). The work of HH and ADH is supported by the Health eResearch Centre Network (HERC-UK), funded by the Medical Research Council in partnership with Arthritis Research UK, the British Heart Foundation, Cancer Research UK, the Economic and Social Research Council, the Engineering and Physical Sciences Research Council, the National Institute of Health Research, the National Institute for Social Care and Health Research (Welsh Assembly Government), the Chief Scientist Office (Scottish Government Health Directorates) and the Wellcome Trust (the views expressed in this paper are those of the authors and not necessarily those of the NHS, the NIHR, or the Department of Health). EWS was supported by The Netherlands Organization for Scientific Research (grant 9120.8004) and the Center for Translational Molecular Medicine (PCMM project, grant 030-203). RDR is supported by the MRC Midlands Hub for Trials Methodology Research (MRC Grant G0800808). DAvdW is supported by the Arthritis Research UK Centre of Excellence in Primary Care.

Competing interests: All authors have completed the ICMJE uniform disclosure form at www.icmje.org/coi_disclosure.pdf (available on request from the corresponding author) and declare: no support from any organisation for the submitted work; no financial relationships with any organisations that might have an interest in the submitted work in the previous three years, no other relationships or activities that could appear to have influenced the submitted work. SS is a full time employee of the BMJ Group but is not involved in deciding which manuscripts are accepted for publication.

Provenance and peer review: Not commissioned; externally peer reviewed. In order to disseminate the output widely, these papers are being published jointly between *BMJ* (PROGRESS papers 1 and 4) and *PLoS Medicine* (PROGRESS papers 2 and 3). As one of the authors is a member of staff at BMJ Group, the handling editor at the BMJ for the manuscripts was an external guest editor, Lucy Chappell (King's College London).

1 Hemingway H, Croft P, Perel P, Hayden JA, Abrams K, Timmis A, et al. Prognosis research strategy (PROGRESS) 1: a framework for researching clinical outcomes. *BMJ* 2013;346:e5595.
2 Hudis CA. Trastuzumab—mechanism of action and use in clinical practice. *N Engl J Med* 2007;357:39-51.
3 Riley RD, Hayden JA, Steyerberg EW, Moons KGM, Abrams K, Kyzas PA, et al. Prognosis research strategy (PROGRESS) 2: Prognostic factor research. *PLoS Med* 2013, doi:10.1371/journal.pmed.1001380.
4 Wolff AC, Hammond ME, Schwartz JN, Hagerty KL, Allred DC, Cote RJ, et al. American Society of Clinical Oncology/College of American Pathologists guideline recommendations for human epidermal growth factor receptor 2 testing in breast cancer. *J Clin Oncol* 2007;25:118-45.
5 Slamon DJ, Clark GM, Wong SG, Levin WJ, Ullrich A, McGuire WL. Human breast cancer: correlation of relapse and survival with amplification of the HER-2/neu oncogene. *Science* 1987;235:177-82.
6 Hamburg MA, Collins FS. The path to personalized medicine. *N Engl J Med* 2010;363:301-4.
7 House of Lords Science and Technology Committee. *Genomic medicine. Volume II: evidence* . Stationery Office, 2009. www.publications.parliament.uk/pa/ld200809/ldselect/ldsctech/107/107ii.pdf
8 Trusheim MR, Berndt ER, Douglas FL. Stratified medicine: strategic and economic implications of combining drugs and clinical biomarkers. *Nat Rev Drug Discov* 2007;6:287-93.
9 Rothwell PM, Mehta Z, Howard SC, Gutnikov SA, Warlow CP. Treating individuals 3: from subgroups to individuals: general principles and the example of carotid endarterectomy. *Lancet* 2005;365:256-65.
10 Steyerberg EW, Moons KGM, van der Windt DA, Hayden JA, Perel P, Schroter S, et al. Prognosis research strategy (PROGRESS) 3: prognostic model research. *PLoS Med* 2013, doi:10.1371/journal.pmed.1001381.
11 Hingorani AD, Hemingway H. How should we balance individual and population benefits of statins for preventing cardiovascular disease? *BMJ* 2011;342:c6244.

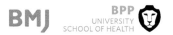

12 Hill JC, Whitehurst DG, Lewis M, Bryan S, Dunn KM, Foster NE, et al. Comparison of stratified primary care management for low back pain with current best practice (STarT Back): a randomised controlled trial. *Lancet* 2011;378:1560-71.

13 Capdeville R, Buchdunger E, Zimmermann J, Matter A. Glivec (STI571, imatinib), a rationally developed, targeted anticancer drug. *Nat Rev Drug Discov* 2002;1:493-502.

14 Mok TS, Wu YL, Thongprasert S, Yang CH, Chu DT, Saijo N, et al. Gefitinib or carboplatin-paclitaxel in pulmonary adenocarcinoma. *N Engl J Med* 2009;361:947-57.

15 Mallal S, Nolan D, Witt C, Masel G, Martin AM, Moore C, et al. Association between presence of HLA-B*5701, HLA-DR7, and HLA-DQ3 and hypersensitivity to HIV-1 reverse-transcriptase inhibitor abacavir. *Lancet* 2002;359:727-32.

16 Flynn MR, Barrett C, Cosio FG, Gitt AK, Wallentin L, Kearney P, et al. The Cardiology Audit and Registration Data Standards (CARDS), European data standards for clinical cardiology practice. *Eur Heart J* 2005;26:308-13.

17 Brennan GP, Fritz JM, Hunter SJ, Thackeray A, Delitto A, Erhard RE. Identifying subgroups of patients with acute/subacute "nonspecific" low back pain: results of a randomized clinical trial. *Spine* 2006;31:623-31.

18 Childs JD, Fritz JM, Flynn TW, Irrgang JJ, Johnson KK, Majkowski GR, et al. A clinical prediction rule to identify patients with low back pain most likely to benefit from spinal manipulation: a validation study. *Ann Intern Med* 2004;141:920-8.

19 Von KM, Moore JC. Stepped care for back pain: activating approaches for primary care. *Ann Intern Med* 2001;134:911-7.

20 Almirall D, Compton SN, Gunlicks-Stoessel M, Duan N, Murphy SA. Designing a pilot sequential multiple assignment randomized trial for developing an adaptive treatment strategy. *Stat Med* 2012;31:1887-902.

21 Hankey GJ, Eikelboom JW. Aspirin resistance. *Lancet* 2006;367:606-17.

22 Clark GM. Prognostic factors versus predictive factors: examples from a clinical trial of erlotinib. *Mol Oncol* 2008;1:406-12.

23 Klein TE, Altman RB, Eriksson N, Gage BF, Kimmel SE, Lee MT, et al. Estimation of the warfarin dose with clinical and pharmacogenetic data. *N Engl J Med* 2009;360:753-64.

24 Early Breast Cancer Trialists' Collaborative Group. Tamoxifen for early breast cancer: an overview of the randomised trials. *Lancet* 1998;351:1451-67.

25 Royston P, Sauerbrei W, Ritchie A. Is treatment with interferon-alpha effective in all patients with metastatic renal carcinoma? A new approach to the investigation of interactions. *Br J Cancer* 2004;90:794-9.

26 Sanderson S, Emery J, Higgins J. CYP2C9 gene variants, drug dose, and bleeding risk in warfarin-treated patients: a HuGEnet systematic review and meta-analysis. *Genet Med* 2005;7:97-104.

27 Kangelaris KN, Bent S, Nussbaum RL, Garcia DA, Tice JA. Genetic testing before anticoagulation? A systematic review of pharmacogenetic dosing of warfarin. *J Gen Intern Med* 2009;24:656-64.

28 Henderson R, Keiding N. Individual survival time prediction using statistical models. *J Med Ethics* 2005;31:703-6.

29 Hlatky MA, Greenland P, Arnett DK, Ballantyne CM, Criqui MH, Elkind MSV, et al. Criteria for evaluation of novel markers of cardiovascular risk: a scientific statement from the American Heart Association. *Circulation* 2009;119:2408-16.

30 Moons KG. Criteria for scientific evaluation of novel markers: a perspective. *Clin Chem* 2010;56:537-41.

31 Lidgren M, Jonsson B, Rehnberg C, Willking N, Bergh J. Cost-effectiveness of HER2 testing and 1-year adjuvant trastuzumab therapy for early breast cancer. *Ann Oncol* 2008;19:487-95.

32 Williams AH, Cookson RA. Equity-efficiency trade-offs in health technology assessment. *Int J Technol Assess Health Care* 2006;22:1-9.

33 Woelderink A, Ibarreta D, Hopkins MM, Rodriguez-Cerezo E. The current clinical practice of pharmacogenetic testing in Europe: TPMT and HER2 as case studies. *Pharmacogenomics J* 2006;6:3-7.

34 Nakhleh RE, Grimm EE, Idowu MO, Souers RJ, Fitzgibbons PL. Laboratory compliance with the American Society of Clinical Oncology/College of American Pathologists guidelines for human epidermal growth factor receptor 2 testing: a College of American Pathologists survey of 757 laboratories. *Arch Pathol Lab Med* 2010;134:728-34.

35 Danese MD, Lalla D, Brammer M, Doan Q, Knopf K. Estimating recurrences prevented from using trastuzumab in HER-2/neu-positive adjuvant breast cancer in the United States. *Cancer* 2010 15;116:5575-83.

36 Li Y, Iakoubova OA, Shiffman D, Devlin JJ, Forrester JS, Superko HR. KIF6 polymorphism as a predictor of risk of coronary events and of clinical event reduction by statin therapy. *Am J Cardiol* 2010;106:994-8.

37 Assimes TL, Holm H, Kathiresan S, Reilly MP, Thorleifsson G, Voight BF, et al. Lack of association between the Trp719Arg polymorphism in kinesin-like protein-6 and coronary artery disease in 19 case-control studies. *J Am Coll Cardiol* 2010;56:1552-63.

38 Fayers PM, King MT. How to guarantee finding a statistically significant difference: the use and abuse of subgroup analyses. *Qual Life Res* 2009;18:527-30.

39 Guillemin F. Primer: the fallacy of subgroup analysis. *Nat Clin Pract Rheumatol* 2007;3:407-13.

40 Sauerbrei W, Royston P, Binder H. Selection of important variables and determination of functional form for continuous predictors in multivariable model building. *Stat Med* 2007;26:5512-28.

41 Sun X, Briel M, Walter SD, Guyatt GH. Is a subgroup effect believable? Updating criteria to evaluate the credibility of subgroup analyses. *BMJ* 2010;340:c117.

42 Willett WC. The search for truth must go beyond statistics. *Epidemiology* 2008;19:655-6.

43 Sauerbrei W, Royston P. Modelling to extract more information from clinical trials data: on some roles for the bootstrap. *Stat Med* 2007;26:4989-5001.

44 Guyatt G, Rennie D, Meade M, Cook D. When to believe a subgroup analysis. In: *Users' guides to the medical literature: a manual for evidence-based clinical practice* . 2nd ed. AMA Press, 2008.

45 Yusuf S, Wittes J, Probstfield J, Tyroler HA. Analysis and interpretation of treatment effects in subgroups of patients in randomized clinical trials. *JAMA* 1991;266:93-8.

46 Riley RD, Lambert PC, Abo-Zaid G. Meta-analysis of individual participant data: rationale, conduct, and reporting. *BMJ* 2010;340:c221.

47 Royston P, Sauerbrei W. A new approach to modelling interactions between treatment and continuous covariates in clinical trials by using fractional polynomials. *Stat Med* 2004;23:2509-25.

48 Assmann SF, Pocock SJ, Enos LE, Kasten LE. Subgroup analysis and other (mis)uses of baseline data in clinical trials. *Lancet* 2000;355:1064-9.

49 Altman DG, Bland JM. Interaction revisited: the difference between two estimates. *BMJ* 2003;326:219.

50 Holmes MV, Shah T, Vickery C, Smeeth L, Hingorani AD, Casas JP. Fulfilling the promise of personalized medicine? Systematic review and field synopsis of pharmacogenetic studies. *PLoS One* 2009;4:e7960.

51 Royston P, Altman DG, Sauerbrei W. Dichotomizing continuous predictors in multiple regression: a bad idea. *Stat Med* 2006;25:127-41.

52 Senn S. Individual response to treatment: is it a valid assumption? *BMJ* 2004;329:966-8.

53 Riley RD, Lambert PC, Staessen JA, Wang J, Gueyffier F, Thijs L, et al. Meta-analysis of continuous outcomes combining individual patient data and aggregate data. *Stat Med* 2008;27:1870-93.

54 Mandrekar JN, Mandrekar SJ. Case-control study design: what, when, and why? *J Thorac Oncol* 2008;3:1371-2.

55 Mandrekar SJ, Sargent DJ. Predictive biomarker validation in practice: lessons from real trials. *Clin Trials* 2010;7:567-73.

More titles in
The BMJ Series

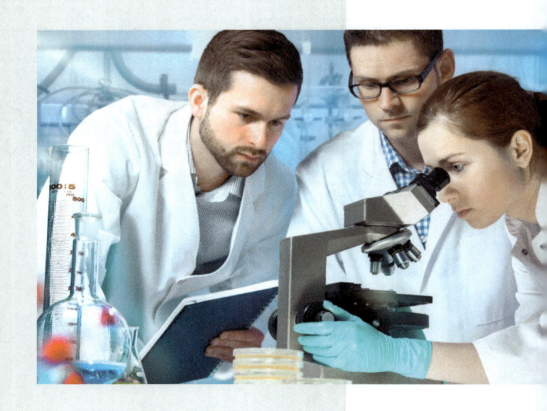

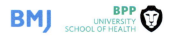

More titles in The BMJ Research Methods and Reporting Series

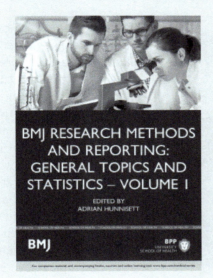

BMJ RESEARCH METHODS AND REPORTING: GENERAL TOPICS AND STATISTICS – VOLUME I

EDITED BY
ADRIAN HUNNISETT

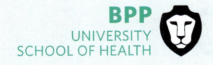

£29.99
February 2016
Paperback
978-1-472745-56-9

This book is the first of two volumes drawing together a collection of articles previously published in the BMJ covering contemporary issues in research. The articles give key messages about the 'nuts and bolts' of doing research, particularly with reference to statistical approaches, methods and interpretation. Each article also provides linked information and explicit evidence to support the statements made. The topics covered answer key questions asked by researchers on subjects such as confidence intervals, p values, same size calculations, use of patient reported outcome measures, conundrums in the application of RCT and more complex statistical analysis. It also highlights implementation research and prognostic research. Each article is written by an expert in the field and the volume brings together a masterclass in research topics.

BPP
UNIVERSITY
SCHOOL OF HEALTH

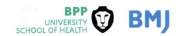

More titles in The BMJ Research Methods and Reporting Series

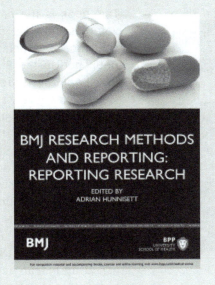

£29.99

February 2016

Paperback

978-1-472745-57-6

This book is the third of three volumes drawing together a collection of articles previously published in the BMJ covering contemporary issues in research. In this volume, the articles give key messages about how the 'nuts and bolts' of doing research, particularly with reference to how research findings should be reported. Each article also provides linked information and explicit evidence to support the statements made. The topics covered take a look at guidelines such as CONSORT, SPIRIT, GPP2, PRISMA and the IDEAL framework for surgical innovation. It also gives some guidance on economic evaluations, policy and service interventions and publication guidelines, as well as providing useful tips on preparing data for publication. Each article is written by an expert in the field and the volume brings together a masterclass in research reporting.

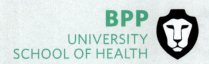

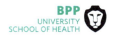

More titles in
The BMJ Easily Missed? Series

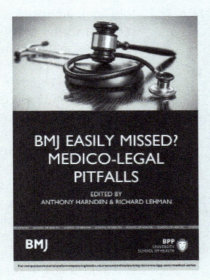

£29.99

January 2016

Paperback

978-1-4-72738-95-0

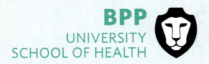

The risk of litigation against clinicians is increasing significantly. Those working in primary care, and whom are often dealing with uncertainty, are at particular risk. This book groups together a series of useful articles on diagnoses that may be easily missed at first presentation in primary care, and which may give rise to clinical negligence claims. The spectrum of conditions which are commonly encountered in claims such as pulmonary embolism, acute leg ischaemia, ectopic pregnancy, inflammatory bowel disease, appendicitis and achilles tendon rupture. All articles describe data to support the assertion that the conditions are often overlooked in primary care and that failure to recognise the diagnosis may have serious implications for the patient. This book provides the reader with:

- Diagnoses that may be encountered in clinical negligence claims
- Evidence that the diagnoses are easily missed in primary care
- Succinct articles with specific learning points and take home messages
- Essential reading to reduce risk of future litigation

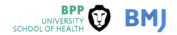
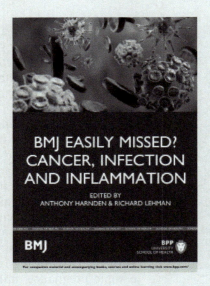
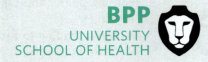

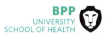

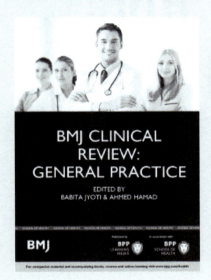
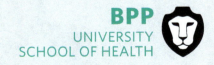

More titles from BPP School of Health

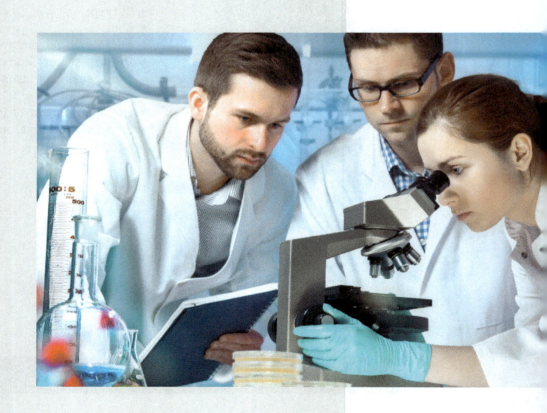

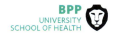
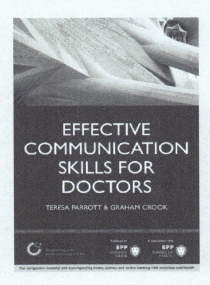
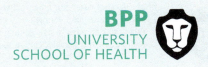

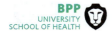

More titles in The Progressing Your Medical Career Series

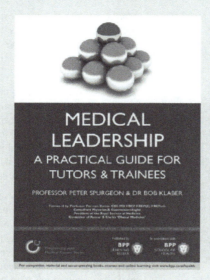

£19.99

November 2011

Paperback

978-1-445379-57-9

Are you a doctor or medical student who wishes to acquire and develop your leadership and management skills? Do you recognise the role and influence of strong leadership and management in modern medicine?

Clinical leadership is something in which all doctors should have an important role in terms of driving forward high quality care for their patients. In this up-to-date guide Peter Spurgeon and Robert Klaber take you through the latest leadership and management thinking, and how this links in with the Medical Leadership Competency Framework. As well as influencing undergraduate curricula and some of the concepts underpinning revalidation, this framework forms the basis of the leadership component of the curricula for all medical specialties, so a practical knowledge of it is essential for all doctors in training.

Using case studies and practical exercises to provide a strong work-based emphasis, this practical guide will enable you to build on your existing experiences to develop your leadership and management skills, and to develop strategies and approaches to improving care for your patients.

This book addresses:

- Why strong leadership and management are crucial to delivering high quality care

- The theory and evidence behind the Medical Leadership Competency Framework

- The practical aspects of leadership learning in a wide range of clinical environments (eg handover, EM, ward etc)

- How Consultants and trainers can best facilitate leadership learning for their trainees and students within the clinical work-place

Whether you are a medical student just starting out on your career, or an established doctor wishing to develop yourself as a clinical leader, this practical, easy-to-use guide will give you the techniques and knowledge you require to excel.

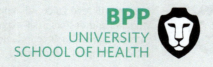

www.bpp.com/medical-series

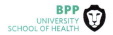

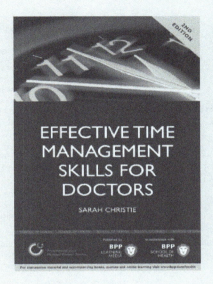

Do you find it difficult to achieve a work-life balance? Would you like to know how you can become more effective with the time you have?

With the introduction of the European Working Time Directive, which will severely limit the hours in the working week, it is more important than ever that doctors improve their personal effectiveness and time management skills. This interactive book will enable you to focus on what activities are needlessly taking up your time and what steps you can take to manage your time better.

By taking the time to read through, complete the exercises and follow the advice contained within this book you will begin to:

- Understand where your time is being needlessly wasted

- Discover how to be more assertive and learn how to say 'No'

- Set yourself priorities and stick to them

- Learn how to complete tasks more efficiently

- Plan better so you can spend more time doing the things you enjoy

In recent years, with the introduction of the NHS Plan and Lord Darzi's commitment to improve the quality of healthcare provision, there is a need for doctors to become more effective within their working environment. This book will offer you the chance to regain some clarity on how you actually spend your time and give you the impetus to ensure you achieve the tasks and goals which are important to you.

£19.99

February 2012

Paperback

978-1-445390-15-4

BPP
UNIVERSITY
SCHOOL OF HEALTH

www.bpp.com/medical-series

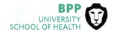

More titles in The Essential Clinical Handbook Series

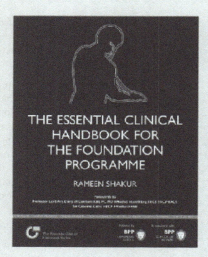

£24.99

October 2011

Paperback

978-1-445381-63-3

Unsure of what clinical competencies you must gain to successfully complete the Foundation Programme? Unclear on how to ensure your ePortfolio is complete to enable your progression to ST training?

This up-to-date clinical handbook is aimed at current foundation doctors and clinical medical students and provides a comprehensive companion to help you in the day-to-day management of patients on the ward. Together with this it is the first handbook to also outline clearly how to gain the core clinical competencies required for successful completion of the Foundation Programme. Written by doctors for doctors this comprehensive handbook explains how to successfully manage all of the common cases you will face during the Foundation Programme and:

- Introduces the Foundation Programme and what is expected of a new doctor especially with the introduction of Modernising Medical Careers

- Illustrates clearly the best way to manage, step-by-step, over 150 commonly encountered clinical diseases, including NICE guidelines to ensure a gold standard of clinical care is achieved

- Describes how to successfully gain the core clinical competencies within Medicine and Surgery including an extensive list of differentials and conditions explained

- Explores the various radiology images you will encounter and how to interpret them

- Tells you how to succeed in the assessment methods used including DOP's, Mini-CEX's and CBD's

- Has step by step diagrammatic guide to doing common clinical procedures competently and safely

- Outlines how to ensure your ePortfolio is maintained properly to ensure successful completion of the Foundation Programme

- Provides tips and advice on how to start preparing now to ensure you are fully prepared and have the competitive edge for your CMT/ST application

The introduction of the e-Portfolio as part of the Foundation Programme has paved the way for foundation doctors to take charge of their own learning and portfolio. Through following the expert guidance laid down in this handbook you will give yourself the best possible chance of progressing successfully through to CMT/ST training.

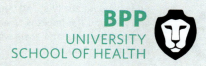

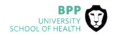

More titles in The Essential Clinical Handbook Series

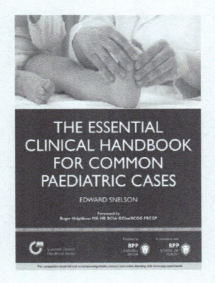

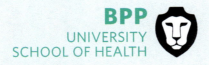

£24.99

September 2011

Paperback

978-1-445379-60-9

Not sure what to do when faced with a crying baby and demanding parent on the ward? Would you like a definitive guide on how to manage commonly encountered paediatric cases?

This clear and concise clinical handbook has been written to help healthcare professionals approach the initial assessment and management of paediatric cases commonly encountered by Junior Doctors, GPs, GP Specialty Trainee's and allied healthcare professionals. The children who make paediatrics so fun, can also make it more than a little daunting for even the most confident person. This insightful guide has been written based on the author's extensive experience within both a General Practice and hospital setting.

Intended as a practical guide to common paediatric problems it will increase confidence and satisfaction in managing these conditions. Each chapter provides a clear structure for investigating potential paediatric illnesses including clinical and non-clinical advice covering: background, how to assess, pitfalls to avoid, FAQs and what to tell parents. This helpful guide provides:

- A problem/symptom based approach to common paediatric conditions

- As essential guide for any doctor assessing children on the front line

- Provides easy-to-follow and step-by-step guidance on how to approach different paediatric conditions

- Useful both as a textbook and a quick reference guide when needed on the ward

This engaging and easy to use guide will provide you with the knowledge, skills and confidence required to effectively diagnose and manage commonly encountered paediatric cases both within a primary and secondary care setting.

BPP
UNIVERSITY
SCHOOL OF HEALTH

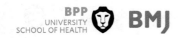